Second Edition

Forensic Psychiatry

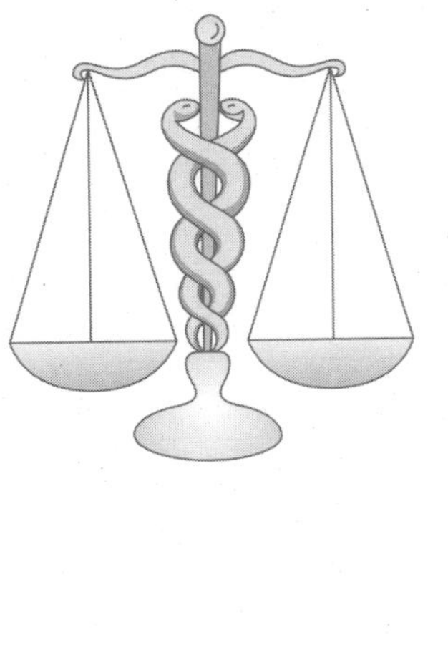

Second Edition

Forensic Psychiatry

Dr BV Subrahmanyam
MD, DGL, FAFM, DYO, MIAFM, AAFS

Professor, Department of Forensic Science
Narayana Medical College and Hospital, Nellore
Former Dean, Medical College, Bhavnagar
Medical Superintendent and
Professor and Head, Department of Forensic Medicine
Medical College and Hospital, Surat

Lt Col (Dr) C Harihar

Professor and Head, Department of Psychiatry
Malla Reddy Institute of Medical Sciences, Hyderabad, AP
Former Professor and Head, Department of Psychiatry
Narayana Medical College and Hospital, Nellore

CBSPD

CBS Publishers & Distributors Pvt Ltd

New Delhi • Bengaluru • Chennai • Kochi • Kolkata • Lucknow • Mumbai
Hyderabad • Jharkhand • Nagpur • Patna • Pune • Uttarakhand

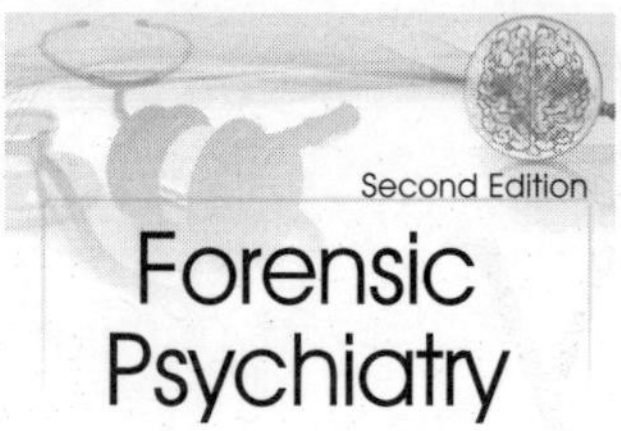

ISBN: 978-93-5466-932-3

Second Edition: 2025

First Edition: 2014

Published by **Satish Kumar Jain** and produced by **Varun Jain** for

CBS Publishers & Distributors Pvt Ltd

4819/XI Prahlad Street, 24 Ansari Road, Daryaganj, New Delhi 110 002, India.

Ph: 011-23266838, 23289259 Website: www.cbspd.com e-mail: delhi@cbspd.com

Corporate Office: 204 FIE, Industrial Area, Patparganj, Delhi 110 092

Ph: 011-4934 4934 Fax: 011-4934 4935 e-mail: publishing@cbspd.com; publicity@cbspd.com

Branches

- **Bengaluru:** Seema House 2975, 17th Cross, K.R. Road, Banasankari 2nd Stage, Bengaluru 560 070, Karnataka, India.
  Ph: +91-80-26771678/79 Fax: +91-80-26771680 e-mail: bangalore@cbspd.com
- **Chennai:** 18/8B, Subbarayan Street, Shenoy Nagar, Chennai 600 030, Tamil Nadu, India
  Ph: +91-044-42032115, 26681266 e-mail: chennai@cbspd.com
- **Kochi:** 42/1325, 1326, Power House Road, Opp. KSEB Power House, Ernakulam 682 018, Kochi, Kerala, India.
  Ph: +91-484-4059061-65,67 Fax: +91-484-4059065 e-mail: kochi@cbspd.com
- **Kolkata:** 147, Hind Ceramics Compound, 1st Floor, Nilgunj Road, Belghoria, Kolkata 700056, West Bengal, India
  Ph: +033-25633055, 033-25633056 e-mail: kolkata@cbspd.com
- **Lucknow:** Basement, Khushnuma Complex, 7 Meerabai Marg (Behind Jawahar Bhawan), Lucknow-226001, UP, India
  Ph: +0522-4000032 e-mail: tiwari.lucknow@cbspd.com
- **Mumbai:** PWD Shed, Gala no 25/26, Ramchandra Bhatt Marg, Next to JJ Hospital Gate no. 2, Opp. Union Bank of India, Noorbaug, Mumbai-400009, Maharashtra, India
  Ph: 022-66661880/89 e-mail: mumbai@cbspd.com

Representatives

- **Hyderabad** 0-9885175004
- **Jharkhand** 0-9811541605
- **Nagpur** 0-8692091830
- **Patna** 0-9334159340
- **Pune** 0-9664372571
- **Uttarakhand** 0-9716462459

Printed at: Shri Prints & Sales, Delhi, India

to

---

the unfortunate humanity
whose unsoundness of mind
leads to actions
not under their check

Foreword

Forensic psychiatry has a vital role to play in helping the courts of law in the administration of justice, and the senior investigating officers and the doctors involved in dealing with cases of alleged unsoundness of mind, behavioral problems, psychopathies, persecutions, harassment, self-poisoning cases and helping the state in arriving at proper justice.

This effort by two well-read authors: Dr BV Subrahmanyam with forty-two years of medico-legal background and writing books in related subjects, and Lt Col (Dr) C Harihar, a disciplined army person and a learned psychiatrist is laudable. This book fills the existing gap in the present scenario where books linking law and psychiatry and the medicolegal issues are not available.

I wish this effort all success as I found this book covers the needed background explanations and court cases.

Dr KSVK Subbarao MS MCh
Director
Jawaharlal Institute of Postgraduate
Medical Education and Research (JIPMER)
Pondicherry

Foreword

This book entitled *Forensic Psychiatry* authored by Dr BV Subrahmanyam, with a professional standing of over forty-two years in various facets of medicolegal practice and Lt Col (Dr) C Harihar, a learned scholar in psychiatry is a good effort for the benefit of judiciary, investigating officers, psychiatrists, forensic medicine experts, and all doctors involved in the assessment of mental status for the benefit of society and administration of justice. This book deals with the basic issues and case law for the benefit of all concerned. I wish this endeavour a grand success.

Dr BA Ramakrishna MD
Principal
Narayana Medical College
Chinthareddypalem, Nellore 524 002, AP
(O) 0861-2303392. (R) 2306659, Fax: 0861-2317962
E-mail: drbaramkrishna@yahoo.co.in, Mobile: 9849400892

Preface to the Second Edition

This small volume on forensic psychiatry is meant for all those interested in the practice, investigation, and in deciding the cases in courts of law, besides the serious-minded students. It provides an overview of various psychiatric problems encountered in a day-to-day practice including adverse effects of psychotropic medications, their diagnosis, treatment and medicolegal implications. Important medicolegal cases have been described at various stages to make the topic easily understood. It is sincerely hoped that the readers would find this book useful whenever they are dealing with legal cases involving psychiatric issues. This edition of the book features addition of a new chapter "Mental Health and Postpartum Psychosis".

Dr BV Subrahmanyam
Lt Col (Dr) C Harihar

Acknowledgments

Thanks are due to our spouses who have tolerated our diminished attention during the preparation of this work.

We sincerely thank the whole team of CBS Publishers & Distributors who have taken the trouble of bringing out this book.

We consulted many books and journals in the preparation of this book and we record our thanks to all the authors and publishers.

We thank Mrs A Karuna who did an immense help in the computation of this work.

Dr BV Subrahmanyam
Lt Col (Dr) C Harihar

Contents

Chapter 1

Introduction

Forensic psychiatry is the branch of medicine that deals with disorders of the mind and their relation to legal principles. The word "forensic" means belonging to the courts of law. Psychiatry and the law intersect when dealing with the social deviants who, by violating the rules of the society secondary to some presumed or proposed mental disorder, adversely affect the functioning of the community.

The social deviant is a potential threat to the safety and the security of other people. The "legalization" of psychiatry has led to increasing practice of defensive medicine. Defensive practice converts patients into litigants. Clinicians have to defend themselves. Patients readily sense the shift from the clinician's interest in the patient to the clinician's self-protection. The patient's feeling triggers litigation. The therapeutic alliance is broken.

On a sheet with his letterhead a psychiatrist typed a warning to the employer that his patient, John Jones, had expressed the desire to kill him (the employer). He sent the letter by first-class mail, not express or registered, and he addressed it not to the employer but to the personnel department of the company. Subsequently liability, suit for breach of confidentiality was faced by him. He wondered, "but I was only doing what the law requires of me"!

HISTORY OF FORENSIC PSYCHIATRY

Indian legal system is by and large based on the British legal system. The role of law in the development of modern psychiatry was extensive, particularly after the 18th century and reflected both a growing public awareness of problems raised by mental disorder and community's need to express and enforce measures to manage the problems. Religion and utilitarian philosophies were influential in English public life during the 19th century and coloured the contemporaneous calls for the reforms of asylums, prisons and the legal system. Thus the English Act of 1774 was replaced sequentially by the Country Asylum Act 1808, then by the English Lunacy Act 1853, then by the Lunacy Act 1891, and later by the Mental Health Act 1959 in order to make fresh provisions for treatment and care of mentally disordered; provisions were made for informal admission of mentally ill to any hospital or nursing home without application or order for detention. Now the primary concern was the welfare and treatment of the individual patient which was left to the doctors, social workers and hospital managers. The Act was further amended in 1983. As far as the European countries are concerned, the literature claims about the relationship between law and psychiatry even in Greece and Rome 2000 years ago in a limited way. By the 14th century, the legal status of the insane person was well defined, two issues central to the forensic psychiatry of today were already being discussed: the responsibility of the mentally ill person and the way he should be dealt with within the community. In the 17th century, a very elaborate medicolegal perception of the individual has been achieved. It was the judge who decided whether the individual was insane and it was his (individual's) relatives who asked that he be placed in custody. In 1808, the term 'Psychiatric' appeared for the first time. Among the achievements at that time, first was the separation of mentally disordered from other prisoners while second was the creation of asylums and reorganization of the existing institutions. By early 20th century, the use of psychiatric experts and the general influence of psychiatry in the criminal justice system were enhanced.

Coming to the Indian scenario, even though diagnosis and treatment of mental illnesses have been well documented in Ayurveda, Charak Samhita and Susruta Samhita, etc. the legal aspects pertaining to the mental illnesses have not been mentioned anywhere in the ancient Indian literature before the arrival of the British. The first lunatic asylum was established by the British at Calcutta in around 1787. The purpose of these asylums was not the care and treatment of the mentally ill but to shut them off in places far away from towns to rid the society of them, while at the same time protecting them against themselves. Law relating to the custody of lunatics and management of their estates was introduced in India through three separate acts viz. Lunacy (Supreme Court) Act 1858, The Lunacy (District Courts) Act 1858, and the Lunatic Asylum Act 1858. The Acts were modified in 1883 and more elaborate instructions and guidelines for admission and treatment of lunatics were outlined. A central supervision of the mental hospital was established in 1906. This was brought out in the form of the Indian Lunacy Act of 1912. In 1920, the names of all lunatic asylums were changed to mental hospitals and the control of mental hospitals was shifted from prison authorities to civil surgeons.

In 1946, the Health Survey and Development Committee, popularly known as the 'Bhore Committee' was asked to survey mental hospitals. As it reported that majority of the mental hospitals in India were quite out-dated and were not designed for curative treatment of the inmates, the Mental Health Act was enacted in 1987 and enforced from 1993. Again after 20 years, it has been revised as the Mental Health Care Act 2010 and its implementation is under process. It aims to provide access to mental health care for persons with mental illness and to protect and promote the rights of persons with mental illness during the delivery of mental health care.

PSYCHIATRISTS AND THE COURTS

The complexity of medicolegal matters is divided into two sides, which pull away from each other trying to place the truth in the hands of the fact finder (the judge or the jury). The clinician gets exposed to merciless cross-examination, feels fear, revulsion, and dismay. These feelings are tempered somewhat by insights into the process. From the clinician's viewpoint an important distinction must be made regarding the clinician's role as a witness.

WITNESS OF FACT

The witnesses' input—the facts—are his direct observations and material from direct scrutiny. A witness of fact may be a psychiatrist who reads portions of the medical record aloud to bring it into the legal record and thus make it available for testimony. Any psychiatrist at any level of training can have that role.

EXPERT WITNESS

In contrast, a psychiatrist under certain circumstances may be qualified as an expert. The qualifying process, however, consists not of popular recognition in one's clinical field but of being accepted by the court and both sides of the case as suitable to perform expert functions. Thus the term "expert" has particular legal meaning and is independent of any actual or presumed expertise the clinician may have in a given area. The clinician's expertise is elucidated during direct examination and cross-examination of the clinician's education, publications, and certifications. In the context of the courtroom, an expert witness is one who may draw conclusions from data and thereby render an opinion—for example, that a patient meets the required criteria for commitment or for an insanity defense under the standards of a jurisdiction. Expert witnesses play a role in determining the standard of care and what constitutes the average practice of psychiatry.

COURT-MANDATED EVALUATIONS

In some cases the judge asks clinicians to be consultants to the court, which raises the issue of for whom the clinicians work. Because clinical information may have to be revealed to the court, clinicians may not enjoy the same confidential relationship with their patients in those situations that they have in private practice. Clinicians who make such court ordered evaluations are under an ethical obligation and, in some states, a legal obligation to so inform the patients at the outset of the examinations and to make sure that the patients understand that condition. Such court-mandated evaluations were supported by the Supreme Court of the United States in Ake *vs* Oklahoma. The Court held that, when a state allows a defense of sanity, it must provide funds for a psychiatric expert for an indigent defense. Such an expert may be part of the defense if appropriate.

COMPETENCE TO BE EXECUTED

A new area of competence to emerge in the interface between psychiatry and the law is the question of the patient's competence to be executed. The requirement for competence is thought to rest on three general principles. First, the patient's awareness of what is happening is supposed to heighten the retributive element of the punishment. Punishment is held as meaningless unless the patient is aware of what it is and to what it is a response. The second element is a religious one; competent persons about to be executed are thought to be inthe best position to make whatever peace is appropriate with their religious beliefs, including confession and absolution. Third, the competent person about to be executed preserves until the end the possibility (admittedly slight) of recalling some forgotten detail of the events of the crime that may prove exonerating.

DURHAM RULE

In the Durham case, Judge Bazelon expressly stated that the purpose of the rule was to get good and complete psychiatric testimony. He sought to release the criminal law from the theoretical straitjacket of the M'Naghten rule. However, judges and juries in cases using the Durham rule became mired in confusion over the terms "product", "disease" and "defect." In 1972, some 18 years after the rule's adoption, the Court of Appeals for the District of Columbia, in United States *vs* Brawner, discarded the rule. The court—all nine members, including judge Bazelon—decided in a 143-page opinion to throw out its Durham rule and to adopt in its place the test recommended in 1962 by the American Law Institute in its model penal code, which is the law in the federal courts today.

MODEL PENAL CODE

In its model penal code the American Law Institute recommended the following tests of criminal responsibility: (1) Persons are not responsible for criminal conduct if at the time of such conduct, as a result of mental disease or defect, they lacked substantial capacity either to appreciate the criminality (wrongfulness) of their conduct or to conform their conduct to the requirement of the law. (2) The term "mental disease or defect" does not include an abnormality manifested only by repeated criminal or otherwise antisocial conduct.

Subsection I of the American Law Institute rule contains five operative concepts: (1) Mental disease or defect, (2) Lack of substantial capacity, (3) Appreciation, (4) Wrongfulness, and (5) Conformity of conduct to the requirements of law. The rule's second subsection, stating that repeated criminal or antisocial conduct is not of itself to be taken as mental disease or defect, aims to keep the sociopath or psychopath within the scope of criminal responsibility.

RESPONDENT SUPERIOR

The Latin phrase respondent superior expresses the axiom, "Let the master answer for the deeds of the servant". That doctrine holds that a person occupying a high position in a chain or hierarchy of responsibility is liable for the actions of a person in a lower position. A typical example is the psychiatric attending physician who supervises a resident. By the same reasoning, when a state hospital, for example, is named in a lawsuit, the list of cited defendants may extend upward to include the commissioner of mental health and the governor of the state. After the traditional first response, the attorneys usually weed out the irrelevant defendants.

Firstly, consultation from outside the line of clinical responsibility often does not fit the model. The consultant is an adviser, not a superior. Secondly, the question of the particular defendant's authority (whether that person can hire and fire, censure, or control subordinates in the system) is relevant to the assignment of blame. Thirdly, as a rule, psychiatrists should remove themselves from situations in which they bear responsibility (liability) for the practice of other professionals but cannot control the activities of those persons or perform their own assessments of the patients. In addition, psychiatrists should clarify ambiguities of responsibility at the point of entry into a system.

SEXUAL RELATIONS WITH PATIENTS

Although maintaining sexual relations with patients is not a common form of malpractice, it is not rare enough. The most common form is heterosexual relations occurring in an outpatient context between a male therapist and a female patient, but all other permutations have come to light and to litigation.

Sexual relations with a patient is considered a breach of the fiduciary (trust-based) relationship of physician to patient and a negligent failure by the physician to work correctly with transference and counter transference issues in a manner consistent with the standard of care. The usual harms identified are the failure to provide treatment during the affair, the misuse of time that might be spent in treatment elsewhere, the creation of severe difficulties for future therapy, and the direct emotional harms of guilt, depression, anxiety, shame, humiliation, and suicidal intent.

Sexual relations with a patient under any circumstances (usually including ex-patients) is unethical, a deviation from the standard of care, and, therefore, proscribed. Many social activities that are not overtly sexual are highly suspect (one famous case involved a therapist's taking tea with a patient). As a form of liability prevention, such activities should also be avoided.

SUICIDE AND SUICIDAL ATTEMPTS BY PATIENTS

Suicide and suicidal attempts are the most frequent causes for lawsuits against psychiatrists. An estimated one out of every two suicides leads to a malpractice action. Psychiatrists may be charged with negligence because they did not properly control a patient under treatment; such negligence causes injury, and the suicidal behavior must have been predictable. The psychiatrist may be judged with malpractice, in decreasing order of culpability, during the patient's hospitalization, while the patient is out of the hospital on a pass, and during outpatient treatment. Supervision is greatest during hospitalization, and supervision is least during outpatient treatment.

NEGLIGENT TREATMENT

Typical claims allege inadequate or insufficient treatment (under-treatment), excessive or overly aggressive treatment (over-treatment), and variations on the theme of improper treatment, such as using the wrong medication, failing to anticipate or respond to side effects appropriately, and creating iatrogenic harms or addictions.

PREVENTING LIABILITY

Preventive approaches: (1) Clinicians should provide only those kinds of care that they are qualified. They should take reasonable care of themselves; they should treat their patients with respect; (2) The documentation of good care is a strong deterrent to liability. A clinician who takes the trouble to obtain a consultation (second opinion) in a difficult and complex case is unlikely to be viewed by a judge careless or negligent; (3) The informed-consent process involves a discussion of the inherent uncertainty of psychiatric practice and helps prevent a liability suit.

Chapter

2

Ethics and Mental Health

VALID CONSENT

The term "valid consent" is preferable to "informed consent" as it implies an accurate and useful parallel between that term and others such as "valid will" and "valid contract". Each of these, in order to be valid, must satisfy three explicit requirements: The patient or client must receive adequate information about what is being proposed; no coercion should be used in obtaining the consent; and the patient or client, must be fully competent to consent or refuse. A wide consensus both in ethics and law is that if any one of these conditions is not met, then the consent or refusal is not valid. It is sometimes justified to treat a patient without having valid consent, but the burden falls clearly on the doctor to justify that treatment.

ADEQUATE INFORMATION

Patients must receive adequate information about the tests, procedures, and treatments suggested to them. How much information should be given to satisfy the criterion of adequacy? A simple general answer is that any information should be given that a rational person would want to know before making a decision, like the significant harms and benefits associated with a suggested treatment, with available alternative treatments, and if no treatment is given.

Harms and Benefits: Harms and benefits must be and explained in a language that the person can readily understand. Technical language should not be employed. Harms and benefits should be explained in terms of the harms that will be caused, avoided, or ameliorated by various courses of action. These include death, pain (both physical and mental), various disabilities and loss of freedom, opportunity, or pleasure.

PROBABILITY OF HARM

Any risk of death beyond a trivial risk (say 1 in 10,000 or less) should be told, because death is so serious that rational persons are always concerned with any non-trivial chance that it may occur.

Alternative treatments: Patients must be told about all alternative treatments for their malady. These should be described in an unbiased manner. To describe treatments that one does not personally favour in a belittling manner makes it difficult for many patients to inquire more fully into them.

Patients should also know the likely harms and benefits associated with electing not to be treated at all. Patients with most maladies are unlikely to choose the option of no treatment.

Absence of coercion: Coercion means the use of such strong negative incentives (for example, threats of severe pain or significant deprivation of freedom) that it would be unreasonable to expect a patient to resist them.

PATIENT COMPETENCE

Competence refers to a patient's cognitive ability to process information. It is specific to a patient's abilities at a given time, so that a patient may be competent to make a treatment decision at one time and not be competent, or be only partially competent, at another time. Competence is also decision-specific; at a given time, a patient may be competent to decide about a relatively simple treatment with easily understood consequences but not adequately competent to decide about some other treatment with a relatively complex set of outcome contingencies.

TREATMENT REFUSALS

Forced treatment: The legal criteria should correctly identify those persons whose decisions or choices we feel morally justified in overruling and also correctly identify those whose decisions or choices should not be overruled.

CENTRALITY OF COMPETENCE

Even if the refusal seems silly, self-defeating, and irrational if the patient is competent, then the refusal holds. One may cajole, argue, and return to argue the issue day after day, but if the patient continues to refuse, one may not treat.

Competence is referred to as "the mental capacity to comprehend the consequences of their decision".

The following factors are considered in evaluating capability to consent or refuse treatment: (1) The person's knowledge that he has a choice to make; (2) The patient's ability to understand the available options, their advantages and disadvantages; (3) The patient's cognitive capacity to consider the relevant factors; (4) The absence of any interfering pathologic perception or belief, such as a delusion concerning the decision; (5) The absence of any interfering emotional state, such as severe depression, mania or emotional disability; (6) The absence of any interfering pathologic motivational pressure; (7) The absence of any interfering pathologic relationship, such as the conviction of helpless dependency on another person; (8) An awareness of how others view the decision, the general social attitude towards the choices and an understanding of his reason for deviating from that attitude if he does.

What is an irrational decision or action? A simple but not very precise way of defining an irrational decision (and some treatment refusals are irrational decisions) is that it involves hurting oneself pointlessly, as in "cutting off one's nose to spite one's face".

An irrational treatment is one from which, on balance, a patient would have much more to lose than to gain, and competent physicians should not suggest such courses of action.

PATERNALISTIC BEHAVIOR

Many instances of paternalistic behavior occur in psychiatric and psychological practice, i.e. giving patients medication against their wishes.

An action is paternalistic if it satisfies four criteria: (1) The action is for the benefit of the subject (the patient, in this context), (2) The action violates a moral rule with regard to the patient, (3) The action is done without the consent of the subject, and (4) The subject is at least partially competent.

TREATING OR HOSPITALIZING AN UNWILLING PATIENT

Several morally relevant criteria must be satisfied:

1. That the treatment will probably avoid death or ameliorate serious physical disability.

2. The harm likely to be caused by the treatment is negligible.
3. The patient's desire not to be treated must be seriously irrational.
4. It must be true that rational persons would always advocate forcing treatment in cases having the same morally relevant characteristics described by the first three criteria.

The forced treatment has to pass the criteria for morally justified paternalism.

DEFINITION OF "MENTAL ILLNESS"

Physical and mental maladies have a great deal in common and belong to the same genus. They differ only in their phenotypic manifestation—what kind of evil the sufferer experiences. Physical maladies are characterized by the predominant suffering of physical symptoms [evils], while mental maladies are characterized by the predominant suffering due to mental symptoms.

Mental illnesses or maladies are no different in type from physical illnesses. Their conceptual status is just the same; they differ only in their symptomatic manifestations. There is no reason to think that mental maladies are any less "real" than physical ones; some mental maladies are far more serious and warrant far more attention and societal resources than do many physical maladies.

DEFINITION OF "MENTAL DISORDER"

The Diagnostic and Statistical Manual of Mental Disorders (DSM-IV) includes this definition.

A clinically significant behavioral or psychological syndrome or pattern that occurs in an individual and that is associated with present distress (i.e. a painful symptom) or disability (i.e. an impairment in one or more important areas of functioning) or with a significantly increased risk of suffering death, pain, disability, or an important loss of freedom. Whatever its original (underlying) causes, it must currently be considered a manifestation of a behavioral, psychological, or biological dysfunction in the individual. The syndrome or pattern must not be merely an expectable and culturally sanctioned response to a particular event. Each of the mental disorders is conceptualized as a clinically significant behavioral or psychological syndrome or pattern that occurs in an individual and that is associated with present distress (e.g. a painful symptom) or disability (i.e. impairment in one or more important areas of functioning) or with a significantly increased risk of suffering, death, pain, disability, or an important loss of freedom. In addition, this syndrome or pattern must not be merely an expectable response to a particular event, e.g. the death of a loved one. Neither deviant behavior (e.g. political, religious, or sexual) nor conflicts that are primarily between the individual and society are mental disorders unless the deviance or conflict is a symptom of a dysfunction in the individual, as described above.

A key point of the psychiatric view is that a legitimate "mental illness" requires underlying "behavioral, psychological, or biological dysfunction in the individual".

Some types of mental illness are characterized by the person's having seriously irrational desires—desires to act in a way that has a high proba bility of causing the person to suffer evils without any adequate reason. Since some mentally ill persons have such irrational desires, and these desires usually disappear after the mental illness is successfully treated, then it follows, using the justification scheme described above, that paternalistic actions toward these persons are sometimes morally justified.

Not all mentally ill persons possess seriously irrational desires of this kind, so the category mental illness is too broad to be used as a criterion. The presence of mental illness correlates with the underlying factors that account for our moral intuitions, but it does not completely or even adequately overlap with them. Judges may find it difficult to clearly designate the dangerous person as to whether he is mentally ill or not, unless explained clearly the ramifications and significance of the symptoms and signs of the mental illness that make him dangerous.

CASE LAW

Medical Ethics: Rights of the Disabled

Reproductive Rights of Mentally Disabled Women

The National Human Rights Commission intervened on the basis of newspaper reports from the State of Maharashtra that mentally ill women were being forcefully sterilized. Their uterus has been removed with only the consent of their parents, with no regard of their reproductive and health rights.

Chapter

3

Mental Health and Law

INTRODUCTION

The mental health sector is governed by, the Mental Health Act 1987 and not a national policy. The law leans heavily on institutionalized care, where ill persons can enter the institution of their own will, but cannot exit on their own volition. There are approximately 10 million persons requiring psychiatric care. The number of qualified psychiatrists in India is very low. Inadequate training capacity, poor or non-existent linkages between community and hospital-based care and weak institutional framework are the problems faced by the psychiatrists.

- What are the different laws that deal with mental health care?
- What are the issues dealt with in the courts regarding mental health?

Under Sec. 328 of the Code of Criminal procedure (CrPC) when an accused is unable to understand the trial due to unsoundness of mind it is mandatory that the magistrate refers the accused for a medical examination. The court postpones the trial only if the accused is not able to understand the proceedings due to unsoundness of mind. The case law shows that further inquiry of incapacity is not undertaken when unsoundness of mind is established, the consequent incapacity is presumed and the trial postponed until the accused regains sanity. Section 330 of the CrPC provides that during the period of postponement, the 'under-trial of unsound mind' should either be released on a bond of safe custody from a relative or friend; or be kept in safe custody in a jail or a mental hospital. There is no guidance in the statute as regards when each of these options is to be utilized. So, an 'under-trial of unsound mind' can obtain the benefit of the less restrictive alternative of being released in the community provided he or she has a relative or a friend who is willing and able to offer security. The statute provides no outer limit for which the trial would remain postponed. The prison authorities must send a medical report every six months on the state of mind of the accused. This is the only safeguard available against indefinite confinement.

Mental health is an issue in connection with laws like:

1. Matrimonial laws where mental illness is a ground for divorce or for nullity of marriage.
2. Mental Health Act (earlier the Lunacy Act) which deals primarily with institutionalization of mentally ill persons. It will soon be replaced by the Mental Health Care Act 2010 draft of which is pending approval by the government.
3. Persons with Disabilities Act which includes the issue of mental disability.

4. Laws dealing with contracts where contractual obligations are contingent upon the contracts having been entered into in sane state of mind.
5. Criminal laws where liability is diminished or extinguished if the person is of unsound mind at the time of committing the crime.
6. Laws dealing with succession of property wherein soundness of mind of one of the heirs is in question.
7. Many other laws wherein a person of sound mind only can take a stand.

Persons suffering from mental illness are treated as persons from whom the society needs to be protected. The Indian Lunacy Act and present Mental Health Act both deal with institutionalization of mentally ill person. The cases involved revolve round the institutional care.

Issues defining mental illness are still a problem. Some acute cases are easy to define but a number of others depend not only on the development of medical science but also the way in which society deals with a particular issue. For instance, in 1851 Dr. Samuel Cartwritght said that *'Drapetomania'* was a mental illness. Drapetomania was defined as tendency of black slaves to run away from their masters. Homosexuality was considered a psychological disorder till very recently and even now many doctors believe it to be so. There is a big debate currently on whether any condition can be called a psychological disorder, as according to many people, we have an image of how people should behave, and if they do not behave in that manner they are branded as having a disorder. Matrimonial litigation is full of cases where insanity is a ground for divorce. Many testamentary depositions or 'wills' are challenged on the ground of unsound mind. There are a number of instances where a person charged with a criminal offence has set up the defense of mental illness.

CASE LAW

Right to Treatment

Dr. Upendra Baxi vs State of Uttar Pradesh (1983) 2 S.C.C. 308

Procedure of Admission, Release and Treatment to be followed for Mentally Ill Inmates by State Protective Homes

Through this public interest litigation, Dr. Baxi and Mrs. Lotika Sarkar sought to enforce the human rights of the occupants of State protective Homes under Art. 21 of the Constitution. The Supreme Court ordered a panel of doctors to examine the inmates at the Agra Home and submit a report to the Court. The report of the psychiatric department incharge showed that 33 out of the 50 inmates had varying degrees of mental retardation and had not been examined at the time of admission into the Home. Despite this report, the Superintendent had released 14 of them, without determining their mental state and with no money to cover even the train fare to their hometowns.

The Court held that firstly it is necessary for the Magistrate ordering the release to ascertain whether the circumstances justify the release of the inmates of State Homes. Thereafter, the Superintendent is required to make relevant entries in the Inmates Register regarding the physical and mental health of the inmates at the time of release. The Court expressed regret that the Superintendent had not personally, as per rules as well as on humane grounds, inquired from the inmates released recently as to where they proposed to go, for which railway tickets ought to have been supplie d. The Court also suggested that the Superintendent in this regard could make an application to the Magistrate.

The court also recommended that psychiatric treatment be provided to the mentally ill inmates, for which a record of the time and place of treatment should be maintained. Further, it was directed that vocational training aimed at rehabilitation ought to be provided and separate accommodation should be made available to these inmates. The State Government and the Superintendent were directed to transfer the mentally ill inmates of the Home to a mental health institute, after consulting a psychiatric doctor for deciding the category. Charges and expenses incurred for providing accommodation in special institutes for these inmates should be borne by the State Government.

Rakesh Chandra Narayan *vs* **State of Bihar** was a case, which arose out of a letter written to the Chief Justice of India by two residents of Patna regarding conditions of mental hospital near Ranchi. The Supreme Court observed "in a welfare state, it is the obligation of the state to provide medical attention to every citizen. Running of the mental hospital is the state's obligation to the citizens and the fact that lakhs of rupees have been spent from the public exchequer (perhaps without inadequate return) is not of any consequence. The State has to realize its obligation and the government of the day has got to perform its duties by running the hospital in a perfect standard and serving the patients in an appropriate way. The reports and affidavits of the Government of Bihar and its officers (not the reports furnished to the Court by the judicial officers) have not given us the satisfaction of the touch of appropriate sincerity in action".

Rakesh Chandra Narayan vs State of Bihar, 1989 Supp (1) S.C.C.

Proper Civic Amenities for Running State Owned Mental Hospitals

Taking cognizance of a letter addressed to the Chief Justice of India, the Court treated it as a PIL under Art. 32 of the Constitution as it spoke of the conditions in the mental health institutions in Bihar. The report submitted by the Chief Judicial Magistrate appointed by the Court to visit the Home revealed shocking and inhumane conditions in the hospital in which a large number of patients were living. The Court observed that it is the obligation of the State to provide attention to every citizen and that it would be difficult for the Supreme Court to monitor the management of a hospital located far away. However, in light of the State Government's indifferent attitude and in spite of several interim Supreme Court orders and assurances held out by the State, defects have still not been remedied. A Committee of Management was appointed with a sitting High Court Judge as its Chairman, with powers to look after all aspects of the institution. Directions were given to the Committee for proper functioning, management, funds, etc. Observing that a hospital is not a place where cured people should be allowed to stay, the Court directed the Committee to take immediate steps to setup a rehabilitation centre at a convenient place around Ranchi, for those who after being cured are not in a position to return to their families or to seek useful employment on their own. Parties including the committee were granted liberty to move the Court from time to time for clarifications or more orders.

The Court also directed that various implementation reports that are furnished by the respondent State from time to time should be placed before the Court. For this purpose, the Court directed that the matter shall be deemed to be pending in order to monitor the progress and also to facilitate passing of further orders.

The Court initially issued the following directions:

1. In respect of each patient in the Ranchi Mansik Arogayashala, the daily allocation for diet will be increased from the existing and adequate articles of that value shall be supplied to each patient.
2. Arrangements should be made forthwith to supply adequate quantity of pure

drinking water to the hospital, if necessary, by engaging water takers to transport potable water from outside.

3. Immediate arrangements should be made for the restoration of proper sanitary conditions in the laboratories and bathrooms of the hospital.
4. All patients in the hospital who are not at present having mattresses and blankets should be immediately supplied the same within 15 days from today. Such of the patients who have not been given cots should also be provided cots within six weeks from today so that no patient shall be thereafter without a cot.
5. The ceiling limit at present in vogue in respect of cost of medicines allowable for each patient will stand removed with immediate effect and the patients will be supplied medicines according to the prescription made by the doctors irrespective of the costs.
6. The State Government shall forthwith take steps to appoint a qualified psychiatrist and a Medical Superintendent for the hospital and they should be posted and take charge of the institution within 6 weeks from today.
7. The Chief Judicial Magistrate, Ranchi to whom a copy of this order is forwarded by the Registry shall visit the hospital once in 3 weeks and submit quarterly report to this Court as to whether the aforesaid directions given by us are being complied with.

There have been repeated allegations that the lady patients who have already been cured are not being released from the hospital. At one stage the explanation offered by the hospital authorities and the State administration was that the relatives, even though notified, are not taking them back. The hospital is not a place where cured people should be allowed to stay. It is, therefore, necessary that there should be a rehabilitation centre for those who after being cured are not in a position to return to their families or on their own seek useful employment. The Committee shall therefore, take immediate steps to have a rehabilitation centre at a convenient place around Ranchi where appropriate rehabilitation schemes may be operated and the patients after being cured, irrespective of being male or female, and could be rehabilitated if they are not being taken back by the members of their families. The funds made available to the Committee may be utilized for such purpose.

In 1994, the Court directed that an autonomous body be set up to manage and run this institution.

HUMAN RIGHTS VIOLATIONS IN INSTITUTIONS

Sheela Barse *vs* Union of India dealt with children who were kept in jails across the country for 'safe custody' as allegedly they are physically and mentally retarded. The Court has clearly observed "there are a few matters which need urgent directions. It seems that there are a number of children who are mentally or physically handicapped and there are also children who are abandoned or destitute and who have no one to take care of them. They are lodged in various jails in different states.

The State Government must take care of these mentally or physically handicapped children and remove them to a home where they can be properly looked after and so far as the mentally handicapped children are concerned, they can be given proper medical treatment and physically handicapped children may be given not only medical treatment but also vocational training to enable them to earn their livelihood. Those children who are abandoned or lost and are presently kept in jails must also be removed by the State Governments to appropriate places where they can be looked after and rehabilitated..."

Another case filed by Sheela Barse dealt with children and women committed to jails as lunatics in Calcutta. The Supreme Court appointed a committee to visit the jails and give its report. Subsequent to this, the Court transferred the matter to the respective High Courts in India asking them to look into the matters.

In Chandan Kumar Banik *vs* State of West Bengal [(1995) supp. 4 SCC 505] the Supreme Court deplored the inhuman conditions of the mentally ill in the Mental Hospital at Mankundu in the District of Hooghli. The Court ordered for discontinuing the practice of tying up the patients with iron chains and ordered drug treatment for them.

The indifference of State and private authorities caused the tragic death of 28 inmates on 06 August 2001 at an asylum in Erwadi (Tamil Nadu) as they were tied to their beds and in the night a fire broke out. In this Rex *vs* Union of India case, the issue of rights of inmates of mental asylum was raised. This petition sought directions for implementation of provisions of Mental Health Act 1987 to prevent another mishap of the kind in mental asylum in Tamil Nadu.

In the light of the provisions of Mental Health Act, Supreme Court issued the following directions for its implementation:

i. Every State and Union Territory must undertake a district-wise survey of all registered/unregistered bodies, by whatever name called, purporting to offer psychiatric/mental health care. All such bodies should be granted or refused licence depending upon whether minimum prescribed standards are fulfilled or not. In case licence is rejected, it shall be the responsibility of SHO of the concerned police station to ensure that the body stops functioning and patients are shifted to government mental hospitals.
ii. Chief Secretary or Additional Chief Secretary designated by him shall be the nodal agency to coordinate all activities involved in implementation of the Mental Health Act 1987, the persons with Disabilities (Equal Opportunities, protection of rights and full participation) Act 1995, and National Trust for Welfare of persons with Autism, Cerebral palsy, Mental Retardation and Multiple Disability Act 1999. He shall ensure that there are no jurisdictional problems or impediments to the effective implementation of the three Acts between different Ministries or Departments. At the Central level, Cabinet Secretary, Government of India or any Secretary designated by him shall be the nodal agency for the same purpose.
i. The Cabinet Secretary, Union of India shall file an affidavit in SC within one month from the date of this order indicating:
   a. The contribution that has been made and that is proposed to be made under Sec. 21 of the 1999 Act which would constitute corpus of the National Trust.
   b. Policy of the Central Government towards setting up at least one Central Government-run mental hospital in each State and Union Territory (UT) and definite time schedule for achieving the said objective.
   c. National policy, if any framed under Sec. 8 (2) (9b) of the 1995 Act.
   d. In respect of the States/UT that do not have even one full-fledged State Government-run mental hospital, the Chief Secretary of the State/UT must file an affidavit within one month from date of this Order indicating steps being taken to establish such full-fledged State Government-run mental hospital in the State/UT and a definite time schedule for establishment of the same.
   e. Both Central and State Governments shall undertake a comprehensive awareness campaign with a special focus to educate people as to provisions of the law relating to mental health, rights of mentally challenged persons, the fact that chaining of mentally

challenged persons is illegal and mental patients should be sent to doctors and not to religious places for treatment.

ii. Every State shall file an affidavit stating:
   a. Whether the state Mental Health Authority under Sec. 3 of the 1987 Act exists in the State and if so, when it was set up.
   b. If it does not exist, the reason thereof and when such an authority is expected to be established and operationalized.
   c. The dates of meetings of those authorities, which already existed, from the date of inception till date and a short summary of the decisions taken.
   d. A statement that the State shall ensure that meetings of the authorities take place in future at least once in every four months or at more frequent intervals depending on exigency and that all the statutory functions and duties of such authorities are duly discharged.
   e. The number of prosecutions, penalties or other punitive/coercive measures taken, if any, by each State under the 1987 Act.

In Saarthak Registered society and another *vs* Union of India, as a continuation to the above order, the Supreme Court passed the following directions:

1. Every State and Union Territory shall undertake an assessment survey and file the report on the following aspects:
   a. Estimated availability of mental health resources including psychiatrists, psychologists, psychiatric social workers and nurses in both public and private sector.
   b. Types of Mental Health Delivery system available in the State including available bed strength, outpatient and rehabilitation services.
   c. An estimate of the Mental Health Services that would be required considering the population of the State and the incidence of mental illness.
2. The Chief Secretary of each State and Administrator/Commissioner of every UT to file affidavit stating clearly:
   a. Whether any minimum standards have been prescribed for licensing of Mental Health Institutions in the State/UT and in case such minimum standards have been prescribed.
   b. Whether each of the existing registered Mental Health Institutions in the State/UT whether private or run by the State meet the basic minimum standards as on date of passing this order and if not, what steps have been taken to ensure compliance of licensing conditions.
   c. Number of unregistered bodies providing psychiatric/mental health care existing in the State and whether any of them comply with minimum standards.
   d. Whether any mentally challenged person is found to be chained in the State.
3. The report on the Need Assessment Survey and affidavit was to be submitted to the Health Secretary, Union of India within a stipulated time. The Health secretary was to compile them and present it to the Court.
4. Further Union of India was directed to:
   a. Frame a policy and initiate steps for establishment of at least one Central Government-run Mental Health Hospital in each State.
   b. Examine the feasibility of formulating uniform rules regarding standard of services for both public and private sector Mental Health Services.
   c. Constitute a committee to give recommendations on the issue of care of mentally challenged persons who have

no immediate relatives or who have been abandoned by relatives.

d. Frame norms for non-government organizations working in the field of mental health and to ensure that the services rendered by them are supervised by qualified/trained persons.

5. All State Governments were also directed to frame policy and initiate steps for establishment of at least one state Government-run Mental Hospital in each state.
6. Two members of the legal aid board of each State were appointed to make monthly visit to such institutions to help the patients and their relatives in applying for discharge if they have fully recovered.
7. Two members of the legal aid and judicial officer would explain their rights to patients and their guardians at the time of admission to the institutions.
8. Form a Board of Visitors as required under the Mental Health Act to every State or private institution at least once a month.
9. Envisage a scheme for rehabilitation process for people who are not having any backing or support in the community.

Sheela Barse (II) *vs* Union of India (1986) 3 S.C.C.

Rehabilitation of Mentally Retarded Children, Abandoned or Destitute Children, Lodged in Various Jails of the Country for 'Safe Custody'

It was observed by the Court that a child is a national asset and it is the duty of the State to look after the child with a view of ensuring full development of its personality. Towards this end, State Governments are to set up necessary remand homes and observation homes where children accused of an offence can be sent if Government has insufficient accommodation in its remand homes or observation homes, and to give directions to ensure the protection of the child in criminal trials.

The Court also clarified that the right to a speedy trial is a fundamental right under Art. 21 and as such the Union Government should endeavour to enact a Central Act for the protection and welfare of children. It should specifically ensure the social, economic and psychological rehabilitation of children, who are abandoned, destitute or lost. Although the Court had already called upon the State Governments by its order dated 5th August, 1986 to bring into force and to implement vigorously the provisions of the Children's Act enacted in various States, it observed that it would be desirable if the Central Government initiates parliamentary legislation on the subject in order to bring about uniformity with regard to various provisions relating to children.

Chandan Kumar Banik *vs* State of West Bengal, 1995 Supp (4) S.C.C.

No Chaining of Mentally Ill Patients in Mental Hospital

A letter, accompanied with a newspaper photograph of a mentally ill patient in chains, in the hospital in question, was addressed to the Chief Justice who issued notice to the State of West Bengal and appointed a Committee to inspect the hospital. In the state's counter-affidavit, it took the plea that the hospital was only under its temporary management, as the same was not being properly managed by the Trust that was entrusted with the property. The Court directed that so long as the State is responsible, no matter how temporary an arrangement, it has to provide adequate facilities. In the context of chaining of inmates, the Court specifically ruled that the practice ought to be discontinued immediately and drug treatment be adopted to treat such patients. The State was also directed to appoint an administrator besides the Chief Medical Officer, so that the management of the hospital can receive due time and consideration.

Sheela Barse *vs* Union of India (1993) 4 S.C.C.

Jailing of Non-Criminal, Mentally Ill Persons is Unconstitutional

The Court held that jailing of non-criminal, mentally ill persons is illegal and unconstitutional, and must be stopped. The report submitted by the Committee appointed by the Court, under its order dated 16th June, 1992 was considered. The directions issued by the Supreme Court inter alia were that the Judicial Magistrate was to get such persons examined by a mental health professional/psychiatrist and on his advice send them to the nearest place of treatment and care. The State Government was to take immediate action and issue instructions for implementation, to order enquiry into the death of such persons in jail and to take remedial action. The Court also directed the State Government to take immediate steps for upgrading the mental hospitals, setting up of psychiatric services in all teaching and district hospitals and integrating mental health care with the primary health care system. Calcutta High Court was requested to appoint a Committee, which will submit its report and detailed recommendations. The recommendations of the Committee appointed on the Court's order dated 16th June, 1992 is to be implemented by the other States as well.

In Veena Sethi *vs* State of Bihar, a letter was sent to Justice Bhagwaty by the free Legal Aid Committee on the basis of an article in a newspaper on 17/12/1981. It was registered as a petition under Art. 32 of the Constitution. The Legal Aid Committee, Jamshedpur, through its lawyer Veena Sethi, directed that all charges be dropped against 16 prisoners kept in the Hazaribagh jail for over 25 years because they were of "unsound mind". The Supreme Court said that there must be an adequate number of institutions for looking after mentally sick prisoners and that the practice of sending persons of unsound mind to jail for safe custody was not a healthy or desirable one because jail was not an appropriate place for treating those who were mentally ill. The Court directed the jail superintendent to have such mentally ill under-trials examined by psychiatrists every six months and submit a report to the district Judge. It said that if, as a result of such examination, it is found at any stage that the prisoner concerned had become sane, the District Judge should immediately order his or her release from the jail. The State Government would provide the necessary funds for meeting the expenses of the journey to his or her native place and his or her maintenance for a period of one week, the court said. The state has to provide legal aid in such cases.

This case has also brought to the fore the cases of individuals who were ordered to be kept in detention after their trials were postponed, as they were incapable of defending themselves on ground of 'unsoundness of mind'. In all cases, the period of detention was longer than what might have been awarded if they had been punished for the offence with which they were charged. The case also showed that this indefinite duration confinement may have continued without remission unless the Supreme Court intervened.

What needs to be understood here is that the provision of medical examination, as also of postponement, has been incorporated ostensibly to ensure that a person with psychosocial disability is accorded a fair trial. What however is not appreciated is that the person with disability pays the cost of this fair process provision with the loss of liberty, which could be of indefinite duration.

This provision of safe custody does not subsist only in relation to 'insane under-trials'. A similar provision exists for 'insane acquittees'. Thus, when a court acquits a person on grounds of unsoundness of mind, acquittal does not mean discharge. The court can under Sec. 335 of the CrPC (Code of criminal procedure) either release the 'insane acquittee' on security of a friend or relative or order the 'insane acquittee' to be kept in safe custody of jail or a mental hospital. Once again, release can be secured only if family support is available. The statute provides no guidelines on the periods for which 'insane acquittees' can be kept in a place of safe custody. Veena Sethi once again provided evidence on the indefinite nature of this confinement and the unwillingness of state authorities to order the release of 'insane acquittees'.

One of the most shocking cases was that of Ajoy Ghosh *vs* State of West Bengal. Ajoy Ghosh was arrested in 1962 on the charge of murdering his brother. Subsequently, he was certified insane. After his mother died in 1968, there was no one to visit him. While he remained an under-trial, the trial judge and all the witnesses died. He could not be acquitted unless tried and since he was declared to be of "unsound mind", he could not be tried. Finally, in November 1999, 37 years after he first stepped into a prison, the Supreme Court ordered his transfer from the presidency jail in Kolkata to a home run by the Missionaries of Charity.

Since the bio-medical approach to mental health equated it with a disease, abnormality and danger, the law and practice in the area of health grounded on this approach generally aim towards prevention of disability and conditions in which treatment to cure disability is to be administered. The Mental Health Act of India is a classic example of this approach.

ELECTROCONVULSIVE THERAPY

It is a well-known fact that mental health institutions in India continue to rely on electroconvulsive therapy (ECT), which is banned in some countries. In S.P. Sathe *vs* State of Maharashtra, the Bombay High Court regulated the prescription of indiscriminate electric shocks to mentally ill persons. The directions included that reports be made whenever electric shocks were given by a prison psychiatrist.

A writ petition in the High Court of Bombay at Panaji challenged the practice of administrating ECT without anesthesia at the Institute of Psychiatry and Human Behavior (IPHB), Panaji, Goa. The petition was filed on the basis of a complaint from a patient's relative recently committed to the IPHB for treatment that patients at the IPHB were administered ECT without anesthesia because no anaesthetist was available and the machine was non-functional and in disrepair. The IPHB administered a minimum of 200 procedures a month, with staff members holding the patient down during the procedure. The practice was considered barbaric, inhuman and hence in violation of Art. 21 of the Constitution; in violation of Sec. 81 (Chapter VIII) of the Mental Health Act 1987, providing that no mentally ill person be subjected during treatment to indignity or cruelty. The use of ECT without anesthesia leads to patient discomfort, fractures of the spine and long bones, and dislocations particularly of the jaw. The ECT is also being administered without the patients' informed consent. The petitioner filed the petition on behalf of patients and their relatives, since patients are in no position to approach the court, and relatives are reluctant to come forward, given the stigma attached to mental illness.

The Institute started modified ECT in 1988. However, it stopped the practice in 1992 after the anaesthetist left. In 1995, the government instructed it not to fill up the post, and that the senior resident in anesthesia attached to the Goa Medical College would be at their disposal. On September 22, 1998, the Goa Medical College deputed an anaesthetist twice a week to the Institute. According to Dr. John Fernandes, Director of IPHB, "Since the inception of the establishment of the Institute in 1980, (it) has been treating patients requiring ECT with direct form without administering anesthesia and without any hazards. Our procedures have been free of incidents of fractures. ECT is conducted after taking the consent of patients or, when appropriate, their relatives". The director attached a list of 11 mental hospitals in India, practicing only direct ECT, and eight practicing both.

Direct ECT is not a medically indicated choice but a practice based on non-medical grounds such as non-availability of anaesthetists. Lack of such facilities is due to socio-political reasons and not germane to sound medical practice and procedure.

At least two of the hospitals listed by the respondent have been severely criticized by the Supreme Court. Also, the High Court of Maharashtra (Shukri *vs* State of Maharashtra, 1989, regarding conditions in the Central Institute of Mental Hygiene and Research, Yervada, Pune) stated:

Hospital authorities should review the effects of direct ECT on the patients and should decide whether the method should be continued in view of the fright taken by the patients. Modified ECT is therefore recommended.

In 1988, Shukri from Bombay filed a writ petition in the Bombay High Court. He complained that his mother, who was an inmate of Yerawada Mental Hospital, died due to negligence of the staff. The High Court appointed a committee to look into the affairs at the Hospital. The Mahajan Committee was appointed to look into the affairs of the Central Institute of Mental Hygiene and Research, Yerawada, Pune; and to submit a report about the improvements to be carried out in the Hospital. The Committee had several meetings and visited to the Hospital, and came out with the Mahajan Committee Report on August 5, 1989. The Report has taken up 8 specific aspects: (i) environment; (ii) patients; (iii) staff for the care of the patients; (iv) method of treatment; (v) conditions at the hospital; (vi) internal control; (vii) orientation; and (viii) arrangement for specialized treatment.

SUMMARY OF MAHAJAN COMMITTEE RECOMMENDATIONS

The following is a summary of all the recommendations of the Mahajan Committee, contained in Chapter 10 of the Report:

i. **Environment:** Immediate steps were to be taken to improve the environmental conditions by creating a more humane and pleasing environment wherein the patients can live with human dignity. The dilapidated buildings were to be repaired or reconstructed, along with additional dormitories or wards. The essential amenities, such as drinking water and toilet facilities were to be provided inside the wards.

ii. **Patients:** No patient should be made to do menial work which is to be done by hospital employees. No patient should be subjected to cruelty. Drab and obnoxious clothing and clothing used by other patients should not be given to patients for use. Patients should be provided with a cot, mattress and sufficient linen, which are frequently changed. Patients should be given a bath daily and should be provided with toiletries. Attention should be paid towards the cleanliness of patients. Medical examination of patients should be conducted on a weekly basis. A wholesome diet should be provided to patients.

iii. **Staff:** The Staff should be provided with orientation and regular in-house training. Medical officers on duty should make rounds of hospitals and record their findings in day record book. They should be available in the duty room in the hospital. Observations about patients should be recorded in the night round book. Employees treating patients in a cruel manner should be strictly dealt with. Special arrangements should be made for emergency cases.

iv. **Method of Treatment:** The individual treatment plan should be prepared by qualified professionals for each patient. Medical professionals should constantly review this individual treatment plan. Patients should undergo a comprehensive physical and mental examination on admission and appropriate treatment for physical illness should be available in mental health institutions.

The case file and medical record of the patient should be maintained. ECT should be given in modified form and in decentralized units. Patients undergoing ECT should not witness shock treatment received by other patients. Code of conduct prescribed in the manual with regard to duties and responsibilities of medical and nursing staff should be strictly enforced. Sufficient number of clinical psychologists should be appointed.

v. **Degrading Condition:** There should not be more than six patients in a room. Each patient should be allocated a minimum of 56 ft floor space. Wards should be periodically treated for pest control. Sufficient toilet and lavatory facility should be provided inside wards, and such facility should ensure privacy to patients. Bathing facilities should be provided in a manner so as to ensure privacy. Both hot and cold water facilities were to be provided. Patients should be provided with proper dining facilities, kitchen should be properly maintained and diet should be constantly changed. The co-operative society of the staff should not be awarded contract for supplying provision or any other material. The system of keeping patients locked up should be discontinued.

vi. **Orientation:** A Comprehensive orientation programme should be conducted for staff at all levels; syllabus of the training course should include legal provisions as well as provisions relating to functioning and management of mental health institutions. Short term and long-term courses are to be conducted. These courses are necessary to acquaint the staff with new approaches in treating patients with mental disorder. Intensive training should be given to the staff to ensure that the staff will perform their respective jobs efficiently. The role of psychiatrists, clinical psychologists and psychiatric social workers should be defined and co-ordinated. Workshops and training programmes should be conducted for specialists in whom their respective roles should be explained.

Even though the petition was disposed of, Malati Ranade presented substantial evidence in her letters dated 25/7/95 and 26/2/96 to the fact that the 'State Mental Authority and Inspector's Board' was a total myth, and that the Government had failed to do its duty towards the mental hospitals. She wrote letters and sent out circulars, and privately circulated several papers to peers and others. She questioned the inability of the State government to implement the mental Health Act 1987 [MHA] within the given time period of two years, thereby proving the invalidity of statements made in the Judgment No. 3128 of Dec. 1995 (pages 5 and 6). She monitored the process by which the mental health authorities were managing the issue by keeping article clippings, official letters, etc. She pointed out the errors, inaccuracies, denials and contradictions in the government response and follow up action. She pointed out how the Visitor's book never reflected their visits for so many years. The Visitor's committee was not even aware of their mandate. Though Malati Ranade urged instruments viz. WHO, to look into the matters, nothing changed. The Government and the Court 'closed' the matter by delivering the final judgement in 1998 disposing of the case.

The Mental Health Act 1987 does not lay down specific guidelines to ensure minimum standards in the mental health institutions. Therefore a number of public interest litigations have been filed by concerned citizens and organizations drawing the attention of the Supreme Court to the appalling conditions that generally prevail in mental health institutions.

In Rakesh Chandra Narayan *vs* Staff of Bihar, the Supreme Court found the conditions in the Ranchi Mental Hospital to be shocking and inhuman and therefore appointed a committee to ensure proper functioning and management of funds. The Court also gave directions for mental health institutions to be modelled on the lines of the National Institute of Mental Health and Neurosciences (NIMHANS) at Bangalore. Similarly, in B.R. Kapoor *vs* Union of India the Supreme Court recommended that the hospital management be taken over by Union of India from the Delhi Administration.

Section 81 (2) of the Mental Health Act bars a "mentally ill person" under treatment to be used for purposes of research except with his consent; if he is incompetent to provide such consent, the consent of his guardian is required. The statute thus allows a mentally ill person to be used as a guinea pig, since the guardian could well be the superintendent of the psychiatric hospital.

Worse, a person wrongfully admitted into a psychiatric hospital cannot engineer her own exit unless she has external assistance. Section 81 (3) does prohibit the interception of correspondence of an inmate. However, this prohibition is not absolute and can be breached if the communication is regarded to be prejudicial to the treatment of the ill person.

The Mental Health Act 1987 has not been premised on the rights of persons with psychosocial disability. The rights based law would unequivocally accept the humanity of the rights holder and allow her opportunity to assert it. Constraints would be the exception and freedom the rule. It is only recently that the Courts have started looking into the issue of mental illness from the point of view of the mentally ill. It may still take more than a decade before a full-fledged understanding of rights of mentally ill develops. The right to health and access to medical services for persons with mental illness has evolved to some extent. However, the law is relatively underdeveloped in respect to a broader right to health for persons. For example, questions of availability, affordability, and accessibility of health services, and participation in planning of health policies by persons with disabilities have yet to form an important part of National and State health policies and programmes and related arrangements for the delivery of health services.

Sharda *vs* Dharmapal (2003) 4 S.C.C

Ordering the Psychiatric Examination of Person for Granting Divorce should be Done Upon being Satisfied that a Strong Prima Facie Case has been Made Out

The parties in this case were married in 1991, according to Hindu rites. In 1995, the respondent filed an application for divorce under Secs. 12 (1) [b] and 13 [1] (iii) of the Hindu Marriage Act 1955, along with an application seeking medical examination of the appellant. The appellant objected on the ground that the Court had no jurisdiction to pass such directions. The Court, however, allowed the application and directed the appellant to submit to medical examination. After unsuccessfully approaching the High Court, she filed an appeal in the Supreme Court. On the basis of her pleadings, the Supreme Court formulated the following questions:

a. Whether a matrimonial Court has the power to direct a party to undergo medical examination?

b. Whether the passing of such an order would be in violation of Art. 21 of the Constitution of India?

The Supreme Court also considered the consequences of the refusal of the party concerned, to comply with such a direction. The Court found that a matrimonial Court has the power to order a person to undergo medical test and that the passing of such an order by the Court would not be in violation of the right to personal liberty under Art. 21 of the Indian Constitution. However, the Court should exercise such a power only if the applicant has a strong prime facie case and if there is sufficient material before the Court. If despite the order of the Court, a party refuses to submit herself/himself to medical examination, the Court will be entitled to draw an adverse inference against such a party.

Social Jurist *vs* Government of NCT of Delhi, Cr. W.P. No. 1174/2002, Delhi High Court, dated 20th February, 2002

State to Provide for the Proper Treatment and Rehabilitation of Mentally ill Persons deserted by Family, as per Law

The petition was moved by a group of socially spirited lawyers for a woman with severe psychiatric disorder, after being deserted by her husband. She suffered bouts of violence and would wander aimlessly on the road. Her mother had started keeping her chained and locked in a room.

The Court directed that she should be moved into the care of the Institute of Human Behavior and Allied Sciences and be provided with proper care and treatment. Subsequent to her treatment, the Government of Delhi was given the duty of providing proper rehabilitation for her as per the mandate of the persons with Disabilities Act 1995.

S. Chattanatha Karayalar *vs* Vaikuntarama Karayalar, AIR 1968 Mad. 346: (1968) 2 M.L.J. 150

Right of Person to litigate not Taken away by a next Kin Reiterating Claim of "Insanity"—Proper Procedure to Determine the Same Ought to be followed

The plaintiff, a deaf and dumb person, approached the High Court to set aside the order of the lower Court by which his son was appointed to represent him as next friend in a pending litigation. This was the resultant order in an application asking for the appointment of a next friend of the plaintiff filed by the defendant, alleging the plaintiff's mental infirmity. Though the plaintiff opposed this claim as being mala fide, his son applied to be next friend reiterating the defendant's claim. Without conducting a judicial inquiry as provided under Order XXXII, Rule 15 of the Code of Civil procedure, the lower Court had appointed the son as the next friend of the plaintiff.

The Madras High Court held that when the procedure for determining the mental sanity of the person being called infirm has not been followed, the right of the person to litigate cannot be taken away, even if the next friend reiterates a claim of insanity.

The Court went on to say that it is clear that a person who is deaf and mute and characterized as suffering from a mental infirmity, cannot be taken for granted as one who should be represented by a next friend. Therefore, the court directed a "proper" enquiry with the assistance of medical experts.

Raj Kumar *vs* Rameshchand (1999) 8 S.C.C.

Who can Make an Application under Sec. 50 of the Mental Health Act 1987?

The appellant, a mentally retarded person, who was the owner of the suite premises, filed an application for eviction of the respondent tenant through a next friend. The respondent objected that a guardian had to be appointed by the District Judge, before the matter could proceed. On an application made under Order XXXII Rule I, CL (15) of the Code of Civil procedure the Rent Controller appointed the father as guardian and next friend. Ultimately, the Rent Controller dismissed the application for eviction. This dismissal was challenged by the appellant in the High Court, but the High Court dismissed the revision petition of the appellant without going into the merits of the case, on the reasoning that the eviction petition was not maintainable without a guardian or next friend appointed under the provisions of Secs. 52 to 55 of the Mental Health Act 1987, hence this appeal.

The Supreme Court allowed the appeal and directed the High Court to decide the revision on merits. It was held that Sec. 50 of the Mental Health Act deals with mental condition of a person who is alleged to be mentally ill and is in possession of property. Such an application can be filed only by the persons or authorities specified in clause (a) to (d) of sub-section (1) of Sec. 50. It is pursuant to the proceedings so initiated that the other provisions of the chapter, including Secs. 52 to 55 would apply. Section 50 does not contemplate any application being made or a contention being raised by a tenant in proceedings for eviction against him.

In this case, what was applicable was Order XXXII Rule I read with Rule 15 of the code of civil procedure and application to this effect was filed before the rent controller. Nothing more was required to be done and the High Court erred in coming to the conclusion that the eviction petition was not maintainable on the grounds that the procedure provided by Secs. 52 to 55 of the Mental Health Act 1987 had not been complied with.

Veena Sethi *vs* State of Bihar (1982) 2 S.C.C.

Illegal Detention of Prisoners in the Hazaribagh Central Jail for Almost three Decades without any Justification

A letter by the Free Legal Aid Committee, Hazaribagh, resulted in a PIL, where the Supreme Court examined the cases of 16 prisoners in Hazaribagh Central Jail, who were "of unsound mind" at the date of their incarceration in jail and were still rotting in jail at the date of filing this PIL although they had been declared "sane" long before.

Stating that it was a matter of shame for society that these persons were detained in jail because there are inadequate institutions for the treatment of the mentally ill, the Supreme Court directed the State Government to drop the cases pending against these prisoners in view of the inordinately long incarceration already suffered by them without justification. Further, it directed to provide them with the necessary funds for meeting the expenses of their journey to their native places, as well as maintenance for a week. However, those prisoners who continue to be of unsound mind were not ordered to be released in the interest of society as well as their own interest.

R.D. Upadhyaya *vs* State of A.P. (2001) 1 S.C.C.

Protracted Incarceration of Mentally Ill Accused

The petitioner, as professor of law, approached the Supreme Court with the case of Ajay Ghosh who had been languishing in the prison for decades, since his trial had been stayed due to his mental state. Since the last order of the Magistrate, which required him to be produced into the Court when he is found fit to stand trial, Ajay Ghosh has been forgotten by the authorities for a total of 27 years. His medical examination to ascertain his mental health had not been conducted till the High Court intervened. The Court directed the proceedings pending against him to be quashed and to be released to the care of Missionaries of Charities. The Court further directed that an inquiry be conducted to explain the protracted incarceration of Ajay Ghosh and the defaulter if any, be identified.

In regard to Inhuman Treatment of Mentally Ill patients at Sultan Alavuden Dargah, Tamil Nadu, Case No. 427/22/1998–99

The Commission acted upon a complaint received about the deplorable condition of mentally ill persons at dargahs in Tamil Nadu, who had been left there by the families in the hope of being cured by faith. A committee was constituted to investigate the situation and the recommendations compiled by the Committee were forwarded to the Government of the State for implementation. These recommendations included the proper assistance and medical supervision of the patients at the dargah by the department of psychiatry, Madurai Medical College. It also strongly cautioned against the improper admission and discharge system with the necessary procedures to provide complete care to the patients.

1998 Cr. L.J. 2237 (Knt) (D.B.)

In **Chandrasekhar *vs* State of Karnataka**, it was held that the accused should be admitted in mental hospital rather than to put in prison in cases where reliable medical evidence shows that the accused was of unsound mind when the offence was committed and also that he cannot be convicted and detained in jail.

Pooja Jha: Mental health in India—Published in Chanakya Civil Services December, 2002

MENTAL DISABILITY AND INSANITY

Though the morbidity rate of mental disorders is surprisingly high in India it is a very recent change that a few people have started acknowledging the relevance of general mental health.

Though the developments in the last few decades are not enough to call major improvements, at the same time, the fact of achieving the developmental milestones cannot be denied, the comparative analysis of the period soon after the independence and the present India gives an account of improvement.

S.C. Talati *vs* A.C. Desai, 1986 (10 H.L.R. 305 (Guj))

A lunatic wife can claim maintenance-the provisions of Secs. 125 to 128 of the code of criminal procedure are self-contained and there is nothing in Secs. 125 to 126 of the code of criminal procedure to show that the application on behalf of the lunatic wife cannot be filed by a next friend or guardians of the lunatic wife. If an application can be filed for or on behalf of a child, who is mentally incapable to initiate and conduct the maintenance proceeding, there is nothing in Indian Lunacy Act 1912, which debars an application being made by a next friend or a guardian of a lunatic claiming maintenance under Sec. 125 CrPC. Thus an application for maintenance under this section can be filed by a lunatic wife through a next friend or a guardian.

Sivasankara Panickar *vs* Ravindranath, 1998 (2) civil L.J. 514 at p.517 (Ker): A.I.R. 1975 Mad. 285: 1917 K.L.T 268: I.L.R. 1976 (20 Ker. 357 referred to

Stigma about Mental Infirmity

When the impression of the Court is that a party has given intelligent answer to the question, there is absolutely no justification for casting on that party a stigma about mental infirmity or of an incapacity for defence in the proceedings. The total absence of materials as presented in the petition and the furnishing of intelligent answers during the personal interrogation should ordinarily put an end to the proceedings under Order XXXII, Rule 15 of the code of civil procedure.

Vidya Devi *vs* Himachal Road Transport Corp. Simla, A.I.R. 1990 H.P. 19:1989 (2) Sim L.R. 215 (H.P.)

Suit by Next Friend

A person of infirm mind may not be a person of unsound mind, hence, he can file petition claiming compensation under the Motor Vehicles Act through his next friend. Even a person of weak mind can sue through next friend provided Court is satisfied that he or she was incapable of protecting his or her right.

CONCLUSION

Mental illness is still a medical problem without adequate recognition of its various kinds, causes and degrees. The law needs to deal with these disabilities by understanding the distinctive nature of each one of them. The law is also underdeveloped in its understanding and recognition of the various levels of autonomy that mentally disabled persons may be able to exercise.

Chapter

4

Legal Insanity—General Principles

1. An unsoundness of mind which may amount to insanity from a medical point of view will not necessarily be legal insanity for the purpose of this section so as to confer immunity on the insane person from criminal liability for any act done by him while he is in that state of mind. AIR 1977 SC 608 (611, 614): 1977 Cri LJ 376** (1997) 13 Orissa CR 186(191).
2. To satisfy the requirement of this section it must be proved that at the time of committing the act, the accused person was laboring under such a defect of reason from disease of the mind as not to know the nature and quality of the act he was doing, or as not to know that what he was doing was either wrong or contrary to law. (1979) 47 Cut LT 197: 1986 Mad LJ(Cri) 201 (204) (DB)(Ker).
3. In order that this section may apply, the unsoundness of mind must have made the accused incapable of knowing either (a) the nature of his act, or (b) what he was doing was either wrong or contrary to law. 1979 Cri LJ 403 (406) (DB) (Bom).
4. The mere fact that on earlier occasions a person had been subject to insane delusions or had suffered from derangement of the mind or had subsequently at times behaved like a mentally deficient person is per se insufficient to bring his case within the exemption provided by Sec. 84. The incapacity must have existed at the time of his doing the act charged as an offence. AIR 1971 SC 778 (781): 1971 Cri LJ 654** 1979 Cri LJ 403 (406) (DB) (Bom).
5. The mere fact that the accused at the time of the alleged offence suffering from fever (but there was no delirium) will not attract the operation of this section. AIR 1927 Mad 688 (688): 28 Cri LJ 543 (DB).
6. Unsoundness of mind is not ipso facto a ground of defence under this section unless in consequence of such unsoundness the accused was incapable, at the time of his committing the alleged offence, of knowing either the nature of his act or that the act was either wrong or contrary to law. 1961 (2) Cri LJ 475(476) (Him Pra)** 1986 Mad LJ (Cri) 417 (421) (DB) (Failure to subject the accused to medical examination immediately after offence would entitle the accused to benefit of doubt).
7. In order that this section may apply, the incapacity to know, referred to in the Section, must be due to unsoundness of mind or insanity and not to any other cause. AIR 1948 Nag 20 (2) (23): 48 Cr LJ 377 ** (1988) 15 Reports 149 (160) (Ker).

TYPE OF INSANITY TO WHICH SECTION 84 OF IPC APPLIES

1. In order to avail of the benefit under this section, it must be shown that the cognitive

faculties of the accused were, as a result of unsoundness of mind, so completely deranged as to render him incapable of knowing the nature of his act or that what he was doing was either morally wrong or contrary to law. AIR 1964 SC 1563 (1572): 1964 (2) Cri LJ 472 ** 1973 Mah LJ (Notes) 24 (DB)**.

2. What may be termed legal insanity under the section is not identical with medical insanity. AIR 1960 Guj 1 (2, 4): 1960 Cri LJ 1200 (DB)**.
3. A distinction must be made between insanity affecting the cognitive faculties of a man and that affecting the will or emotions. It is only the first type of insanity that is within the purview of the section. AIR 1948 Nag 20 (2) (23): 48 Cri LJ 377 (DB)**.
4. When the accused was a lesbian and had possible homosexual relationship with the deceased, Sec. 84 cannot be invoked. Lesbianism is a perversity which is a pathological condition distinct from insanity (In insanity there is total loss of control of the mind and inability to distinguish right and wrong). (1996) 2 Ker LT (739) (742): (1996) 2 Ker LJ 417.
5. Where the accused, a young boy who had great interest in his studies and extra-curricular activities went abroad for further studies but his parents who visited there completely ignored him by avoiding to see him and his grandfather's death was also communicated to him much later and he thus being neglected by his parents returned back to his native country and committed offences of brutal nature which a normal man of his status could not do and thereafter he again joined his parents and continued his studies and became a normal individual, accused in such facts and circumstances would be entitled to benefit of Sec. 84. 1993 Cri LJ 2554 (2564) (Kant): 1993 (3) All Cri LR 181.

LUCID INTERVALS—FITS OF INSANITY

1. The section will apply even in cases in which the accused is subject to periodic fits of insanity. But in such cases it must be proved that at the time when he committed the alleged offence, he was suffering from such a fit of insanity. (1976) 42 Cut LT 958 (961): 1977 Cri LJ NOC 21 (DB) ** 1977 Cri LJ 985 (DB).
2. Even in the case of a person subject to fits of insanity the law will presume that he did the act alleged to be the offence during a lucid interval, until the contrary is established. AIR 1969 Madh Pra 203 (205): 1986 Cri LJ 1222 (1225) (DB).
3. When the FIR lodged by the mother of the victims showed that the accused was suffering from fits of lunacy and he killed the kids during those fits and the accused did not conceal the bodies of the victims, nor did he attempt to destroy any evidence, and he had not prepared for the killings, then all these factors would indicate that there could be no mens rea on his part and he killed his grandchildren in fits of lunacy hence benefits of Sec. 84 have to be extended so as to acquit him. (1991) 2 Recent LR 484 (488) (DB) (Bom).
4. Over sensitiveness of mind or character cannot be equated with insanity or automatism. Epileptic insanity must exist at the time of commission of act. 1985 Cri LJ 844 (848) (DB): (1985) 1 Bom CR 508 (DB).

"INCAPABLE OF KNOWING THAT HE IS DOING WHAT IS EITHER WRONG OR CONTRARY TO LAW"

1. Where, at the time of committing the alleged offence, he is aware that his act is wrong (whether from the moral or legal point view), he will not be entitled to the benefit of this section 1962 (2) Cri LJ 135 (140,141) (DB) (Ker) (1945) 47 Punj LR 158 (160).

2. Where a person commits a murder knowing that it is legally an offence but believing that the act is necessary to appease the Gods, or that he has been divinely ordered to commit the murder, he will not escape criminal liability by reason of this section. AIR 1917 pat 503 (503): 1931 Mad WN 719 (721, 722) (DB).
3. The benefit of the section is available to an accused person where owing to insanity, he was not aware, at the time of the commission of the alleged offence, either that the act was wrong or that it was contrary to law. AIR 1949 Cal 182 (183): 50 Cri LJ 255 (DB). 1990 Cri LJ 97 (99) (DB).
4. Although the accused was aware at the time of committing the alleged offence, that he was doing something which was contrary to law, he would be exempt from criminal liability if, owing to his insanity, he believed that his act was ethically or spiritually justified and right. 27 St. Trials 1281, R. V. Hadfield.

   [See 1887 Pun Re (Cr) No. 42. P.99 (102) (DB)].
5. Where an accused kills another person under the insane belief that he will thereby earn spiritual merit and that his act is morally not wrong, although his act may be contrary to law, he will not be criminally liable by reason of this section. AIR 1949 Cal 182 (183): 50 Cri LJ 255 (DB).
6. Murder or other offence committed under the influence of an insane delusion for redressing or revenging some supposed or imaginary grievance will be an offence punishable under the law where the accused was not incapable of knowing that his act was contrary to law. AIR 1918 Pat 179 (181): 19 Cri LJ 135 (SB) AIR 1939 Lah 355 (355): 40 Cri LJ 907.

HALLUCINATION

Where a person is not insane but is unbalanced and excited and is probably laboring under some kind of delusion or hallucination, this section cannot be invoked in his favour.

1963 Mah LJ (Notes) 24 (DB). (Murder of wife and children)

IRRESISTIBLE IMPULSE

Irresistible impulse is not insanity in the sense of this section and is no defence under it. 1978 Ker LT 177: 1978 Cri LJ NOC 182 (DB).

SOMNAMBULISM

Somnambulism, if proved, will constitute unsoundness of mind attracting the application of this section. AIR 1959 Mad 239 (241): 1959 Cri LJ 724 (DB).

PARTIAL MENTAL DERANGEMENT

1. Mental derangement of a partial type which at the time of commission of the alleged offence, does not affect the capacity of the accused to understand the nature of his act or that he is doing what is morally or legally wrong, is not within the section. AIR 1932 All 233 (236): 33 Cri LJ 714 (DB).
2. For pleading insanity and bringing the case within the purview of this section, history of earlier mental derangement is not by itself sufficient. 1993 Cri LJ 3450 (3453) (DB) (Bom).

ABERRATIONS OF MIND

Mere aberrations of mind not amounting to insanity of the degree and type described in this section (i.e. incapacitating the accused at the time of committing the alleged offence from understanding what he is doing or that his act is morally or legally wrong) will not make this section applicable. (1972) 2 Malayan LJ 178 (181).

ECCENTRICITY OF BEHAVIOR

Mere eccentricity of behavior will not prove that the person concerned was insane in the sense of this section, i.e. so as not to be able to understand the nature of his act, or that his act is wrong or contrary to law. 1979 Cri LJ 403 (Pr 9) (DB) (Bom) 1992 Cri LR (Raj) 154 (159, 160) (DB). (Court has also to take into consideration the circumstances which preceded, attended and/or followed the crime.)

ANNOYANCE, FURY, ETC.

The mere fact that the accused had become highly excited and flew into a fury would not bring his case within this section and operate as a defence to a charge of murder committed by him in that state of mind. (1886) ILR 10 Bom 512 (518) (DB) AIR 1955 NUC (Assam) 2852 (DB).

MENTAL AGITATION, DEPRESSION, ETC.

The mere fact that the accused was in a state of acute mental agitation, depression or despondency or that he was, for some time before the act extremely moody, taciturn and so on will not prove that he was suffering from such unsoundness of mind as to make him incapable of knowing what he was doing or that his act was morally or legally wrong. Hence, in such cases the accused will not be entitled to protection under this section merely on the proof of facts of the above nature. 1974 WLN (UC) 102 (104) (DB).

INCAPACITY TO FORM PARTICULAR INTENTION REQUIRED FOR OFFENCE

1. The unsoundness of mind of the accused may, in certain cases, make him incapable of understanding that his act is " dishonest" so as to constitute the offence of criminal breach of trust. In such a case, he will not be criminally liable at all. AIR 1939 Mad 407 (409): 40 Cri LJ 642.
   [See also AIR 1937 Nag 386 (387): 39 Cri LJ 72 (DB)]
2. When the issue of insanity of accused was raised by prosecution itself and the FIR showed that he was mentally disbalanced and there was absence of motive and the accused did not run away from the spot and he was under treatment for mental illness, all these factors establish that the accused had no mens rea and he was utterly unaware of the nature and quality of the act he was doing at the time of incidence, therefore he is entitled to be acquitted under Sec. 84 1990 Sc Cri R 246 (253) (Cal).

POINT OF TIME AT WHICH ACCUSED SHOULD BE SHOWN TO HAVE BEEN INSANE

1. The crucial point of time under this Section, at which the insanity of the accused in the sense of the section must have existed, is the time when the alleged offence was committed by the accused. AIR 1964 SC 1563 (1572): 1964 (2) Cri LJ 472 ** 1997 Cri LJ (NOC) 168 (DB)**.
2. Unsoundness of mind—Accused suffering from schizophrenia—Behavior of accused found to be strange before and after the incident prosecution unable to provide requisite mens rea when accused stabbed the deceased. Held accused was entitled to benefit of Sec. 84 and for acquittal under Sec. 302. 1996 Cri LJ 4186 (4193, 4194) (DB) (Bom).

EVIDENCE OF INSANITY

1. Insanity in the sense of this section is a question of fact. (1973) 39 Cut LT 1289 (1295) (DB)** AIR 1929 Cal 1 (7): 30 Cri LJ 494 (DB).
2. Scientific evidence of insanity is not necessary to sustain a defence under this section and the plea of insanity may be proved from inference of facts and circumstances of each case. AIR 1961 SC 998 (999): 1961 (2) Cri LJ 43 **1997AP LJ (Cri) 40. (Accused killing his 14 month old nephew without any enmity with his parents in a state of insanity.) **
3. Evidence as to the conduct of the accused shortly prior to the offence and his conduct

at the time of or immediately after the crime, his mental condition, family history and so forth will be relevant on the question of the accused's insanity at the time of the offence. AIR 1969 SC 15 (17): 1969 Cri LJ 259 ** 1993 Cri LJ 3450 (3453) (DB) (Bom) **.

4. When it was positively proved by the evidence of the doctor that the accused was suffering from chronic schizophrenia which was incurable and had developed homicidal tendencies then the insanity defence set up by him would be established and he would be entitled to benefit of Sec. 84. (1988) 1 Ker LT 547 (551) (DB).
5. The desire to commit suicide is not necessarily proof of insanity within the meaning of this section which would afford a ground of defence under this section to a charge of murder. 8 Car and P 418: 173 ER 557 (559) **1994 Cri LJ 1173 (1179, 1180) (DB): (1993) 2 Ker LT 852 ** (1848) 3 Cox Cr 275 (276).
6. Homicidal tendency is only a sign of insanity. AIR 1971 SC 778 (780): 1971 Cri LJ 654.
7. Where accused, after raping a 6 years old girl murdered her out of sheer nervousness and fear of being exposed and it was not pre-planned, premeditated or determined action, such act would be said to lean towards a kind of insanity and hence he was awarded life imprisonment instead of death sentence. 1993 All LJ 973 (994) (DB).
8. Where an accused took a girl of four years on his bicycle to a lonely place near the canal and sexually assaulted her and then threw her into the canal, the action was a carefully thought out action and not an act of insane person. 1994 Cri LJ 774 (777) (DB): (1994) 1 Bom LR 575.
9. If at that time the accused was aware that he was doing something wrong or contrary to law, he would not get the benefit of the section. Hence, evidence throwing light on this aspect of the question is relevant for the purpose of showing whether the case is covered by this section. AIR 1961 SC 998 (999): 1961 (2) Cri LJ 43. 1992 Cri LJ 176 (179, 180) (DB) (Ker).

   [See 1978 Ker LT 177: 1978 Cri LJ (NOC) 182 9DB).(Mere presence of circumstances).]
10. The test is to see whether at the time when the accused did the alleged act, he would have done it if a policeman was by his side and the accused was aware of the presence of the policeman. AIR 1959 Madh Pra 259 (261):1959 Cr LJ 844 (DB) **.
11. The fact that after committing a murder the accused tried to run away to conceal himself or otherwise tried to avoid detection and punishment would be evidence to show that he was conscious of his guilt and hence was capable of knowing, in spite of his insanity, if any, that his act was wrong or contrary to law. 1978 Raj LW 230 (233): 1978 Cri LJ (NOC) 264 (DB) ** 1993 Cri LJ 1159 (1161) (DB): 1993 (1) Crimes 430 (DB) (Orissa) **.
12. Where an act of the accused of pushing a young child of 4 years into fire resulting in his death, was accompanied by manifestation of unnatural brutality which was committed in open space and there was no material to show that there was any preparation to commit crime and there was no evidence of a desire to conceal and he also did not show consciousness of guilt by running away or trying to avoid detection, accused would be entitled to benefit under the provisions of this section. 1993 Cri LJ 1201 (1205): 1993 Orissa CR 41 (DB).

INSANITY DURING TRIAL—EVIDENTIARY VALUE

1. Insanity of accused during the trial or during the investigation or preliminary enquiry into the offence is by itself

irrelevant for the purpose of this section. But such insanity may give rise to a suspicion that the accused might have been insane at the time of the commission of the offence and might be a relevant fact in that context. 1961 (1) Cri LJ 811 (812, 813) (Cal) (DB) ** 1954 All LJ 293.

MOTIVE FOR CRIME

1. The absence of an adequate motive for a serious crime like murder is not by itself proof of insanity on the part of the accused in the sense of this section. 1982 Cri LJ 2158 (2162): (1982) 54 Cut LT 195 (DB) **1994 Cri LJ 450 (454, 455) (DB).
2. Accused killing his own mother during epileptic insanity—Complete absence of motive or provocation, the nature and multiplicity of weapons used, the duration of the attack, the maniacal fury with which the attack was delivered and his subsequent conduct were all indication that the accused was acting under some insane impulse and therefore (his act) was saved under Sec. 84. AIR 1960 Ker 24 (26, 27): 1960 Cri LJ 73 (DB).

HEREDITARY INSANITY

1. A history of insanity in the accused's family will be a relevant piece of evidence to support a plea of insanity under this section. 1953 BL JR 606 ** AIR 1923 All 327 (2) (328): 24 Cri LJ 225 (DB).
2. The opinion of a medical man as to the state of mind of the accused at the time of the commission of the alleged offence is not conclusive and binding on the Court and it is for the Court to decide the question whether at that time the accused was, by reason of unsoundness of mind incapable of knowing what he was doing or that he was doing something wrong or contrary to law. AIR 1969 Orissa 222 (223): 1969 Cri LJ 1147**.
3. A mere medical certificate of insanity is not enough as proof of insanity under this section. The Medical Officer who issued the medical certificate must be asked to appear personally as a witness in the case and be examined carefully. AIR 1955 NUC (Madh Bha) 2993 (DB) ** AIR 1934 Lah 123 (126): 35 Cri LJ 869 (DB).

EXCESSIVE OR UNUSUAL VIOLENCE AS PROOF OF INSANITY

1. The insanity of the accused, in the sense of this section at the time of his committing the act constituting the alleged offence cannot be established merely by the brutality or the ferociousness of the Act.AIR 1964 SC 1563 (1572): 1964 (2) Cri LJ 472 ** 1979 Cri LJ 403 (407) (DB) (Bom) **.

   [See also 1978 Ker LT 177: 1978 Cri LJ (NOC) 182 (DB) ** 1974 MPLJ 203: 1974 Jab LJ 302 (307) (DB).]

BURDEN OF PROOF

1. The law presumes every person to be sane and quite capable of distinguishing between right and wrong, till the contrary is proved. 1978 Ker LT 177: 1978 Cri LJ (NOC) 182 (DB) ** 1986 Cri LJ 1222 (1225) (DB).
2. The rules of burden of proof in the context of plea of insanity are: (a) The prosecution must prove beyond reasonable doubt that the offence was committed by the accused, (b) It is rebuttable presumption that the prisoner was not insane when he committed offence, (c) The accused may rebut the presumption of sanity at the relevant time bringing the case within Sec. 84 by producing oral, documentary, circumstantial and other materials and he may discharge the burden by establishing a reasonably probable case and (d) Even if the accused fails to establish affirmatively

or conclusively that he was of unsound mind and committed the act under the circumstances set out in Sec. 84, but raises a reasonable doubt in the mind of the Court as regards presence of essential ingredients of the offence, which includes 'mens rea,' the requisite criminal intention, the Court would be entitled to acquit the accused on the ground that the general burden of proof resting on the prosecution was not discharged. 1997 Cri LJ 1461 (1463) (DB): 1996 (3) Rec Cri R 334 (Gauhati).

3. Where the accused pleads insanity at the time of the commission of the offence the burden of proof of such plea is entirely on the accused. AIR 1974 SC 216 (217, 218): 1975 Cri LJ 305 ** 1994 Cri LJ 450 (453) (DB): (1992) 1 Ker LT 544 ** 1994 Cri LJ (NOC) 110 (DB): 1994 Cri LJ 1897 (1900) (DB): (1994) 1 Raj LW 1. **

PLEA OF INSANITY

Where the defence wishes to rely on the plea of insanity of the accused at the time of the offence, it is for the defence to raise the plea and where there is no indication at all that the accused was suffering from unsoundness of mind at the time of the offence, it cannot be contended that the trial is vitiated by the failure of the Court to try as a preliminary issue the question of the accused's sanity (1931) 32 Cri LJ 816 (817) (DB) (Lah).

SENTENCE

1. Where at the time of committing the offence the accused was laboring under some form of insanity, but, at the same time, was aware of the nature of his act and that it was wrong or contrary to law, it would not be appropriate to award the extreme (death) penalty of the law, but it would be more in accordance with justice to pass a sentence for imprisonment for life. AIR 1967 Ker 92 (94, 95): 1967 Cri LJ 494 ** [See also 1957 Madh BLJ 1008 (1015) (DB).]
2. An accused, who is insane, especially if he is undefended, is naturally thrown on the mercy of the Court whose duty is then to offer him all reasonable assistance. The first thing is to place the prisoner suspected of insanity under medical observation promptly so that when the case comes up for trial, there would be reliable medical evidence of the state of mind of the accused immediately after the incident. AIR 1960 Ker 241 (243): 1960 Cri LJ 1086.
3. Where the defence of diminished responsibility is raised and the Judge is satisfied on the balance of probabilities that the accused was suffering from "abnormality of mind" from one of the causes specified in Exception 7 of S 300 of the Penal Code, the crucial question that arises for the Judge to decide is whether or not the abnormality was such as substantially impaired the accused's mental responsibility for his acts in causing the death or being a party to causing the death. (1981) 1 Malayan LJ 1 (3).

SCOPE AND APPLICABILITY OF SECTIONS

1. Sections 85 and 86 deal with cases in which an offence is committed by a person while he is in a state of intoxication. Where there is no evidence of intoxication, these sections do not apply. AIR 1970 Pat 303 (304): 1970 Cri LJ 1245 (DB).
2. Section 85 deals with cases in which, by reason of intoxication, a person is incapable of knowing the nature of the act or that he is doing what is either wrong or contrary to law. In these cases, the accused will not be criminally liable provided that the thing which intoxicated the accused was administered to him without his knowledge or against his will (1912) 13 Cri LJ 167 (167, 168) (DB) (Nag).
3. Under both the sections, the defence that the alleged criminal act was done under the influence of intoxication will not be available if the intoxication was "volun-

tary", i.e. was the result of the accused's own voluntary act. (1978) 45 Cut LT 533: 1978 Cri LJ (NOC) 259 (DB) ** 1982 Cri LJ (NOC) 39 (DB) (Gau).

4. Section 86 is an exception to Sec. 85: the degree of intoxication demanded is the same and the Sec.86 cannot be construed to mean that it permits intoxication of a lesser degree. 1987 Cri LJ 1416 (1417) (DB): (1987) 2 Bom CR 46.
5. Habitual and excessive drunkenness or the taking of drugs or smoking of narcotics may lead to insanity. There is no difference between insanity caused by drink, etc. like delirium tremens and insanity resulting from other causes. AIR 1941 Lah 454 (457): 43 Cri LJ 332 (DB) ** AIR 1937 Nag 386 (387): 39 Cri LJ 72 (DB).
6. Voluntary drunkenness will save a person from criminal liability for his acts only where such drunkenness has led to his insanity and he is unable by reason of such insanity to understand what he is doing or that his act is wrong or contrary to law. AIR 1957 All 667 (670, 671): 1957 Cri LJ 1056 (DB) ** AIR 1941 Lah 454 (456): 43 Cri LJ 332 (DB) ** AIR 1937 Nag 386 (387): 39 Cri LJ 72 (DB) ** (1912) 13 Cri LJ 164 (165) (DB) (Nag).

"LIABLE TO BE DEALT WITH..."—MEANING

1. In case of voluntarily intoxication it is left to the discretion of the Court to deal with the accused person as if he had the same knowledge as a sober person and does not make it obligatory on the Court to do so. AIR 1929 All 260 (260): 30 Cri LJ 340 (DB).

OFFENCE REQUIRING PARTICULAR KNOWLEDGE

1. If the accused did the act while in a state of voluntary intoxication, he will be presumed to have known that it was so imminently dangerous that it must in all probability, cause death, and if the presumption is not rebutted, the accused will be held guilty of murder. AIR 1953 Raj 40 (42): 1953 Cri LJ 434 (DB).

INTENTION AND KNOWLEDGE—DISTINCTION IN MODE OF TREATMENT UNDER SECTION 86

1. Section 86 makes a distinction between offences requiring a particular knowledge and those requiring a particular intention. While under Sec. 86 presumption as to the knowledge possessed by the accused at the time of commission of offence can be raised there is no provision in Sec. 86 for presuming intention. AIR 1942 pat 420 (421): 43 Cri LJ 883 (DB) ** AIR 1939 Mad 407 (408, 409): 40 Cri LJ 642 ** 1931 Mad WN 113 (114).

   [See AIR 1942 Pat 427 (429): 43 Cri LJ 544 (DB) ** AIR 1917 Lah 226 (230): 18 Cri LJ 868 (DB) ** AIR 1916 Mad 489 (490): 16 Cri LJ 627.]

   (See also 1937 Mad WN 1329 (1330, 1331) (DB).]

CASE LAW

Bhikari *vs* State of UP, Supreme Court Cr App No. 263 of 1964

The way in which the accused used to conduct himself before the incident, the manner in which he acted during the incident and his subsequent conduct are the factors to be considered.

R *vs* Podola (1960) QB 235

GF Podola, aged 40, while in detention was charged for the murder of Detective-Sergeant Purdy by shooting and then escaped. He was actually rearrested four days after the murder. It was pleaded by the defence that Podola was unfit to plead, as he was suffering from hysterical amnesia and had lost all memory regarding his arrest and alleged shooting. The presiding judge held that the onus of proof of amnesia was with the defence.

One of the experts for the defence said that in hysterical amnesia, skill is virtually never lost, but memory of identity, place where one lives, is lost. What one normally does is apt to go. Thus, a person suffering from hysterical amnesia may be able to drive a car or play chess. He emphasized that the functional loss of memory is a selective matter and that a malingerer would produce a blanket loss of memory. Another expert opined that it is the tremendeous continuous fear that triggers off all potential explosive anxiety in his personality and drives the man out of his mind.

Dr. Brisby, the senior medical officer of the prison, said that he had never seen or found a recorded case where there was complete loss of memory without some impairment of the personality or other signs of hysteria. According to another expert who disagreed, his essential consciousness of his own identity was lost and with it there was loss of general knowledge and essential skills. Finally, the jury decided that he was fit to stand the trial, convicted, and sentenced to death; since then, there had been considerable criticism against the sentence of death.

(1892) 8 TLR 559

Even in England, there is little authority to show whether a person of unsound mind is liable for torts committed by him. Justice Esher in Hanbury *vs* Hanbury stated that 'I am prepared to lay down as the law of England that whenever a person does an act which is either a criminal or a culpable act, which act, if done by a person with perfect mind, would make him civilly or criminally responsible to the law, provided the disease of the mind of the person doing the act be not so great as to make him unable to understand the nature and consequence of the act which he is doing'.

(1952) 1 all ER 925

In Morris *vs* Marsden, a person suffering from mental disease attacked and injured the plaintiff who then recovered damages against the mentally diseased person, since that defendant knew the nature and quality of his tortious act even though he did not know that what he was doing was wrong. The McNaughton Rules were held not to apply to this tort in the circumstances. The question that arose was where the defendant knew the nature and quality of his act, was it a defence that owing to mental infirmity, he was incapable of knowing that his act was wrong? Mr. Justice Stable said:

"If the basis of liability be that it depends not in the injury to the victim, but on the culpability of the wrong doer, there is a considerable force in the argument that it is, but I have come to the conclusion that knowledge of the wrong doing is an immaterial averment, and that where there is the capacity to know the nature and quality of the act, that is sufficient, although the mind directing the hand that did the wrong was diseased".

Law of Torts, 12th edn, PP 88–89 quoted in Anand and Sastri, Law of Torts, fifth edn, pp 195–196

Clerk and Lindsall made the following observation.

There is no reported instance of an action of tort ever having been brought in this country against a lunatic, but it is apprehended that lunatics are liable for torts to the same extent as sane persons, provided that the torts are committed by them while in that condition of mind which is essential to the liability in sane persons.

(1894) 42 Am St Rep 743

In Williams *vs* Hays, the defendant a co-owner of the ship was held liable to his co-owners for negligent wrecking of the ship owing to his insanity. It was held that an insane person is just as responsible in tort as a sane person except where malice and hence intention, actual or implied, is necessary.

Hanbury *vs* Hanbury 8 TLR 559

In summing up the law, it may be stated in the words of Justice Esher M.R. that 'a lunatic' is liable unless the disease of his mind is so great that he cannot understand the nature and consequences of his act.

Munishwar Dutt *vs* Indra AIR 1963 Punj 449

Before the 1976 amendment, when the statutory description of insanity was extremely limited, it was once held that though medical evidence had its importance, the question was for the courts to decide, and not for experts.

Kuttappan *vs* State of Kerala 1986 Cr LJ 271 (Ker) (DB)

Criminal Responsibility: The law presumes every individual at the age of discretion, to be sane and to possess a sufficient degree of reason to be responsible for his criminal acts, unless the contrary is proved to the satisfaction of the court. Defence of insanity is mostly raised in charges of murder.

Leaders, 17 September 1925

In an appeal to the High Court of Allahabad, one Lockmani, who had been convicted of murdering his wife and sentenced to death under Sec. 302 of Indian Penal Code 1860, by the Sessions Judge of Kumaon, the High Court set aside conviction and the sentence, as there was no motive for committing the murder. The accused admitted the crime before the magistrate, and when asked why he did it, he said it was the will of the God. It was concluded that, by reason of unsoundness of mind, he was incapable of knowing the nature of the act.

1929 Cr LJ 1924; KE *vs* Sankappa Setty (1941) 42 Cr LJ 558

In another case, where one Jalal killed a young woman of 26 years with a 'toka', it was held that the mere want of a motive and the fact that the accused showed some sign, that he suffered from a certain hallucination are not sufficient to attract the application of Sec. 84 of the Indian Penal Code 1860. He was convicted of murder under Sec. 302 of the Indian Penal Code 1860, and was sentenced to transportation for life.

KE *vs* Ghungar Mal Chania Lal (1939) 40 Cr LJ 907

In an appeal before the Lahore High Court, where the accused had been sentenced to transportation for life under Sec. 302 of the Indian Penal Code 1860, for having murdered a boy by beating him on the head till he died, the plea of insanity was raised on behalf of the appellant, as he was certified insane and was admitted to the Punjab Mental Hospital from which he was discharged as cured after a certain period. He then stood his trial.

(1929) 30 Cr LJ 247

One Karma Urang, accused, had a dream in which the Goddess Kali appeared before him and told him that his father was a descendant of Kali and that if the accused did not kill his father, his father would kill him. The accused honestly believed this and cut his father's head the next day and was coolly proceeding with it to the court with the object of producing the head before the court, when he was arrested. The medical evidence showed that he was under a definite delusion. It was ruled in an appeal in the Calcutta High Court that the accused must, under the circumstances, be held to have been incapable at the time of the doing of the act by reason of unsoundness of mind of knowing the nature of the act or that he was doing what was either wrong or contrary to law within the meaning of Sec. 84 of the Indian Penal Code 1860 and that he could not be convicted of murder.

Leader, 23 September 1933

It was, therefore, found that the accused did stab the boy with a knife and caused his death, but he was acquitted on the ground that at the time when he committed the act, he was, by reason of unsoundness of mind, incapable of knowing the nature of the act. Under Sec. 471 of the Code of Criminal Procedure 1973, the accused was directed to be detained in safe custody in such place and manner, as the sessions judge might think fit.

State *vs* Balu Narain Sessions Case No. 161 of 1971

In another case, Balu Narain took her one and a half year old daughter Soni, by her legs and after spinning the child dashed her head against a wall, thereby, breaking open her head. The child died on the spot. On the evidence of Dr. Franklin, the Police Surgeon, it was held that at the time of the incident, she was of unsound mind and incapable of knowing the nature of the act or what she was doing was either wrong or contrary to law. She was acquitted by the judge from the charge of murdering her own daughter under Sec. 302 of the Indian Penal Code 1860: However, she was ordered to be kept detained in safe custody.

Abdul Latif *vs* state 1981 Cr LJ 1205

It is not justice to demand proof of insanity from a person who has just recovered from mental derangement to establish his mental faculties at the time of offence. In such cases, insanity may be established by preponderance of probabilities on the basis of some features flowing from the conduct of the accused, which point to a reasonable doubt that he had acted under circumstances set forth in Sec. 84 of the Indian Penal code 1860.

Dahyabhai Chaganbhai Thakkar *vs* State of Gujarat AIR 1964 SC 1563,(1964) 2 Cr LJ 472 relied on in Sheralli Wali Mohammed *vs* State of Maharashtra (1973) SCC (Cr) 726, (1973) 4 SCC 790; Kuttappan *vs* State of Kerala 1986 Cr LJ 271, 1986 KLT 64 (DB); Shama Tudu *vs* State 1987 Cr LJ 618

Subba Rao J, as he then was speaking for the court said: "The prosecution must prove beyond reasonable doubt that the accused had committed the offence with the requisite mens rea, and that the burden of proving always rests on the prosecution from the beginning to the end of the trial".

There is a rebuttable presumption that the accused was not insane, when he committed the crime, in the sense laid down by Sec. 84 of the Indian Penal Code 1860; the accused may rebut it by placing before the court all the relevant evidence—oral, documentary or circumstantial, but the burden of proof upon him is no higher than that which rests upon a party to civil proceedings.

Even if the accused was not able to establish conclusively that he was insane at the time he committed the offence, the evidence placed before the court by the accused or by the prosecution may raise a reasonable doubt in the mind of the court as regards one or more of the ingredients of the offence, including mens rea of the accused on the ground that the general burden of proof resting on the prosecution was not discharged.

M Parvaiah *vs* State of Andhra Pradesh 1985 Cr LJ 1924 (AP) (DB)

In a case, where the conduct of the accused in committing an act demonstrates an abnormality, the prosecution should place, before the court, some evidence to indicate that the accused was in a proper state of mind at the time when he committed the alleged offence.

Kusa Majhi *vs* State 1985 Cr LJ 1460 (Ori) (DB)

An accused person does not have to prove his case beyond reasonable doubt and it is sufficient if his plea of insanity is established by preponderance of probabilities as in a civil case.

State *vs* J Gaspar AIR 1971 Goa 3 at 7; Balwant Rao Bajirao *vs* Emperor AIR 1949 Nag 66; State *vs* Kaji Jeeram AIR 1955 Sau 105, 1955 Cr LJ 1628

Where the opinion of the medical witness is based on the testimony of the witnesses and not on his own observations, in such a case it is only the presumption of the medical witness and no importance can be attached to it.

Onkar Lal *vs* State of Madhya Pradesh 1987 Cr LJ 1289 at 1292–93

For the purpose of criminal law, the emphasis is, therefore on that degree of unsoundness of mind, which incapacitates a person from knowing the nature of the act or that, he is doing what is either wrong or contrary to law.

Keshav Rao *vs* State of Maharashtra 1979 Cr LJ 403 (Bom); Sudhir Ch Biswas *vs* State 1987 Cr LJ 683 (Cal) (DB); Narayan Chandra Dey *vs* State 1988 Cr LJ 387 (Cal) (DB)

Unsoundness of mind implies a state of mind in which an accused is incapable of knowing that he is doing anything wrong or anything contrary to law. Mere eccentricity or strange behavior of the accused is not enough to constitute his unsoundness of mind.

Ramswarup Thakur *vs* State of Bihar 2000 Cr LJ 426

Ramswarup Thakur, the accused killed his three year-old son and was sent for treatment at Manasik Arogyashala, Ranchi where he was treated for two years and thereafter was declared fit. The trial court did not examine the doctors of Mansik Arogyashala and convicted him, assuming him to be of sound mind at the time of commission of the crime. The Patna High Court, in appeal, set aside the conviction, citing Chhaganbhai Thakkar where it was held.

When a plea of legal insanity is set up, the court has to consider whether at the time of commission of offence, the accused, by reason of unsoundness of mind, was incapable of knowing the nature of the act or the act he was doing was either wrong or contrary to law. The crucial point of time for ascertaining the state of mind of the accused is the time when the offence was committed. Whether the accused was in such a state of mind as to be entitled to the benefit of Sec. 84 of the Indian Penal Code 1860, can only be established from the circumstances which preceded, attended and followed the crime. In the present case, it was essential to examine the doctors who had treated the appellant at Ranchi. The conviction was set aside after getting reports from the doctors of the Ranchi Manasik Arogyashala. (Dahyabhai Chhaganbhai Thakkar *vs* State of Gujarat 1964 Cr LJ 472.)

1993 Cr LJ 3149

In Brushabha Digal *vs* State of Orissa, the accused killed a girl of two years of age and oral evidence along with the doctor's report when he visited the jail, gave evidence about unsoundness of mind of the accused. The Orissa High Court set aside the conviction by the trial court on the ground of insanity.

1998 Cr LJ 4325

In Raval Mohanbhai Laxmanbhai *vs* State of Gujarat, the accused killed his wife and the testimony of witness established that the accused had some effect on his mind about 10 days prior to incident and was intended to be treated by a sorcerer. The conduct of the accused prior to, at the time of and subsequently showed that he was not in a fit state of mind. The Gujarat High Court setting aside the conviction of trial court and extended the benefit of Sec. 84 of the Indian Penal Code 1860 to the accused.

1997 Cr LJ 772

In SK Nair *vs* State of Punjab, the appellant was convicted by the trial court for the offence of murder which was upheld by the Punjab and Haryana High Court and the same was further confirmed by the Supreme Court by observing that:

We are, however, unable to accept the submission of the learned counsel that being paranoid, the appellant must be presumed to have committed the said offence being seized of sudden impulsive feeds of passion for which temporarily, he was completely incapable to understand as to what he had been doing with what consequences. Even if it is assumed that in the case of paranoia, the ordinary test of lucid interval as applicable in case of patients with unsound mind is not to be applied, and if paranoia is likely to be seized of sudden bouts of impulsive feeds for which temporarily he becomes completely incapable to understand the implication of his activities and such sudden bouts may also disappear within a very short time. In the instant case, it has been revealed from the evidence adduced that at the time of the commission of the said offence, the appellant did not completely lose his sense of understanding. When the deceased caught hold of him and told him that he would be taken to the officers, he retorted that the deceased could do that if he was alive then and so saying inflicted khukri blows on him. Such words and acts only demonstrate that at the time of commission of the offence, he could explain his intended action with logic. Hence, it is not necessary to consider the probabilities which may happen with a paranoid. In the facts of the case, it has been clearly established that the accused was not incapable to understand the implication of his acts. Hence, no interference is called for in this appeal. Appeal dismissed.

Hazara Singh *vs* State, AIR 1958 P & H

Criminal Liability of Mentally Unsound Persons and Imposition of Death Penalty

The trial court had found the appellant Hazara Singh guilty of having murdered his wife, and sentenced him to death after having considered the defence plea of mental insanity. The appellant was laboring under strong delusions that his wife being unfaithful and previously his son had attempted to admit him for treatment. The medical testimony presented in defence stated clearly that apart from the delusions under which he grievously hurt his wife, the appellant was conscious of his surroundings and had an ordinary conception of right and wrong.

The High Court did not confirm the death penalty upon reference from the District court. While it had not found the case as one fit for the extreme form of punishment since the crime was a result of mental delusions, the court stated that not every kind of mental condition would form part of defence from criminal sanctions. Since the medical expert was clear on the fact that barring the indelible delusions, the accused knew his bearings, the court did not rid him of the criminal liability of his actions, instead, the sentence was reduced to life imprisonment.

The commentary of criminal liability of the mentally unsound contained in the judgment is of immense relevance in ascertaining the legal understanding of mental illnesses while determining culpability and punishment or protection. The courts in reducing the sentence of the condemned to life imprisonment have duly considered both the nature and degree of insanity as well as the capacity of the person to make his defence, thereby laying down a principle. The case also assumes immense significance on both subjects—culpability of the mentally unsound and the death penalty.

Vivian Rodrick *vs* State of West Bengal (1969) 3 SCC

Postponement of Court Proceedings in Case of Unsoundness of Mind

Vivian Rodrick was convicted of several offences and sentenced to death under Sec. 302 of the Indian penal Code. The High Court confirmed the sentence. In the special leave petition filed before the Supreme Court by Rodrick, one of the contentions raised by him was that at the time of the proceedings of the appeal before the High Court, he was of unsound mind and hence an inquiry should have been made under Sec. 465 of the Code of Criminal Procedure about the unsoundness of his mind before proceeding on the merits of the case.

The Apex Court held that when a medical report states that an accused-appellant is of unsound mind, it is reasonable to infer that he is incapable of making his defence. If the manner, in which the accused behaves or answers questions, raises doubts in the mind of the Court, the proceedings may be postponed.

1996 (1) Civil LJ 857: AIR 1996 SC 1002: 1996 (1) SCC 720: JT 1996 (1) (SC) 205

Mental Illness

In Karumanda Gounder *vs* Mithuswami Gounder, it was held that a person of weak intellect or who is unable to managing his affairs should not be called lunatic, rather to be adjudged as a mild lunatic.

AIR 1992 Ker 257: 1992 (1) Ker. L.J. 482

Mental Illness

In Mytheen Kunju Abdul Salem *vs* Mohammed Kasim Ismail, it was held that the application can be dismissed for want of directing inquisition as application for adjudging a person to be lunatic ought to be decided only on inquisition.

AIR 1994 Gau. 99

Mental Illness

In Jyotindra Bhattacharjee *vs* Mrs. Sona Bala Bora, the sale deed was vitiated because at the time of execution of the deed the person was not of sound mind.

1968 2 S.C.R. 572

In Ram Chandra Arya *vs* Man Singh, it was held that decree against a person of unsound mind is to be treated as without jurisdiction and void.

1994 Cr.L.J. 1173 (Ker)

In Sankaran *vs* State it was held that minor deviations from regular and usual human conduct do not render a person insane.

AIR 1979 S.C. 15 1968 Cr. L.J. 259; 1996 Cr.L.J.2582 (A.P.) (D.B.)

In Jai Lal *vs* Delhi Administration, and in Shaik Ahmed *vs* State of AP it was held that it is not the duty of prosecution to establish the fact that the accused was capable of knowing the nature of the act or of knowing that what he was doing was either wrong or contrary to law, in cases where plea of insanity is raised.

2000 Cr.L.J. 426 (Pat) (D.B.)

In Ram Swarup Thakur *vs* State of Bihar, the accused had killed his 3 years old minor son for no apparent reason, pleaded insanity, and was in mental hospital for 2 years. His plea of unsoundness of mind was accepted and he was acquitted.

AIR 1977 S.C. 608:1977 Cr. L.J. 376;1996 Cr.L.J. 3363 (Ker) (D.B.)

In Amrit Bhusan *vs* Union of India and Venugopalan Venu *vs* State of Kerala, it was held that as at the time of occurrence and thereafter, the accused was in normal state of mind, so the plea of unsoundness of mind was rejected.

AIR 1997 SC 1537:1997 Cr. LJ 772

In S.K. Nair *vs* State of Punjab, the plea of insanity under Sec. 84 of the Indian Penal Code, 1860, was not accepted because the evidence shows that the accused fully knew the implications of his act when he committed the offence.

1994 Cr.L.J. 1173 (Ker)

The word "insanity" does not connote any definite medical entity. It is solely a legal and sociological concept used to designate those members of the society who are unable on account of mental disease, to adapt themselves to ordinary social requirements.

The word "insanity" has no technical meaning in law or medicine. In Sankaran *vs*

State, Kerala High Court has defined the word 'insanity' as follows quoting the cases noted below:

Surati Abdul Sattar *vs* Hajee Md. Abdul Rahim Surati, 1982 (1) Civil L.J. 1 at p. 4 (Knt)

Some are born insane and some become insane. In both the cases it suggests some derangement of the mind, which is not to be confused with or taken as analogous to a mere mental weakness or lack of intelligence.

Majaharuddin Khan *vs* Serajuddin Khan, (1906) 4 C.L.J. 115

Unsoundness of mind taken by itself is not sufficient to bring a person within the term "lunatic", unless it would incapacitate him from managing his own affairs; nor on the other hand will a person who is incapable of managing his affairs be a lunatic, unless that incapacity is produced by unsoundness of mind.

Karumanda Gounder *vs* Muthuswami Gounder, 1996 (1) Civil L.J. 857 (S.C.)" AIR 1996 S.C.1002: 1996 (1) S.C.C. 720: J.T. 1996 (1) 205 (S.C.)

A person has to be adjudged a lunatic whereafter certain consequences may follow but since there was no such thing as a "mild lunatic", therefore, it was held that a person may be of weak intellect, incapable of managing his affairs, but that per se would not make him a lunatic.

Jyotindra Bhattacharjee *vs* Sona Bala Bora. AIR 1994 Gau. 99

Execution of sale deed by person of unsound mind—sale deed executed by a person not of sound mind at the time of execution of the deed stands vitiated.

Devkoo *vs* Rama Dogra, 1993 (1) Civil L.J. 145 (H.P.)

Unsoundness of Mind—Test for

Person pleading unsoundness of mind has to prove unsoundness.

H.S.trivedi *vs* Namdeo Vishnu Kanalekar, 1985 (20 Civil L.J. 576 at p. 583 (Bom)

Unsound Mind—Burden of Proof

A person may prove to have fits of epileptic insanity and can also plead the same as defence to a criminal charge but the cause of the whole question is whether the man was suffering from epilepsy at the time he committed the act. It is the moment of the act that is important and it will have to be shown that the person was incapable of knowing that what he was doing was wrong.

Najir Ahmed *vs* Haneefa, AIR 1974 J & K. 43:1973 J & K.L.R. 247: 1973 Kash L.J. 211

Compromise decree against person of unsound mind—Compromise decree against person of unsound mind without leave of Court as required by Rule 7(1) of Order XXXII of the Code of Civil procedure is not invalid or void. It is only voidable at the instance of the person under infirmity.

Johni *vs* Mahila Draupadi alias Dropadi, AIR 1991 M.P. 340: 1991 M.P. L.J. 217 (M.P.)

Where the transferee knew that the owner was lunatic, the transfer in his favour will be rendered void.

Jhabarmal Panda *vs* Bhagwati Kedia., AIR 1990 Gau. 95

Insanity—Determination of

Inquiry—Order XXXII, rule 15 of Civil procedure insists an inquiry to be made in respect of persons who are incapable, by reason of any mental infirmity, of protecting their interest. As held in the instant case, for determination of the question of alleged insanity of a party, it is necessary that the party alleged to be insane may be got examined by a medical expert and a certificate obtained from him as to whether he is mentally fit. To protect his interest, the court must conduct an inquiry into the alleged mental infirmity of the person and come to a definite conclusion that the alleged information is well founded before proceeding to appoint a guardian for him.

S. Murthy *vs* State (1988) 1 Crimes 326 (Mad); Shama *vs* State (1986) 61 Cut L.T. 649; venkatraj *vs* State, 1985 M.L.J. (Cr.) 394

A person suffers from legal insanity where his cognitive faculty of mind is destroyed as a result of unsoundness of mind to such an extent as to render him incapable of knowing the nature of the act or that what he was doing was contrary to law.

Venugopalan Venu *vs* State of kerala, 1996 Cr. L.J. 3363 (Ker); 1996 (2) I.L.R. 818 (Ker)

Insanity—Unsound of Mind—Nature of

In other words, the unsoundness of mind should be of such a nature, which will blind or affect the perception of facts by the accused person so that he does not know the nature of the act he is doing or that what he is doing is wrong or contrary to law. To express in a more abstract language his cognitive faculties must, be affected by the unsoundness of mind to such an extent that he does not know the nature of the act he is doing or that what he is doing is wrong or contrary to law. This has to be arrived at by the court from the medical evidence in the case and from the other evidence adduced.

Bhan Singh *vs* State of M.P. 1990 Cr.L.J. 1861 (M.P.)

In a plea of insanity the antecedents and subsequent conduct of the accused is relevant, but, such conduct is not per se enough to show, the state of mind of the accused at the time of the commission of the act, in absence of materials to show that what he was doing was wrong or contrary to law. The mere circumstance that without apparent motive he has committed at least two murders and in all, four ghastly murders, in itself does not lead to a reasonable inference that he suffered from insanity. In absence of proper materials, such defence if treated as part of our judicial system would be subversive to life and property.

Govind Ram Chandra Jadhav *vs* State of Maharashtra 1996 Cr. L.J. 4186

Plea of Insanity—Proof of

The accused was not feigning insanity nor could it be said with any certainty of definiteness that the accused was absolutely sane on the date and at the time, when he assaulted the deceased with a knife. It has to be borne in mind that the burden on accused is not to prove or establish his defence beyond a shadow of doubt, as in the case of prosecution but, he has only to establish it with preponderance of probability. The said doctor could not categorically state that the accused had capacity or not to understand the nature of his act at the time of alleged incident, or that the accused was suffering from his mental abnormality prior to or at the time of the incident. In that case, the benefit must, go to the appellant accused.

Narayana Chandra Dey *vs* State, 1988 Cr. L.J. 387(Cal)

History of Earlier Mental Derangement

Section 105 of the Evidence Act places the burden of proving such a plea upon the accused. The burden on the accused is not as heavy as the burden lying on the prosecution to prove its case. Where the evidence adduced fails to satisfy the court of the existence of circumstances bringing the case within the exception pleaded, the accused is entitled to be acquitted if upon a consideration of the evidence on both sides the Court is left in a state of reasonable doubt as to whether the accused is or not entitled to benefit of the exception pleaded.

Amrita *vs* State of Maharashtra, 1996 Cr.L.J. 1916 (Bom) (D.B.)

Defence of Insanity—Rejected

On the day of the occurrence, the accused was found dancing with a dog on his head with a broken bottle. The plea of insanity under Sec. 84 IPC was found to be afterthought and rejected in view of the medical opinion.

Nathu Bapu Mhaskar *vs* State of Maharashtra, 1996 Cr. L.J. 2120 (Bom) (D.M.)

When the accused at the time of the occurrence and thereafter was not abnormal the plea of unsoundness of mind was an afterthought and rejected.

Ramdhin *vs* State of M.P. 1996 Cr. L.J. 3708 (M.P.) (D.B.)

The mere fact that the murder was committed by the accused on a sudden impulse will not be sufficient to accept the plea of insanity under Sec. 84 of the Indian Penal Code.

K.Madhavan *vs* State, 1994 Cr. L.J. 450

The accused stabbed the deceased and thereafter ran away, never had history of mental illness earlier. The plea of insanity was rejected.

S.K. Nair *vs* State of Punjab AIR 1997 S.C. 1537: 1997 Cr. L.J. 772

The evidence showed that the accused fully knew the implications of his act, when he committed the offence; hence the plea of insanity under Sec. 84 of the Indian penal code, 1860, was rejected.

Sankaran *vs* State, Cr.L.J. 1175 (Ker)

Procedure in case of person of unsound mind tried before court

When the accused did not show sign of unsoundness of mind during trial of the case or during examination under Sec. 313 of the Code of Criminal procedure but gave certain strange answers, the Court invited the report of the Psychiatrist who reported that the intellectual functions of the accused were within normal limits and that no delusion or hallucination was detected; thereafter sessions Court proceeded with the trial of the case as there was substantial compliance of Sec. 329 of the Code of Criminal Procedure.

State of Manipur *vs* Saikham Ramo Singh, 2004 (2) Crimes 385

Insanity—Accused, a person of unsound mind—Report of Medical Officer—Admissibility

The fact that the report of the medical officer is admissible in evidence does not necessarily mean that it is conclusive proof regarding mental condition of the concerned individual.

Gulab Manik Surware *vs* State, 2001 Cri LJ 4302 (Bom)

Unsoundness of mind: The conduct of the accused at the time of assaulting the deceased, i.e. his own father's aunt in broad daylight in front of his own and the house of his uncle and within the sight of his relatives and leaving the blood stained axe on the spot demonstrate abnormality.

Ashis Dey *vs* State, 2004 (1) Cri. 501

Legal insanity is different from medical insanity — each and every unnatural behavior does not fall within the purview of legal insanity. To prove legal insanity, it has to be shown that his cognitive faculty of mind is destroyed as a result of unnatural mind to such extent so as to render him incapable of knowing the nature of the act he has committed.

Raval Mohanbhai *vs* State, 1998 Cri L.J. 4325 (Guj)

Insanity: Absence of medical evidence: Even if the accused was not able to establish conclusively that he was insane at the time he committed the offence, the evidence placed before the Court by the accused or by the prosecution, may raise reasonable doubt in the mind of the Court about the mental condition of the accused.

Kushiyaramadiyil Madhavan *vs* State, 1992 (1) Crimes 1227 (Ker).

Insanity as a plea of defence and plea of insanity—One important factor to be remembered is minor mental aberration, hot temperament, lack of self-control or getting easily provoked are not sufficient to absolve one from the liability of his act. When there was nothing in the evidence to show that the accused had a history of mental disease or that he was under treatment for the same, it could not be held that the accused was insane.

Saratnaik *vs* State of Orissa, 1990 Cri L.J. NOC 72

Plea of insanity: Act done by a person by fatal blows on the head of the deceased by an axe —The plea of insanity will fail when there is no material to show that the accused lost his cognitive faculty at the time of occurrence.

Basanti *vs* State of Orissa, 1989 Cri L.J. 415

Plea of Insanity: Where a woman who jumped into a well with her children, immediately after rescue confessed that her mind was not working properly. It was held that she was conscious of her acting improperly and the fact was clear when she offered explanation immediately on being rescued. Plea of insanity not accepted.

Patreswar *vs* State of Assam, 1986 Cri L.J. 196

Insanity as a plea of defence: Where the accused in his dream felt throttled by someone, took the duo and dealt a blow resulting in the death of deceased. Due to the state of semi sleep, it could not be said that the accused had criminal intention or motive of killing. Benefit of doubt given to the accused.

Anurugham *vs* State of Tamil Nadu, 1989 (2) Crimes 597 (Mad)

Plea of insanity—Murder of a child of seven years of age by thrashing—The accused was identified by the witness—Medical Evidence available on record coupled with the post-mortem report, amply corroborating the testimony of eye-witnesses from the act of the accused in catching hold of the legs of the deceased and dashing him against the ground thrice, clearly establish that though he might not be having the requisite intention of causing death, it cannot be said that while doing so he was not in his senses—The plea of insanity, therefore, rejected.

Murthi *vs* State of Tamil Nadu, 1988 (1) Crimes 326

Plea of insanity—It is not sufficient to prove that a person was not of sound mind at the time of commission of offence—It must also be proved that by reason of such insanity he was incapable of knowing the nature of the act or that he was doing what was either wrong or contrary to law — Such state of mind can be ascertained from the circumstances that preceded, attended and followed the crime.

Onkar Lal *vs* State of MP, 1987 Cri L J 1289

Insanity—Legal and mental form of insanity —A person may be fit subject for confinement in a mental hospital but that fact alone will not be sufficient to permit him to enjoy exemption from punishment—Incurable perversions, hypersensitivity, excitability, stupidity, gross eccentricity and idiosyncrasy are forms of insanity and mental deficiency.

Budhiyabhai Kayabhai *vs* State of Gujarat, 1987 (1) Crimes 594

Insanity as plea of defence—The accused murdering his mother-in-law and causing grievous hurt to his wife—The accused admitted the offence but pleaded insanity—To prove that accused was insane at the time of commission of the offence, the evidence produced found to be not reliable—Plea of insanity not accepted.

Kuttappan *vs* State of Kerala, 1986 Cri L J 271

Insanity—In law every person is presumed to be sane and accountable for his acts unless the contrary is proved—The burden to prove insanity is upon the accused for setting the defence of insanity.

Gurit Singh *vs* State of Punjab 1986 Cri L J 1505 (P & H)

Insanity—Proof of insanity—The procedure for the trial of the fact of unsoundness of mind and consequent incapacity to make a defence by the accused postulates the recording of evidence in support of and in rebuttal of it—The accused cannot be permitted to get away from the punishment by malingering unsoundness of mind.

Satish Kumar Sharma *vs* Smt Meera Sharma, 1986 Marr. L J 120 P & H

Insanity—Medical evidence regarding schizophrenia and mental disorder.
The strained relation existing between the spouses and the medical evidence was not sufficient to prove that the wife was suffering from mental disorder—In the circumstances, the mental disorder of the wife not proved—Held, on facts that it was the husband who was guilty of cruelty towards wife.

Kusamjhi *vs* State, 1985 CriL J 1460 (Orissa)

Insanity—Proof of Insanity: An accused person need not to prove his case beyond reasonable doubt and it is sufficient if his plea of insanity is established by preponderance of probabilities as in a civil case.

Ramachandran *vs* State of Kerala, 1985 Ker. LT 1175

Insanity as a plea of defence: Plea of insanity: The question for consideration would be whether there is evidence in support of plea of insanity — As is clear from the terms of Sec. 105 of Evidence Act, it is for the accused to establish the fact of insanity.

Budha *vs* State of Maharashtra, 1985 Cri L J 844.

Insanity as a plea of defence: Premeditation on the part of the accused was writ large on his conduct in fetching the axe from his cousin and sharpening it on the grinding wheel and delivering a forcible blow on the helpless and defenceless brother who was sleeping with a blanket over his head—It cannot be equated with insanity.

Ruduil Sah *vs* State of Bihar, AIR 1983 SC 1086: 1983 SCC Cri 798: 1983 (4) scc 141

Plea of insanity—Medical evidence regarding insanity—When no medical opinion was produced in support of diagnosis that he was insane nor indeed is there any record to show as to what kind of medical treatment was prescribed—If he was insane, at least skeletal medical report could have been produced to show that he was being treated for insanity.

Lata Seikh *vs* State of West Bengal, 1983 Cri L J 1675: 1983 (2) Crimes 166: Parapuzha Thamban *vs* State of Kerala, 1989(2) Crimes 250: 1989 Cri. L.J. 1372 (Ker)

Plea of insanity: Only legal insanity furnishes the ground of exemption from criminal liability—Unless the defect in cognitive faculty of the accused is a result of unsoundness of mind, there can be no legal insanity.

Dhani Ram *vs* State of HP, 1982 Cri L J 1546 (HP)

Insanity: Duty of the Court—When the court is of the opinion that the accused is of unsound mind not capable of understanding the trial, provisions of Sec. 329 of CrPC should be invoked but court cannot convict or acquit an accused merely on the basis of medical report.

Surya Prasad *vs* State of Orissa, 1982 Cri L J 931; Gour Chandra *vs* State of Orissa, 1990 (1) Crimes 168: 1989 Cri. L J 1667

Plea of insanity—Insanity to be recognised as an exception to criminal liability must be such as to disable the accused person from knowing the nature of act, when he commits the criminal act—If by committing the offence, the accused knew the nature of the act, he cannot take benefit of the plea of insanity.

Keshav Rao *vs* State of Maharashtra, 1979 Cri L J 403; Naraincha ndra Dey *vs* State, 1988 Cri L J 387 (Cal)

Insanity—Unsoundness of mind implies a state of mind in which an accused is incapable of knowing that he is doing any wrong or anything contrary to law—Mere eccentricity or strange behavior is not enough to constitute insanity or unsound mind. **Insanity**—It must be such as to disable accused person from knowing nature of the act—If at the time of committing the offence the accused knew the nature of the act, he will be guilty of the offence.

Amrit Bhushan Gupta *vs* Union of India and another, AIR 1977 SC 608: 1977 (1) SCC 180: 1977 SCC (Cri) 66: 1977 Cri L J 376: 1977 (2) SCR 240

Insanity as a plea of defence: Staying of the execution of death sentence sought on the ground of insanity of the accused—If at the time of commission of offence, the prisoner knew the nature of the act he committed, he could not be absolved of the responsibility of grave offence of murder—Legality of sentence of death cannot be questioned in appeal on the ground of insanity.

Ram Lal *vs* State of Rajasthan, 1977 Cri L J NOC 168

Plea of insanity—Epileptic patient: The report of the doctor, that the accused was having epileptic fits in jail—It will not necessarily demolish the fact that accused was sane at the time of commission of the offence.

1977 Hindu L R 149 (pb)

Insanity—Duty of the court: Court has to hold inquiry into the unsoundness of mind but the inquiry need not be elaborate and the court can be satisfied on affidavits.

Tuba Chetia *vs* State of Assam, 1976 Cri L J 1416

Insanity as plea of defence—Unsoundness of mind as contemplated under Sec. 84 of IPC is legal insanity which means the state of mind in which an accused is incapable of knowing the nature of his act or he is incapable of knowing that he was doing what is either wrong or contrary to the law—In other words he does not know what he has done or what will follow his act.

Shiv Raj Singh *vs* State, 1975 MP L J 98

Insanity—Mere abnormal behavior is not sufficient: Abnormal behavior shown by the accused such as indifference to food, removing or tearing clothes, smearing cow dung on the body, might be in order to get relief from the stomach pain, heat, irritation which he was feeling—After the arrest, the doctor observing him in the jail opined that he suffered from depressive psychosis based on want of proper sleep, indifference to food, etc.—Held, the accused failed to prove insanity and would be guilty of the offence committed.

Oyami Ayatu *vs* State of MP, AIR 1974 SC 216: 1974 (3) SCC 299: 1974 Cri LJ 305: 1973 SCC (Cri) 925; Kusa Majhi *vs* State, 1985 Cri LJ 1460

Insanity—Everyone is presumed to know the natural consequences of his act, however, there is rebuttable presumption that the accused was not insane when he committed the crime—Mere fact that the accused made a clean breast of the matter and admitted the various allegations would not go to show that he was of unsound mind.

Sheralli Wali Mohammed *vs* State of Maharashtra, AIR 1972 SC 2443: 1972 Cri LJ 1523: 1973 (4) SCC 79: 1973 SCC (Cri) 726

Insanity as a plea of defence—State of mind before and after the commission of offence of the accused is relevant to determine as to whether he was insane at the time of commission of offence—To establish that the acts done are not offences within the meaning of Sec. 84, it must be proved that at the time of commission of the act the appellant by reason of unsoundness of mind, was incapable of either knowing the nature of the act or that the acts were either morally wrong or contrary to the law.

Rattan Lal *vs* State of MP, AIR 1971 SC 778: 1971 (3) SCR 251: 1971 Cri. L.J. 654: 1971 SCC (Cri) 139

Insanity—Determination of unsoundness of mind—Crucial point of the time at which unsoundness of mind has to be proved is the time when the crime was actually committed—This burden can be discharged by the accused from the circumstances before and after commission of the crime.

I.V. Shivaswamy *vs* State of Mysore, AIR 1971 SC 1638: 1971 Cri LJ 1198

Insanity—Plea of Insanity: In view of section 465 CrPC there should be an inquiry and if it appears to the court that accused was insane, it will not be necessary to conduct a regular inquiry—If on examining the accused the court is of the opinion that he is not insane, it is not necessary to go for further medical examination.

Ratan Lal *vs* State of MP, AIR 1971 SC 778: 1971 Cri LJ 654: 1971 MP LJ 677: 1971 (3) SCR 251: 1970 (3) SCC 533

Insanity as a plea of defence—Crucial point at which unsoundness of the mind has to be proved is the time when crime was actually committed and the burden to prove the same will be on the accused which can be discharged from the circumstances preceding, attendant and following the crime.

A.S. Mehta *vs* Vasumat, AIR 1969 Guj. 48

Insanity—Determination of Insanity—It is not essential to call medical witness or lunacy expert to support or to rebut the plea of insanity—The final responsibility of medical witness is simply to make a clinical appreciation of the facts at his disposal—When history, examination and result of special investigation are available, the doctor must draft his report in such a way that the court can understand clearly the nature of the opinion as to the mental state of accused person—A mere production of medical certificate of insanity is not enough unless it is supported by a clear statement of what the doctor noticed and on what he based his opinion.

Makhanmal *vs* Pritam Devi, AIR 1961 pb. 411

Insanity—Test of soundness of the mind: Where the testator lived for three years after execution of the will and the attesting witnesses deposed that he was of sound mind when the will was executed, the fact that testator was almost blind and the person to whom the property was bequeathed were living, it can be held that there was no undue influence or unsoundness of the mind of the testator.

State of MP *vs* Ahmedulla, AIR 1961 (2) 197

Insanity—Burden of proof of insanity— Burden is on the accused, who claims the benefit of exemption—Where the crime was committed not in a sudden mood of insanity but one that was preceded by careful planning, the accused could not claim acquittal on the ground of insanity.

Chenna Bassappa *vs* The State of Mysore, AIR 1957 Mysore 68; 1957 Cri L J 985

Plea of insanity—Medical and legal insanity: There is clear distinction between medical and legal insanity—a man may be suffering from some form of insanity in the sense in which the term is used by medical man but may not be suffering from unsoundness of mind within the meaning of Sec. 84 IPC.

Desouza *vs* Desouza, AIR 1956 MB 227

Insanity—Criteria of sound disposing mind: The test of a sound disposing mind in the testator involves the requirement that he should have sound disposing mind.

Baswantrao Bajirao *vs* Emperor, AIR 1949 Nag. 66: 50 Cri L J 181

Insanity—Duty of the medical expert: The medical expert called to prove insanity of the prisoner at the time of commission of offence, must offer to keep the prisoner under observation—He cannot base his opinion on the summary of evidence at the trial supplied to him—The opinion of the medical witness however eminent he may be must not be read as conclusive of the fact which is to be adjudicated by the court—The opinion however, may be invited in exceptional circumstances.

Baswantrao Bajirao *vs* Emperor, AIR 1949 Nag. 66

Insanity—Medical evidence of insanity. A medical witness who considered it unnecessary to examine a person, however sane at the moment, for suspected lunacy is not of much value—when the doctor attempted to substitute his judgment for that of the court, held, such course was not permissible.

AIR 1949 Nag. 66

Insanity—Legal and medical insanity: In dealing with the case involving defence of insanity, distinction must be drawn between cases in which insanity is more or less proved and the question is only as to the degree of irresponsibility and the cases in which insanity is sought to be proved in respect of a person who for all intents appears to be sane —It would be a dangerous doctrine to lay down that because a man committed a desperate offence with the chance of instant death and the certainty of future punishment before him, he was, therefore, insane as if the perpetration of the crime was to be excused by their very atrocities.

AIR 1946 Nag. 321

Insanity—Evidentiary value of statement of medical man—A medical man cannot in the strictness be asked his opinion regarding state of mind of prisoner at the time of commission of offence—The question whether the accused was of unsound mind at the time of commission of the act or by reason thereof he was incapable of knowing the nature of the act or that he was doing what was either wrong or contrary to law, will not be relevant for the opinion of the expert.

Chapter

5

Behavior of Criminal Offenders

- Nature and type of offender
- Types of Rapists' behavior
- Child victimizers
- Types of child molesters
- Child abductors
- Parents as murderers and abusers
- Stacking
- Homicide

The law enforcement or the medical/health community can properly deal with violent, predatory, and often repeat or serial criminals or even evaluate the critical question of their current or future level of dangerousness, only when efforts are made to understand the nature and type of offenders.

Family history of alcoholism and psychiatric disorders, instability of residence, mother as the dominant parent, and negative relationship with father or male caretaker, all of these factors come into play in significantly more than half of the instances. Other important indicators like family members with criminal histories, father leaving before the subject's twelfth birthday, negative relationship with the mother, the subject's ongoing perception of unfair treatment, and no older sibling (good) role model all show up in roughly 50% of the cases.

This type of upbringing leads to a tendency to fail in interpersonal relationships, aggressiveness and other antisocial behavior patterns, inappropriate emotional responses, including absence of guilt or conscience, chronic lying, and rebelliousness, underperformance in school and underemployment, active fantasy life and preoccupation with fantasies of violence, domination, and control. It is therefore not difficult to see the type of background, combined with whatever is inherent in the child's physical/neurologic/emotional makeup, as part of a template for the adult violent offender.

Once the antisocial behavior begins (often with acts such as starting a fire or causing cruelty to animals and other children), a series of "feedback filters", come into play: the subject justifies the act in his own mind; he sorts out errors in his performance of the act so that he can do it "better" and more efficiently next time; he finds that in performing the act he experiences an increased state of arousal; he discovers increased areas of dominance, power, and control in his life; he learns how to continue these acts without detection or punishment; he progresses to a larger, more elaborate, and harmful acting out of his fantasies.

Why do serial predatory offenders do what they do? It is because this act of manipulation, domination, and control—be it rape, murder, arson, or any other criminal enterprise—gives them feelings of power, satisfaction, and fulfilment that they cannot obtain anywhere else in life.

A girl who appears to have a background identical to that of a boy who goes on to a troubled life of crime will almost never develop into the same type of sexual predator. Girls and women from dysfunctional and abusive backgrounds tend to direct their rage, anger, and despair inward. Rather than being outwardly aggressive toward others, they often engage in self-destructive or self-punishing behaviors, such as alcohol or drug abuse, suicide attempts, prostitution, and attraction to abusive men.

Regardless of family background and all other formative influences and regardless of intelligence or level of emotional stability, the overwhelming numbers of predatory criminals choose to do what they do because of the way it makes them feel. They are fully aware of what they are doing, often plan it, and understand that it is wrong and contrary to societal rules. They simply do not care. Or if they do care, that care is outweighed by the desire to do it anyway.

The more times he is able to get away with a particular offense, the better will be his ability to refine his modus operandi to continue to get away with the same crime. In any given case, this may be because the offender is above average in intelligence, despite his records of under achievement. Many serial offenders, particularly of the organized variety are reasonably bright. However, avoiding detection and capture can also be related to the amount of time and energy the offender puts into fantasizing, planning, and evaluating the crime.

THE POWER-REASSURANCE RAPIST

The power-reassurance rapist (numerically, the most common type of rapist) feels inadequate, not being the type with whom women would voluntarily become involved. He compensates for these feelings of male inadequacy by forcing women to have sex with him.

Although he is physically the least dangerous type of rapist, if he is successful over a series of attacks, his confidence may be boosted and he may become more physically aggressive.

THE EXPLOITATIVE RAPIST

The exploitative rapist (the second most common type of rapist) is a more impulsive predator. His crimes result from seizing an opportunity that presents itself rather than by fantasizing about the act ahead of time.

Once he has a woman under his control, his only concern is getting her to submit sexually to him. That is the real thrill for him—the sex act is satisfying as an act of domination and control rather than providing what we think of as sexual gratification. Once he has forced submission, as far as he is concerned, the experience is over.

He wants a macho reputation, to be known as a man's man, and therefore is likely to have some physically oriented employment. He is interested in sports. His vehicle reflects that image, too.

THE ANGER RAPIST

The anger rapist is also referred to as the anger retaliatory rapist. Sexual assault is a displaced expression of rage and anger. The offender hates either his mother, wife, or girlfriend, even women in general. His anger and resentment need not be rooted in an actual or legitimate wrong ever perpetrated against him.

He is driven by rage, the consequences of the anger rapist's attack can be anything from verbal abuse, to severe beating, to murder, although the fact that his conscious or subconscious intention is to get the anger out of his system means that this type usually will not kill.

This type accounts for about 5% of rapists.

THE SADISTIC RAPIST

The sadistic rapist is the least common type of rapist. He is the most dangerous. The purpose of his attack is to live out his sadistic sexual fantasies on the unwilling victim. With this type, sexual fantasy and aggression merge, which is why he is also referred to as an anger-excitation rapist. Aggression and sadistic fantasy feed on each other, so as the level of aggression rises, his level of arousal rises accordingly. Various forms of mental and physical torture may be directed particularly at sexually significant parts of the body such as mouth, breasts, genitals, buttocks, and rectum. His weapon of choice is frequently a knife, because it is so intimidating and causes mental anguish on the part of the victim. He often cuts or tears off his victim's clothing because he figures she will not need it after he has finished with her. Depending on his preferences, there may be much sexual activity, probably highly perverse in nature, or even none. He could, for example, prefer to penetrate with a sharp object rather than with his penis. His language can be commanding and degrading, but impersonal.

CHILD VICTIMIZERS

If there is any crime more odious than sexual violence against women, it would be sexual violence against children. Offenders display varying personality types and a continuum of behaviors, all of which go into the evaluation of the individual case. They themselves may have been victims of abuse as children, and their young victims may, in turn, either become future victimizers or be chronically victimized by others. A shy, timid individual without social skills or deep, peer-oriented personal relationships may seem "creepy". He would not steal a child from a public environment and attempt to take him or her away with him.

Predators of children use their advantages. They are bigger and stronger than their victims. They may impersonate police officers, teachers, or priests to legitimatize themselves. They may manipulate a child's emotions by showering him or her with attention and then threaten to isolate the child from parents and others.

It is critical for parents to teach children age-appropriate safety skills and to take careful note of any changes in their child's attitudes, behavior, or self-confidence. These changes include withdrawal or fearfulness; sleep disturbances, such as nightmares or bed-wetting; sexual "acting out" or unusual interest in sex; aggressiveness or rebelliousness; regression or infantile behavior; fear of specific people, places, or activities; and/or pain or injury in private regions.

TYPES OF CHILD MOLESTERS

It is also important to note that not all pedophiles molest children; Pedophiles may have sexual relationships with adults and satisfy their urges in other ways, such as fantasy, masturbation with dolls, or choosing lovers who are childlike, such as a small and/or flat-chested woman or one who engages in baby talk or similar behavior. **Three types of child molesters** have been described: the Situational, the Introverted, and the Sadistic molester.

FBI's Behavioral Science Unit outlines four types of **Situational child molesters**: repressed, morally indiscriminate, sexually indiscriminate, and inadequate. Situational child molesters behavior is insidious in nature and they may be involved with children as a popular teacher, coach, or scout or youth group leader.

The Introverted molester, the closest to the stereotype of the creepy stranger in a raincoat, does not possess the interpersonal or social skills to lure or con potential victims. His sexual activity is limited to brief encounters, and he usually targets strangers or young children.

Sadistic molester is physically the most dangerous type because, like the sadistic rapist of adults, his satisfaction derives from having total control and seeing the victim's response to the suffering inflicted. He causes physical and/or psychological pain to become sexually aroused. This molester uses trickery or force to obtain victims and then tortures them when they are under his control. He is likely to abduct and murder his victims.

CHILD ABDUCTORS

They are often social misfits who would have shown signs of trouble even as children. Usually unmarried, too incompetent socially to maintain a relationship with a woman, even as a cover, they have no regular contact with children. Their poor social skills make it difficult for them to manipulate, lure, or seduce a child, so they might carry weapons to intimidate or control a victim. They are also likely to harm the victim.

Four phases of child abduction: build-up, abduction, post-abduction, and recovery/ release. In the **build-up** and **abduction** phases, the fantasy creates the need, and the precipitating stressor or stressors fuel the action. The level of planning and the chances of success depend on the type of abductor. The thought-driven abductor plans ahead, weighs risks, and exercises discipline in selection of the victim, whereas the abductor answers his specific emotional needs and follows his own ritual, although this might increase his risk of being caught.

The treatment of the child depends on the motivation for the abduction and on the competence of the offender. As pressure grows, the abductor must somehow rid himself of the victim. The longer a child is missing, the smaller the chances of a positive outcome.

Incestuous molesters can cross the spectrum of types. An **introverted paedophile** may marry with the intent of producing children whom he can molest. A **seduction molester** may marry a woman with children so as to become a "father figure" and have access to them. Incestuous molesters are not only fathers. They can be grandfathers, uncles, or any other relative also.

When a molester is accused, particularly for the first time, there are certain behaviors seen frequently. He will deny, acting shocked, surprised, and indignant. He may blame the accusation on the child's misunderstanding, saying something like, "Is it a crime to hug a child?" Depending on his social support structure, he may bring in character witnesses to back him up. He will try to minimize events and may be aided in this strategy inadvertently by the victim's reluctance to admit the extent of the molestation because of embarrassment or discomfort. The molester often attempts to justify or reinterpret what happened or patently falsify the truth. He may pursue a strategy to lessen the impact or punishment, such as agreeing to plead to a lesser crime or claiming temporary insanity. Accused molesters in this phase tend to be high suicide risks.

PARENTS AS MURDERERS AND ABUSERS

Some parents kill their children. The behavioral indicators of parental involvement in a homicide are often clear to a trained investigator. Parents are not usually as detached about body disposal as strangers are, taking care with the body, wrapping it up, and showing it tenderness. Parents are also far more likely than strangers to feel remorse, leading investigators to recover the body for proper burial.

DOMESTIC VIOLENCE: STALKING

This is a crime where anybody can be an offender or a victim—people of all races and socioeconomic backgrounds and of either gender. Approximately one-third of men undergoing counselling for physically abusing a wife or girlfriend, held respectable, professional occupations and often enjoyed high status in their community as executives, doctors, or even ministers.

The offender's criminal behavior grows out of a need to control and dominate his victim to boost his own self-esteem. This offender suffers from extreme insecurity and is often unable to develop and maintain personal and love relationships.

To increase his control, the abuser tries to put his victim in a situation in which she is economically dependent on him. If there is a child involved, this makes it even easier for him to keep her under control because she may not feel capable of supporting herself and her child on her own. She may also be afraid that if she leaves he will get custody of—or outright kidnap her children, and she will never see them or be able to protect them from him again.

In the offender's mind, violence occurs not because he is unable to cope with his emotions and lacks self-control, but because the victim did something wrong that set him off.

When a woman escapes such a relationship, the abuser may rationalize subsequent stalking behavior as efforts to win her back—often trying first the charm, flowers, and candy routine he used to win her the first time—or as the punishment she deserves for leaving him and treating him so unfairly.

As the stalker grows more frustrated by what he perceives as his victim's unwillingness to give him what he needs, he becomes increasingly harassing and threatening, in keeping with the abusive behavior he is accustomed to inflicting. If the victim tries to remove him permanently from her life at this stage, he may become violent in a last-ditch effort to reassert control over the relationship.

Stalking is a terribly difficult crime for a victim to deal with because it can be long term and unpredictable. Unlike any other domestic crime, stalking can involve the perpetrator and victim for years rather than minutes, hours, or days.

HOMICIDE

Behavior reflects personality. This is one of the guiding principles of criminal investigative analysis. It is equally true that behavior often reveals the true nature of the crime.

Group cause homicide pertains to two or more people with a common ideology that sanctions an act, committed by one or more of its members, that results in death. This category is divided into cult murder, extremist murder (paramilitary extremist murder and hostage extremist murder), and group excitement homicide such as a gang attack, fed by its own momentum and peer reinforcement, that escalates into murder.

- Criminal offending behavior depends upon many factors alcoholism, dominant parent, under performance, etc.
- Various types of rapists and their behaviors are noted
- Domestic violence: Parents and relatives as stalkers and murderers are also known.

Chapter 6

Physical Treatment Modalities

INTRODUCTION

Restraint, seclusion and physical punishment are non-biological physical treatments sometimes applied to young people. Electroconvulsive therapy (ECT) is a nonpharmacological biological treatment which may be considered on occasion in specific cases. It is a biological intervention which in some circumstances can also be regarded as an integral part of the medical treatment for a mental disorder, particularly severe depression with suicidal risk. Specific pharmacological agents can be instrumental in major improvements in a young person's behavior, emotions, cognitions and overall level of functioning when used appropriately to treat particular disorders.

GENERAL PRINCIPLES OF TREATMENT

- It is based upon an appropriate assessment and formulation
- It is based on diagnosis and evidence for efficacy of treatment.
- It should be at the least interventionist level
- It should be based upon appropriate informed consent
- All prescriptions must be accompanied by arrangements for monitoring and review of treatment efficacy, side effects, and use of appropriate rating scales.

CONSENT

For consent to be valid it is necessary that the individual giving that consent is able to understand the nature, purpose and likely effects of the proposed treatment.

RESTRAINT

Physical punishment has no place in the management of psychiatric disturbance at any age. **Physical containment** and ensuring of safety play an important part in the management of a disturbed patient. The separation of the young person from others, and from any instrument with which the individual might self-harm or injure others, is done by **seclusion**.

ANTIPSYCHOTIC MEDICATIONS

Antipsychotic medications are specifically indicated in the treatment of schizophrenia and manic disorders, and in the symptomatic management of acute organic brain syndromes including drug-induced psychotic states.

ANTIDEPRESSANTS

In adults the efficacy of antidepressants in treating major depressive disorders is well established. However, randomized controlled trials of a variety of tricyclic antidepressants amongst children and adolescents have consistently failed to demonstrate any clinically significant benefit.

MOOD STABILIZERS

Both lithium and carbamazepine are used extensively in adult practice in the treatment of bipolar affective disorder in both its acute phases and as prophylaxis, and sodium valporate is finding increased usage—despite continuing controversy about the effectiveness of all three drugs.

Lithium therapy requires close therapeutic monitoring with regular assessment of serum levels (at least every 2 months) if toxic levels are to be avoided. Blood levels should be kept at 0.5–1.0 mmol/L. Additionally, serum urea and creatinine levels should be regularly checked while thyroid function should be checked annually.

Its prescription is inappropriate for some individuals where non-compliance can be anticipated, whether with the treatment itself or with the accompanying monitoring. In these cases prescription of carbamazepine or valproate may be safer and more appropriate. These have greater safety in over dose, and whilst serum levels can be informative they are not essential to monitoring of treatment. Typical carbamazepine dose is 100–200 mg three times daily.

It would appear that lithium plus valproate is probably the safest and most effective combination, although further research is needed.

HYPNOTICS AND ANXIOLYTICS

Initially, use of sleep hygiene measures (regular routines, avoidance of alcohol, nicotine and stimulants, appropriate conducive environment) should be encouraged as an alternative to use of medication (Stores 1996).

Benzodiazepines, antidepressants and low-dose propranolol have all been used although without proven benefit. Psychological approaches should remain first choice.

Benzodiazepines may occasionally be useful in providing a **short-term** interim additional sedative effect in the treatment of psychotic disorders when used adjunctively to antipsychotic medication. Low regular doses of diazepam (up to 5 mg thrice daily) or of lorazepam (up to 2 mg four hourly) (Clark and Lewis 1998), are given to start with.

ELECTROCONVULSIVE THERAPY

Electroconvulsive therapy (ECT) is generally accepted as an effective treatment of severe depressive disorders in adults. It is also used on occasion in certain types of schizophrenia and in resistant manic disorder. Its effects and side effects have been extensively studied in a range of populations and disorders. In childhood and adolescence, however, its usage remains infrequent.

Involvement of mental health professionals in the administration of the ECT is mandatory. Regular review of the mental state of the young person should take place between treatments, and applications should not be prescribed as a set course or number of treatments to be completed.

FOOD

Food is not usually regarded as a medicine and the giving of food is not usually regarded as physical treatment. In certain circumstances, however, the giving of food by artificial means is defined as medical treatment. This is true in respect of anorexia nervosa, in cases of persistent vegetative state and in rare instance of psychopathic disorder with total food refusal. Decisions regarding nasogastric feeding, even in severe and life-threatening situations and particularly those without the individual's consent must be carefully considered and regularly reviewed.

Chapter

7

Psychotherapy Dynamics

INTRODUCTION

Young offenders have been particularly in the news in recent years. They stir strong emotions within society, with polarizations of views from extreme demands for more and more punishment to the frankly sentimental.

Minor acts of delinquency are part of normal adolescence (and for that matter adulthood), and 'the delinquent' or juvenile offender needs to be seen in this context. Social and political policy tends towards defining core high-risk groups.

To work with juvenile offenders is necessarily to become involved in the politics of our response—politics with a small 'p', but also, particularly at the present time. The individuals working with these children achieve great success through their devotion, however, they often work in poor conditions with low pay and with little recognition from the public, and the children suffer as a consequence.

The populations of young offender institutions, as well as adult prisons, have a high incidence of having been in "care". It is an interesting question why we tend to be punitive to this already disposed group rather than rehabilitative, habilitative or therapeutic. Possibly, they are further 'hated' because of their very 'failure' and vulnerability which confronts society with the unbearable.

The long-term criminal outcome of adolescent sex offenders is very poor, if we try to correlate with adult sexual offending. This is also true for future adult non-sexual violent offending (for example, murder, kidnapping, robbery and assault compared with adolescent non-sexual offenders).

PSYCHODYNAMIC SCHEME OF DEVELOPMENT

According to Freud, the father of psychoanalysis, adolescence is a predominantly genital stage of psychosexual development as a sequel to 'oral', 'anal' and 'phallic' stages. Adolescence is divided into four sub-stages.

Pre-adolescence

Pre-adolescence, or onset of puberty, is characterized by increased instinctual pressure tending to the indiscriminate investment of the libidinal and aggressive model of early and infantile life. The fact is that 'aggression' can no longer be thought of simply as instinctual and unitary. Erotic life is not developed; physical manifestations like erections and nocturnal emissions occur in male.

Precocious sexualisation by adults (i.e. sexual abuse) during adolescent development can have disastrous consequences for the very active psychological changes—progression, digressions and regressions—which are partly flexible and pliable organic series of stages of development.

Early Adolescence

The emotional life becomes wider and richer. Friendships are formed and tend to be idealized and narcissistic. It is not common that, he or she experiences 'lows of mood'.

Adolescence Per Se

In adolescence proper, a turn occurs towards heterosexual object choice with renunciation of the incestuous, parental, 'Oedipal object'. It is also a phase of increased intellectualization, asceticism and religiousness with concern for philosophical and social issues in age range, for boys between 14 and 16 years, and for girls somewhat lower in age.

Late Adolescence and Adulthood

In late and post-adolescence, momentous new departures are put through 'trials' and experimentations towards the eventual establishment of a fairly coherent structure of character by the end of adolescence—around 21 years: Not a finished product but a formed one.

DEVIATIONS FROM NORMAL

Failure of attachment, or of normal 'attachment' and reciprocity', between infant and caregiver, and of the later building up of 'affiliative bonds' of affection, etc., leads to deficient development of self-esteem and a failure of the development of a capacity for empathy for others, and generally to failed socialization.

Failure of attachment is a common denominator of many young and adult offenders. Frequently these young people have spent most of their lives 'in care', with serial placements and numerous substitute parents. They suffered from different types of parents—foster parents, house parents, and various surrogate parents — and so the growth of attachment could not reasonably proceed.

Williams (1978) distinguished between two types of adolescent 'acting out' or offending. Both, however, can become overladen with secondary gain, whereby the initial 'cause' (the primary 'gain') becomes established, and lends certain additional (secondary) psychological advantages. Put in other words, the 'acting out' may become part of an individual's identity, and 'ego-syntonic' rather than causing distress (ego-dystonic).

First Type of 'Acting Out'/Offending

A child may, steal money from his mother's handbag. The child steals in symbolic form only what once belonged to him by right. The child is unwittingly trying to make up for a deprivation experienced from the original domain of his or her relationship with mother.

The Second type 'Acting out'/Offending is More Serious

Adolescent offenders with libidinal and 'aggressive' (destructive) drives come together in a dramatic and catastrophic way. We do not need to enter the debate of whether the aggressive drive is 'primary' (innate), or 'secondary' (consequent upon the internalization of trauma), or a mixture of both. We may be shocked and horrified, but so much as the offending adolescent: post hoc, it is frequently not difficult to understand the mental state behind the escalation—from apparently minor acts of destruction to the possibly cataclysmic.

Most delinquents are troubled children, but they do not know it and deny the same. The psychoanalytic or psychodynamic approach allows us to know it by a particular form of listening—with a 'third ear'—to the communication behind the act.

The age of locking up young offenders in our system, from 12 to 21 years, corresponds quite precisely with the stages of development in adolescence, which have been detailed above. Young people are locked up, frequently for 23 hours a day in the worse scenarios, and have little hope of 'practising' the tasks of relatively successful separation from parental figures—both real (objective, parents) and the internal images of them. They have no opportunity for developing attachments of new 'heterosexual' objects, and of negotiating (and resolving) adolescent homosexual anxieties and experiences.

CONCLUSION

For a forensic population of serious offenders, forms of compulsory detention are unavoidable. There are major difficulties in establishing a therapeutic community where young people are compulsorily detained, and the whole idea may thereby be seriously diluted. The alternatives to such attempts at therapeutic facilities have grown largely 'piecemeal'.

CASE STUDIES

1. Michael was first seen the day after he had been charged with attempted murder: he was a white, British, 16 year old secondary school pupil and had no previous records of offending behavior, although later he was able to tell him-shame-faced-of perverse, quasi-psychotic sexual experimentation in his early teens with a male infant cousin.
   On the day of the offence he picked up a man from the same public lavatory and took him home. During sexual 'play' he attacked the man viciously. Only the proximity of a casualty department prevented the man's death. The patient/client felt horrified by what he had done, but he was no longer tormented by his sexual conflict: He felt relieved and remained so for a longer time. He was desperate to talk and try to understand how he could have done such a thing. However, after some six weeks, the same persecuting dilemma returned and with it a rage at the therapist which was hardly bearable and which continued—mutas mutandi—some years on. This young man illustrates—in the crudest and most concrete way—the fantasy of 'cure' by the psychodynamically described mechanism of projective identification".
2. Robert has nightmares. He has a long history of violent assaults, first on teachers, then on staff in a residential home. He has not assaulted staff in the penal institution-he has not been allowed the opportunity. Instead he breaks up his cell from time to time and sometimes cuts his own arms or thighs with any sharp instrument that comes to hand. This is not uncommon behavior in violent young men who lose the psychologically stabilizing opportunities of 'acting out 'in the community, and frequently of violence towards others.

   Robert has an extreme and clear version of what is common to many of these boys. They are very much victims as well as perpetrators. The description by Herbert Rosenfeld of the 'internal mafia gang' in the persecuted, paranoid mind is an accurate description of the internal world of these superficially 'normal', antisocial adolescents.

   A boy who had killed but denied that it had happened: 'It was a dream'. 'Tell me the dream'. I suggested. He responded with a long and accurate narrative of the sequence of events preceding, during and after the homicide. Only later was he able to accept—albeit partially, and with editing of the most horrific detail—the reality of his mostly accurately registered and remembered 'dream'. Those who live in such awful, persecuted internal worlds —and who sometimes act it out in fact—potentially know far more than they can fully bear to acknowledge.

Chapter

8

Behavior Modification

BEHAVIOR DIFFERENCES

What is Behavior?

Behavior is the way an individual acts towards people, society or objects. It can be either bad or good. It can be normal or abnormal according to society norms. Society tries to correct bad behavior and tries to bring abnormal behavior back to normal, religious or traditional by ethical or legal means.

Root Causes of Behavioral Differences

1. Individual differences
2. Differences in family patterns
3. Impairment/disabilities
4. Environmental factors
5. Psychological factors

1. Individual Differences

a. Sex differences
b. Intellectual differences
c. Physical differences
d. Personal and emotional differences.

a. *Sex differences:* Most instances of human behavior is sex-specific, either masculine or feminine.

b. *Intellectual differences:* We are all aware that there are intellectual differences amongst individuals. Some are bright; others dull, while some are geniuses.

c. *Physical differences:* People differ in
- Physical appearance
- Facial features
- Growth and development rate
- Energy
- Posture
- Height, weight and volume.

d. *Personal and emotional differences*

2. Differences in Family Patterns

a. Maintenance of large families
b. Socio-economic status of the family
c. Structure of the family

3. Impairment/Disabilities

There are some biological factors which contribute to some of the behavior problems summarized as follows:

a. *Genetic accidents*
- Genes have been suggested as the causes of behavioral difficulties, from hyperactivity to criminality. Environmental factors, particularly social learning, play an important role in modifying inherited behavioral predispositions.

b. *Brain damage or dysfunction*
- The brain can be traumatized in the following different ways before, during or after birth.

- During birth, in an accident, prolonged high fever, infectious diseases (such as meningitis), toxic chemicals (such as drugs or poisons taken by the child or by the woman during pregnancy), or hypoxia (reduced oxygen availability).

c. *Nutritional errors*

- Severe malnutrition in young children leads to retardation in brain growth, irreversible brain damage and mental retardation often leading to apathy, social withdrawal and scholastic backwardness.

d. *Physical illness or disability*

A child who is physically ill is more prone to irritability, withdrawal or other behavior problems. Some physical illnesses are transitory.

Physical illnesses believed to be caused by an individual's psychological state are called psychosomatic or psycho-physiological. Disorders that are assumed to be psycho-physiological involve disruption of normal biological processes, e.g. breathing disorders such as asthma. The following are examples of disorders which have an impact on an individual's behavior:

- *Eating disorder:* e.g. Anorexia nervosa—self-starvation; bulimia—binges of overeating followed by purging, vomiting or extreme dieting; pica—eating non-nutritional substances like paint, paper and cloth.
- *Elimination disorders:* e.g. enuresis or encopresis—releasing urine or faeces at inappropriate times or places, a lack of control of the bladder or bowel function.
- *Movement disorders:* e.g. tics—sudden, repetitive and involuntary movements.
- *Sleep disorders:* e.g. sleep walking and night terrors.
- *Difficult temperament:* Classroom research does not indicate that temperament is the direct result of biological factors, but it suggests that students exhibit consistent behavioral styles that teachers recognize, and should consider, when planning instructional materials.

4. Environmental Factors

Environment has a significant influence on the development of the individual and on his/her subsequent behavior and attitudes.

a. *Physical environment:* This may consist of geographical factors: climate, physical features, urban or rural environment—all affect the development of the individual. They affect personality, character and outlook. They affect ways of talking, ways of dressing and even ways of walking, behavior and attitudes.

b. *Social environment:* This is provided mainly by the people around the child. The voices the child hears, the food he/she takes or drinks all have an influence on the way the child develops. Good care will make a child feel that he/she belongs to somewhere and is secure. A poor social environment, on the other hand, contributes to maladjustment in child behavior.

5. Psychological Factors as Causal Explanations of Behavior

The most important factor is motivation. Motivation is channelling or directing behavior towards satisfying a need or needs. It is a drive or urge to do something. Every individual has motives, driving forces behind his or her actions, needs or intentions. The needs can take different forms.

Behavior may be considered normal, abnormal, or disordered. The difference between normal and disordered behavior is usually of degree rather than kind. No sharp line can be drawn between them sometimes.

Causes of Behavioral Problems

There are three major causes of behavioral problems:

1. Cultural factors
2. School factors
3. Religious factors

Each of these is discussed in detail below.

1. Cultural Factors

The following pressures on teenage girls to become sexually active and to become pregnant (i.e. the presence of sugar daddies) and the penalties teenage mothers must pay, must be taken into account.

a. Child abuse
b. Ambitions/aspirations
c. Rural-urban migration
d. Parental separations, broken homes/divorces
e. Being homeless and orphaned
f. Lack of information on sex
g. Living with people of the opposite sex
h. Racism
i. Recognition of minority groups

2. School Factors

There are six ways in which the school can contribute to the development of disordered behavior and academic failure:

a. Insensitivity to students' individuality
b. Mismatch with the (inappropriate) student expectations
c. Inconsistent management of behavior
d. Instruction in non-functional and irrelevant skills
e. Destructive contingencies of reinforcement
f. Undesirable models of school conduct

3. Religious Factors

Most religions tend to maintain a belief in the inferior status of women and this has implications for girls' self-confidence and striving for excellence on equal terms with boys. It affects their aspirations to enter careers where they have to compete with men.

a. *Stealing:* This is an undesirable behavior. It includes stealing money and school property or stealing fellow students' belongings. In many schools, stealing is a punishable offence and can easily lead to dismissal.

   A number of factors lead to stealing. They are:

   - The child is not satisfied with what he has, while at school.
   - Some family members steal.
   - His/her peers encourage it.
   - He/she is not aware that stealing is wrong.

b. *Truancy:* This includes staying away from school for no justifiable reason and loitering or wandering. This leads to losing valuable study time and may ultimately lead to failure. Dissatisfaction with a school programme, for example, can lead to this.

c. *Disobedience and insubordination:* It can be disobedience, rebelliousness, sarcasm, etc. towards teachers and school authorities (very common in urban schools). It may also lead to dismissal from school. Rigid or poor relationships between teachers and pupils can cause disobedience.

d. *Lying:* Lies are told to classroom teachers, head-teachers and prefects. Sometimes parents report cases of lying. A rude teacher (or parent) who gives unfair punishment is likely to face more lies from his/her pupils.

e. *Fighting:* This may be common in schools. Fighting can be over food or over a boyfriend or girlfriend. Pupils, who have not been taught the value of respecting others, or living in harmony as a group, are likely to fight.

f. *Cheating:* You may have found pupils cheating in your schools. Young people cheat at examinations, tests, and in many school activities.

g. *Lateness:* Late comers are penalized. Coming late is a failing you pay for. Pupils usually come late when schools start a new term, when the classes are boring or when the teachers are missing from the class. Inability to value and observe programmes results in pupils coming late.

h. *Rudeness:* This includes rudeness to teachers, prefects, servants in the dining-hall, watchmen, and others. Rudeness can be copied from people in the community. It is also traceable to hereditary factors though it can be controlled.

i. *Destructiveness:* This includes malicious destruction of school property during strikes or unrest, or even on ordinary school days. Pupils' dissatisfaction with school rules, welfare, etc. usually causes strikes. Some pupils may also be rebellious by nature and motivate others to strike.

j. *Sex offences/harassment:* This includes hitting girls, attempted rape (for boys), rape and sexual acts with teachers. This can lead to dismissal from school, sexually transmitted diseases and becoming pregnant. Pupils who have not had enough, or any, sex education are at greater risk.

k. *Cruelty:* This includes bullying younger boys and girls, cruelty to animals and children who trespass in the school compound. Pupils who lack information on the value of the environment or life do this.

l. *Smoking and drinking alcohol:* No child is born smoking cigarettes or opium, drinking alcohol and taking other drugs. Selling and buying drugs is something you may know about. Pupils who involve themselves in this 'business' may end up as thieves, robbers, idlers, etc. Pupils who become involved are usually those who are dissatisfied with, or fail in, family relationships, and may have been encouraged by peers or adults who do such things.

Chapter

9

Growing up in Prison

INTRODUCTION

Staff in young-offender institutions is faced with the challenge of building an environment which at the least does no further damage and at the most offers young people a genuine opportunity to stop and think.

Along with the fractured family relationships, lack of parental supervision, low income, poor health and interrupted schooling which so many share, all young people in prison have in common the fact that they are intransition from childhood to adulthood. They are growing up in an institution.

We are faced with two imperatives. The first is to use prison as a place of absolute last resort for the young, if we are to avoid the confirmation of criminal identities at an early age. The second is to ensure that young-offender institutions operate to the highest possible quality and standards if we are to avoid further alienation and more disordered lives.

BASIC TENETS OF GOOD-QUALITY CARE

- The creation of a safe, healthy environment with clear objectives and firm boundaries.
- The maintenance of family ties and links with education, employment, outside agencies and friends.
- A purposeful and active regime which provides opportunities for young people to confront their offending behavior and to plan for the future.
- Stable, consistent leadership and professional staff committed to the respectful treatment of young people coupled with a belief in their capacity to change.

AGE-APPROPRIATE REGIMES

All prisoners aged 18 and above are being considered as adults. Young offenders constitute a significant and separate group in terms of policy, research and provision. Their reconviction rates are much higher than the reconviction rates for older prisoners, at 75% within two years for young men and something slightly less for young women. Their behavior in prison is also generally more challenging than that of older adult prisoners. They are responsible for a disproportionately high percentage of assaults. Self-harm is much more common among this group, as are cell damage and 'smash ups'.

AN EFFECTIVE SAFER PRISON STRATEGY SHOULD FOLLOW

- Management commitment to develop a safe environment for everyone.
- Respect for the humanity and individualism of every prisoner.
- Effective communications.

- Ensuring that no incident is allowed to go un-investigated and action is taken which demonstrates the staff's attitude against bullying.
- Involvement of the whole community—staff and prisoners.
- Continuous and imaginative monitoring.
- Development of a positive and supportive environment.
- Improved arrangements for reception and induction, and the introduction of first night in custody centres.

RESETTLEMENT OR REHABILITATION

Resettlement is the most difficult area of work for a young-offender institution. The high rate of reconviction amongst young offenders is alarming. Many of them leave prison well-intentioned but ill-prepared. They lack support in the community and are heavily influenced by a criminal peer group. Drug taking has exacerbated these problems.

The most successful resettlement initiatives for young offenders have involved some form of mentoring support on discharge. The ultimate measure of the success of a young offender institution remains a reduced rate of reconviction. The transition period following release is particularly difficult, and often success is dependent upon the support available to the young person in the community. Many have little family support that they can rely on. It is clear that a reduction in the use of custodial remand, an improvement in remand conditions and a sustained focus on resettlement would all make a positive difference. It is thus possible, to create healthy secure conditions for children and young people.

Chapter

10

Genetic and Environmental Influence on Behavior

- An interaction between genes and the environment predicts criminal behavior
- Genetic predisposition for criminal behavior alone does not determine the actions of an individual.
- If they are exposed to criminals, their chances are greater for engaging in criminal or antisocial behavior.

Criminal justice system appears to be a new home for individuals with psychological problems. Some psychological problems are heritable and if given the right circumstances; individuals with these genes start engaging in criminal activity.

In the late nineteenth and early twentieth century, the role of genetics in crime received wide acceptance. Many researchers believed that genes are fully responsible for criminal activity and criminals can be identified by their physiological features. This information and the idea of a eugenics movement lead to sterilizations to remove from society "criminals, idiots, imbeciles, and rapists" (Joseph, 2001).

Early family studies showed a predisposition for criminal behavior as a result of inherited characteristics, but that an individual's characteristics and personality can still be modified by the environment (Joseph, 2001). Although these studies were void of high validity and reliability, it still raised the question of whether the environment can also influence individuals to act in a criminal manner. The debate between genetics and environment continues today with much more reliable research and data. Consequently, this chapter will examine the various roles in which both genes and environmental factors influence criminal behavior.

DEFINITION AND MEASUREMENT OF CRIMINAL BEHAVIOR

To fully understand the nature of how genes and the environment influence criminal behavior, one must first know how criminal behavior is defined. Law in our society is defined by social and legal institutions, not by biology. Therefore determining what constitutes criminal behavior envelopes a wide variety of activities and researchers tend to focus on the wider context of antisocial behavior. Morley and Hall (2003) investigated the genetic influences on criminal behavior and pointed out three different ways to define antisocial behavior. First is equating it with criminality and delinquency, which both involve engaging in criminal acts. The second approach that is often used in genetic studies is to use diagnostic criteria for various personality disorders that are associated with an increased risk of criminal activity, namely, Antisocial Personality Disorder (ASPD). A third approach to antisocial behavior has been to investigate personality traits that may be risk factors for engaging in criminal behavior. Aggressiveness and impulsivity have been the most heavily researched traits, usually assessed by personality questionnaires (Rhee and Waldman 2002). These two traits have been implicated in criminal behavior. Criminality can lead to arrest, conviction, or incarceration for adults, while delinquency is related to juveniles committing unlawful acts.

TWIN, ADOPTION, AND FAMILY STUDIES

Twin studies are conducted on the basis of comparing the rates of criminal behavior of monozygotic (MZ) or identical twins with that in dizygotic (DZ) or fraternal twins. Ordinarily these studies are used to assess the roles of genetic and environmental influences.

A study conducted looked at thirty two MZ twins reared apart, who had been adopted by non-relatives a short time after birth. The results showed that for both childhood and adult antisocial behavior, there was a high degree of heritability involved (Joseph, 2001). This study is of particular importance because it examined the factor of separate environments. Another researcher studied eighty-five MZ and one hundred and forty-seven DZ pairs and found that there is a higher concordance rate for the MZ pairs.

Adoption studies are critical in examining the relationship that exists between adopted children and both their biological and adoptive parents because they assume to separate nature and nurture. Studies were conducted to test for the criminal behavior of the adopted-away children, if their biological parents had also been involved with criminal activity. In Iowa, the first adoption study conducted looked at the genetics of criminal behavior. The researchers found that as compared to the control group, the adopted individuals born to incarcerated female offenders had a higher rate of criminal convictions as adults. Therefore this evidence supports the existence of a heritable component to antisocial or criminal behavior (Tehrani J and Mednick S et al, 2000). Another study in Sweden also showed that if a biological background existed for criminality, then there is an increased risk of criminal behavior in the adopted children. In Denmark, one of the largest studies of adopted children was conducted and found similar results to the previous studies. The defining feature of the Denmark study is that the researchers found a biological component for criminal acts against property, but not for violent crimes (Joseph, 2001). Children whose biological fathers are convicted of property crimes are more likely to engage in similar behavior, when compared to those biological fathers who had been convicted of violent crimes. According to an article by Jay Joseph (2001), who studied all of the minor and major adoption studies, the majority of researchers found and agreed upon the non-significance of genes in violent crime. This re-establishes the findings from the studies mentioned already in that there may be a genetic component to antisocial behavior or that genes influence criminal behavior, but specifically for property offenses.

Family studies are the third type of instrument used to assess the relationship between genetics and environmental influences on criminal or antisocial behavior. Research in this field has probably been the least accepted by psychologists and other scholars because of the degree of difficulty in separating out nature and nurture in the family environment. Children experience both the influence of their parents' genes and also the environment in which they are raised, so it is difficult to assign which behaviors are influenced by the two factors. Twin studies have this flaw. It is more prevalent in family studies. An additional concern with family studies is the inability to replicate the results, therefore leading to a small number of studies. Regardless of these drawbacks, one family study in particular should be acknowledged for its findings.

Brunner HG et al (1993) conducted a study utilizing a large Dutch family. In their study they found a point mutation in the structural gene for monoamine oxidase A (MAOA), a neurochemical in the brain, which they associated with aggressive criminal behavior among a number of males in that family (Alper, 1995). These males were reported to have selective MAOA deficiency, which can lead to decreased concentrations of 5-hydroxyindole-3-acetic acid (5-HIAA) in cerebrospinal fluid. Evidence suggests that low concentrations of 5-HIAA can be associated with impulsive aggression. These results have not been confirmed in any additional family studies, which lead to a need for more studies to determine if other families share similar results (Brunner et al., 1993). However, this one family study does seem to suggest that genetics play an important role in antisocial or criminal behavior.

NEUROCHEMICALS IN CRIMINAL AND ANTI-SOCIAL BEHAVIOR

Neurochemicals are responsible for the activation of behavioral patterns and tendencies in specific areas of the brain (Elliot, 2000). As seen in the Brunner et al. study, there have been attempts to determine the role of neurochemicals such as monoamine oxidase (MAO), epinephrine, norepinephrine, serotonin, and dopamine in influencing criminal or antisocial behavior.

Monoamine oxidase (MAO) is an enzyme that has been shown to be inversely related to antisocial behavior. Specifically, low MAO activity results in disinhibition which can lead to impulsivity and aggression (Elliot, 2000). The Brunner et al. study is the only one to report findings of a relationship between a point mutation in the structural gene for MAOA and aggression, which makes the findings rare. There is other evidence that points to the conclusion that deficiencies in MAOA activity may be more common and as a result may predispose individuals to antisocial or aggressive behavior (Brunner et al., 1993). MAO is associated with many of the neurochemicals that already have a link to antisocial or criminal behavior. Norepinephrine, serotonin, and dopamine are metabolized by both MAOA and MAOB (Elliot, 2000).

Serotonin is a neurochemical that plays an important role in the personality traits of depression, anxiety, and bipolar disorder (Larsen and Buss, 2005). It is also involved with brain development and a disorder in this system could lead to an increase in aggressiveness and impulsivity (Morley and Hall, 2003). As Lowenstein (2003) states, "studies point to serotonin as one of the most important central neurotransmitters underlying the modulation of impulsive aggression". Low levels of serotonin have been found to be associated with impulsive behavior and emotional aggression. In addition, children suffering from conduct disorder show to low blood serotonin (Elliot, 2000). Needless to say, there is a great deal of evidence that shows serotonin is inversely related to aggression, which can be further associated with antisocial or criminal behavior.

Dopamine is a neurotransmitter in the brain that is associated with pleasure and is also one of the neurotransmitters that is chiefly associated with aggression. Activation of both affective (emotionally driven) and predatory aggression is accomplished by dopamine (Elliot, 2000). Genes in the dopaminergic pathway have also been found to be involved with attention deficit hyperactivity disorder (ADHD). Morley and Hall (2003) found a relationship between the genes in the dopaminergic pathway, impulsivity, ADHD, and violent offenders. Obviously the study of MAO, serotonin and dopamine suggests that there is a genetic component to antisocial or criminal behavior.

PERSONALITY DISORDERS AND TRAITS

Attention deficit hyperactivity disorder (ADHD), conduct disorder (CD), and oppositional defiance disorder (ODD) are three of the more prominent disorders that show a relationship with later adult behavior (Holmes, Slaughter, and Kashani, 2001).

ODD is characterized by a recurrent pattern of negativistic, defiant, disobedient, and hostile behavior toward authority figures that is clearly more frequent, more intense, and more persistent across the child's development than is typically observed in individuals of similar age and developmental level. Symptoms generally begin early in life and are usually more prevalent and severe at home in the child's interactions with the parents. Only with more severe and pervasive oppositional defiant disorder and later in the course of illness does the disorder tend to generalize out of the home with hostile and defiant symptoms expressed toward authority figures at school and in the community. (Daniel F. Connor, 2009) Not all children of ODD develop CD. Current research suggests that about 30 percent of children with ODD will eventually develop CD while only about 10 percent will grow up to meet the criteria of anti-social personality disorder (ASPD).

ADHD is associated with hyperactivity-impulsivity and the inability to keep attention focused or concentrated on a particular thing (Morley and Hall, 2003). Holmes et al (2001) stated that, "impulse control dysfunction and the presence of hyperactivity and inattention are the most highly related predisposing factors for presentation of antisocial behavior". They also point to the fact that children diagnosed with ADHD have the inability to analyse and anticipate consequences or learn from their past behavior. Children with this disorder are at risk of developing ODD and CD, unless the child is only diagnosed with attention deficit disorder (ADD), in which case their chances of developing ODD or CD are limited. The future for some children is made worse when ADHD and CD are co-occurring because they will be more likely to continue their antisocial tendencies into adulthood (Holmes et al., 2001).

Conduct disorder is characterized by an individual's repetitive and persistent violation of societal rules and norms beginning in childhood or adolescence. These behaviors fall into four main groupings: Aggressive behaviors that cause harm to or threaten harm to others, nonaggressive property destruction, covert aggressive behaviors of deceitfulness or theft, and rule violations. What is even more significant is the fact that ODD, ADHD, and CD are risk factors for developing ASPD. Current research suggests that of the adolescents with ODD, ADHD or CD, about 10, 13 and 40 per cent respectively would eventually develop ASPD.

ASPD can only be diagnosed when an individual is over the age of eighteen and at which point an individual shows persistent disregard for the rights of others (Morley and Hall, 2003). ASPD has been shown to be associated with an increased risk of criminal activity. Therefore, it is of great importance that these early childhood disorders are correctly diagnosed and effectively treated to prevent future problems.

Two of the most cited personality traits that can be shown to have an association with antisocial or criminal behavior are impulsivity and aggression (Morley and Hall, 2003). According to the article written by Holmes et al. (2001), antisocial behavior between the ages of nine and fifteen can be correlated strongly with impulsivity and that aggression in early childhood can predict antisocial acts and delinquency. One statistic shows that between seventy and ninety per cent of violent offenders had been highly aggressive as young children (Holmes et al., 2001). These personality traits are shown to be heritable.

ENVIRONMENTAL INFLUENCES

Family environment influences the hyperactivity of children (Schmitz, 2003). Family risk factors are poverty, education, parenting practices, and family structure. Prior research on the relationship between family environment and child behavior characterizes a child's well-being with a positive and caring parent-child relationship, a stimulating home environment, and consistent disciplinary techniques (Schmitz, 2003). It seems obvious to conclude that those families who are less financially sound, perhaps have more children, and who are unable to consistently punish their children will have a greater likelihood of promoting an environment that will influence antisocial or delinquent behavior. Another indicator of future antisocial or criminal behavior is that of abuse or neglect in childhood. A statistic shows that children are at a fifty percent greater risk of engaging in criminal acts, if they were neglected or abused (Holmes et al., 2001). This has been one of the most popular arguments as to why children develop antisocial or delinquent behaviors.

Genetic and environmental influences on antisocial or criminal behavior have to deal with the age of the individual.

One significant factor in the development of antisocial or delinquent behavior in adolescence is the influence of peer groups. Garnfeski et al (1996) stated that there is a correlation between the involvement in an antisocial or delinquent peer group and problem behavior.

Interaction between family members and disciplinary techniques are influential in creating antisocial behavior. Children who were raised in an aggressive family environment would most likely have experienced a lack of parental monitoring, permissiveness or inconsistency in punishment, parental rejection and aggression.

GENE-ENVIRONMENT INTERACTIONS

Personality psychologist Eysenck created a model based on three factors known as psychoticism, extraversion, and, neuroticism, or what is referred to as the PEN model (Eysenck, 1996). Psychoticism is associated with the traits of being aggressive, impersonal, impulsive, cold, antisocial, and unempathetic. Extraversion is correlated with the traits of being sociable, lively, active, sensation-seeking, carefree, dominant, and assertive. Finally, neuroticism is associated with being anxious, depressed, low self-esteem, irrational, moody, emotional, and tense (Eysenck, 1996). Eysenck found that these three factors could be used as predictors of criminal behavior. He believed this to be especially true of the psychoticism factor and that measuring it could predict the difference between criminals and non-criminals. Extraversion is a better predictor for young individuals, while neuroticism is a better predictor for older individuals (Eysenck, 1996). An important point about these factors and the personality traits associated with them is that most of them have already been found to be heritable (Miles and Carey, 1997).

The premise of the general arousal theory of criminality is that individuals inherit a nervous system that is unresponsive to low levels of stimulation and as a consequence, these individuals have to seek out the proper stimulation to increase their arousal. Under this theory, the proper stimulation includes high-risk activities associated with antisocial behavior, which consists of sexual promiscuity, substance abuse, and crime (Miles and Carey, 1997). A significant fact that must be pointed out though is that not every individual with low arousal levels or those who are extraverts will seek those high risk activities just mentioned. It takes the right environment and personality to create an individual with antisocial or criminal tendencies and that is why this theory can be considered to take into account both factors of genetic and environmental influences.

Genetics play an important role in the outcome or behavior of an individual.

Environmental factors account for what cannot be explained by genes. An individual's antisocial or criminal behavior can be the result of both their genetic background and the environment in which they are raised.

A primary sociopath is lacking in moral development and does not feel socially responsible for his actions. This type of sociopath is a product of the individual's personality, physiotype, and genotype. A secondary sociopath develops in response to his or her environment because of the disadvantages of social competition. Living in an urban residence, having a low socio-economic status, or poor social skills can lead an individual to being unsuccessful in reaching their needs in a socially desirable way, which can turn into antisocial or criminal behavior. The first type of sociopath is dependent on their genetic makeup and personality, while certain factors of the second type can also be heritable. Notwithstanding, the second type has a greater dependence on environmental factors (Miles and Carey, 1997). Both genetic and environmental factors support the idea of a secondary type of sociopaths. An individual can inherit certain genes and when combined with the right environmental factors can lead them to engage in antisocial or criminal behavior.

Women should not be entirely eliminated from the spectrum of criminality just because of their smaller predisposition toward aggression. Women are as capable as men of committing a violent act. Jones discussed how certain neurochemicals are associated with criminal behavior. These neurochemicals might be more active in men, but women can still grow up in environments in which certain tendencies are brought on.

Whether one is male or female, growing up in an environment in which one is beaten or neglected is going to cause serious traumatic repercussions. The aggressive tendencies in males head them to become more aggressive in adulthood, which in turn is why they are more apt to commit violent crimes. Men have committed more crimes and are known to be more violent, yet women should not be eliminated from the discussion. It has not been shown that genes or environment alone determine criminal behavior, as Jones mentioned in her paper, so there should be no reason why only men are mentioned, whether directly or by implication.

Research has indicated that the single DRD4 gene may account for 10% of the genetic variance in relation to novelty-seeking (Sloan, 2000).

Some studies have demonstrated a genetic link among ADHD, CD, and ODD and criminality. It has been shown that people evoke certain responses from their environment. It is plausible that children suffering from these disorders are treated in a different manner than normal children due to the responses that evoke, and it is because of these environmental differences that they are more prone to criminal behavior.

A Swedish study found that the occurrence of major mental disorders in prisoners to be 5%, as well as a 20% occurrence of personality disorders (Rasmussen, 1999).

Leonard Heston in 1960 examined children of schizophrenic mothers that were removed after birth and raised by foster parents. Out of a total of 47 children examined, Heston found that nine of them were diagnosed with sociopathic personalities and antisocial behavior, and four of the 47 children developed schizophrenia.

KEY LEARNING POINTS

- If environment affects the regulation of gene expression and, in turn, the activity of neurotransmitters that modulate behavior, this kind of interaction may be a significant factor in the development of criminal and antisocial behavior.

- An adult's personality is the combination of traits and learned behavior patterns that have been established throughout childhood.
- A eugenic approach to preventing antisocial behavior is immoral and impinges on human rights, but taking an active approach to ensure positive environmental influences would be appropriate.

CASE LAW

GS Eveseef, EM Wisniewski, A Psychiatric Study of Violent Mass Murder, JFS, 1972, 17:371 and A Potential Young Murderer, JFS, 1976, 21: 441

Traumatic childhood experiences of being abandoned, of being beaten and of being sexually abused may lead many persons to 'homicide proneness'.

Chapter

11

Court Decisions: Diminished or Partial Responsibility and Murder

EXPLANATION

In State *vs* Byrne—(CCC 1959), the Irish labourer Patrick Byrne, 27 years was charged to have committed sadistic murder of Stephanie Baird 29 years in YWCA hostel in Birmingham, when he, after being ordered off from his work, made his way to the hostel, attacked the girl in her room, strangled her to death and mutilated her body parts. In the trial, though it was admitted that Byrne was not insane as per Mc Naughten's rule, as he was quite aware of his act and its consequences, the psychiatrists opined that, he was suffering from some disease or abnormality of mind, which would absolve him from charge of murder as per Homicide Act. In the Court of Appeal it was successfully pleaded that he was suffering from abnormality of mind with sadistic sexual propensity and he was sentenced to life imprisonment.

Similarly, in Rex *vs* Matheson (1958) IWLR 474, the accused was found guilty of capital murder of Gordon Lockhart, aged 15 years. He was found to be not truly insane in normal sense, but was a psychopathic personality; was once a voluntary patient in a mental hospital, his mental age was that of a child of 10 years. The defence psychiatrist successfully pleaded that he suffered from such abnormality of mind as to substantially impair his criminal responsibility. He was sentenced to 20 years of imprisonment.

PLEA OF IRRESTIBLE IMPULSE IN MURDER

In case of State *vs* Sher Singh vide Lahore High Court Criminal Appeal No. 1046 of 1922, the Court found Sher Singh guilty of murder charge. He, in a highly excited and unbalanced state of mind, attempted to kill his wife and mother-in-law, killed his 10 years old brother-in-law and set fire to the hut of his mother-in-law. He was quite conscious of his act to be wrong and illegal, and his plea of irresistible impulse was of no avail.

i. Every person is presumed to be sane and to possess a degree of reason sufficient to be responsible for his acts, unless the contrary is proved.

   Vide State of Madhya Pradesh *vs* Ahmadulla AIR 1961, SC 998.

ii. To prove that the accused is an insane, it will have to be proved that at the material moment, the accused was in such defective state of mind that he did not know the nature and quality of the act he was doing; and even if he knew that, he did not know that it was wrong and against law—Vide State of Madhya Pradesh *vs* Ahamadullah AIR 1961 SC 998.

iii. If the evidence shows that the accused was conscious of the nature of the act, he must also have been conscious of its criminal nature too.

Vide Queen *vs* Lakshman ILR 10, Bombay 50; Ambi *vs* State of Kerala 1962; 2 Cr. Leg Jl 135 (Ker).

iv. The mere fact that the act was done unpremeditated without any apparent motive is not by itself sufficient to establish insanity—Vide—Ambi *vs* State of Kerala 1962, 2 CRC. IJ (Ker) 135–141; State *vs* Kanda Sami Mudali, AIR 1960, Madras 316

v. The previous history and the subsequent conduct of the alleged lunatic are relevant only to show what the state of mind of the accused was at the material moment. The Court is only concerned with the state of mind of the accused at the time of committing the criminal act—vide Kaubi Kurji Duba *vs* State AIR 1960 Guj I.

vi. Peculiar and abnormal behavior by itself will not suffice to amount to insanity as per Sec. 84 IPC—Vide re-Kandaswami Mudali AIR 1960, Madras 316.

SOMNAMBULISM AND CRIMINAL RESPONSIBILITY

Explanation

Rex *vs* WE Boshears (Essex Assizes, 1961). An American staff Sergeant Willis Eugene Boshears 29 years married with 3 children was charged for having murdered Jean Constable 20 years whom he met in a pub with another man on new year's eve. All of them came to his flat, the man had intercourse with the girl, and then she went to sleep on the mattress on the floor. The other man left and Boshears lay down beside her very drunk. He said later "The next thing I remember is that I felt something pulling at my mouth. I was not awake but this woke me and I found that I was over Jean and I had my hands around her throat. Jean was dead and I panicked". He took the body to the spare room, dressed her up and again went to sleep: On awakening, and that not before 2 days after she died, he took her body in his car and dumped it in a ditch. In the trial, the jury accepted the plea of defence that the act was accidental and was done inadvertently during sleep. The accused was found not guilty and discharged.

SOMNOLENTIA AND CRIMINAL RESPONSIBILITY

Explanation

In Hungary, one lady inflicted serious injuries on her daughter in the middle of a night in a state of dream, when she fancied to have seen her daughter arrested against public morals; unconsciously she gave way to an overpowering impulse to kill her and thus did hit her. The court believed her version and discharged her—Times, Jan 2, 1937,9.

HYPNOTISM AND CRIMINAL RESPONSIBILITY

Explanation

In Rex *vs* Eyrand, when Mr. Gouffe was murdered by homicidal hanging by Eyrand in collusion with Miss Bompard. Miss Bompard took the plea that she was hypnotised by Eyrand to take part in the crime. The Court did not accept this defence.

The law relating to drunkenness and criminal responsibility has been dealt with under Secs. 85 and 86 IPC.

DELIRIUM AND CRIMINAL RESPONSIBILITY

Delirium was earlier defined as "a perversion of mental processes manifested in speech or action". However, delirium now means sudden severe confusion and rapid changes in brain function that occur with physical or mental illness (Pub Med Health). The disturbance is characterised by incoherent speech, hallucinations, illusions, delusions, restlessness, watchfulness, apparently purposeless actions, inability to fix the attention, etc."—vide Tuke, Dict. of Psych. Medicine.

Because of hallucinations and delusions, the patient may commit some criminal acts. Such a person will not be held liable for his act committed during the state of delirium, if it could be proved that the subject in this state, lost his power of understanding the nature of the act or power of distinguishing between right or wrong vide Section 84 IPC.

CASE LAW

Leader, 25 September 1933

One Martin Ali with a friend of his, engaged a taxi from Nagpur for Chindwara, and while returning shot the owner and the cleaner of the car at night. He was absconding and was arrested on the fourth day of the occurrence. He was sentenced to transportation for life by the Session Judge of Chindwara for the double murder. On an appeal preferred by him, the judicial commissioner, in the course of his judgment, observed that the case did not fall within Section 84 of the Indian Penal Code 1860, because the mental faculties of Martin, distinguishing right from wrong from moral point of view, were absolutely clear. The applicant fully believed that taking life of another was not only illegal, but immoral. The appellant divided himself into two parts, viz Martin Ali and Rumi Safa (freelance). According to him, there resided in his physical body both good and evil spirits and in spite of his control, the evil spirit forced him to kill useless persons like himself to make the world better. Martin did not commit suicide as the world would have taken him to be a coward. The present crimes were committed in a fit of impulsive insanity without any motive or premeditation; nevertheless they did come under purview of Section 302 of the Indian Penal Code 1860, but necessitated indulgent consideration. Having regard to the fact that the appellant belonged to a respectable family and had received higher education, the judicial commissioner directed that the case be laid before the local government for such indulgent consideration, as they may be pleased to show to the appellant under Section 401 of the Code of Criminal Procedure 1973.

DK Henderson and RD Gillespie, A Textbook of Psychiatry, 1956, eighth edn, Oxford Medical Publications, University press, London, 714–715

The unwritten law in this relation stated by J Alness in the case of Rex *vs* Savage is as follows:

'Formerly there were only two classes of prisoners—those who were completely responsible, and those who were completely irresponsible. Our law has now come to recognize in murder cases a third class—those who, while they may not merit the description of being insane, are nevertheless in such a condition as to reduce the quality of their act from murder to culpable homicide. There must be aberration or weakness of mind; there must be some form of mental unsoundness; there must be a state of mind bordering on, though not amounting to, insanity; there must be a mind so affected that responsibility is diminished from full responsibility to partial responsibility; the prisoner in question must be only partially responsible for this action.

R *vs* Byrne 1963 WRL 440

DJ Power, MSL, October 1967, 189–191

In the case where a middle aged man suffering from alleged 'chronic anxiety', who had a delusion concerning his wife's infidelity, shot his sister-in-law and her husband in an erroneous belief that they were trying to break up his marriage, the plea of diminished responsibility was accepted.

It was also accepted in the case of an epileptic in R *vs* Candy who strangled a woman but claimed complete amnesia for the crime.

In the case of an appeal by Byrne, who had strangled a young girl at Birmingham YMCA, and mutilated her body, a plea for diminished responsibility within Section 2 of the Homicide Act 1957, was put forward with a view to be charged for manslaughter and not murder.

Bai Ramilaben *vs* State of Gujarat 1991 Cr LJ 2219

In Bai Ramilaben, the accused killed her four children of various ages and the plea of insanity was taken after recording of prosecution evidence. The trial court convicted the accused. However, the Gujarat High Court in appeal extended the benefit of Section 84 of the IPC to the accused and observed that having regard to the facts and circumstances of this case that the accused had killed her four children of various ages, at the same time it was the duty of the prosecution to subject the accused to medical examination and obtain opinion as regards her mental state. It may not be possible to know the state of mind of the accused at the time of the commission of the offence, but the state of mind, immediately after the incident could have been known. This would have thrown some light on the state of mind of the accused at the time of commission of offence. No evidence has been laid by the prosecution on this point and therefore, adverse inference is required to be drawn. On this short ground alone, the accused is entitled to benefit of doubt.

Namu Ram Bora *vs* State of Assam, AIR 1975 SC 762: 1975 SCC (Cri) 98: 1975 Cri LJ 646

Plea of insanity: Accused suffering from mental disorder, since after he suffered a dog bite and committed murder in such state of mind—The triple murder committed by him was not preplanned but as a result of mental imbalance—In the circumstances, the extreme penalty of death, converted to life imprisonment.

Ram Bharose *vs* State of MP, 1974 MP LJ 406

Plea of Insanity: A child was throttled to death in the Puja room under some delusion and that the child would come to life after three days—Held, though it was not a case of feigned insanity but was affected by some mental disorder the accused was entitled to benefit of Section 84 IPC as he was incapable of knowing that he was doing something wrong.

Gopalan Nayar *vs* State of Kerala AIR 1973 SC 806: 1973 Cri U 583: 1973 (1) SCC 469: 1973 SCC (Cri) 408

Insanity—Plea of unsoundness of mind: Where the accused has some sort of mental trouble prior to the date of occurrence and there was nothing to show that he was not suffering from mental obsession, which may not amount to insanity it will not be a case in which death penalty could be justified.

Francis Aleal Ponnan and another *vs* State of Kerala, AIR 1974 SC 2281: 1974 Cri LJ 1310.

Insanity as a plea of defence—Plea of insanity is easily taken to escape capital punishment in the charges of murder—However, every sort of mental disorder will not absolve the sufferer from criminal liability or justify a less severe punishment—A mere possession of a twisted mind which could not absolve him from criminal liability can mitigate his crime, if proved fact disclosed that something even falling short of either legal insanity satisfying the test laid down in Mc Naghten Rules, which will negate criminal liability, or 'insane impulse' which is receiving increasing jurisprudential recognition for absolving its victim from criminal liability or grave and sudden provocation which will reduce a culpable homicide from murder to one which is not murder.

Chapter

12

Dementia of the Alzheimer's Type

Alois Alzheimer first described the condition that later assumed his name: in 1906 he described a 51 year old woman with a 4½ year course of progressive dementia. The final diagnosis of Alzheimer's disease is based on a neuropathological examination of the brain; nevertheless, dementia of the Alzheimer's type is commonly diagnosed in the clinical setting after other causes of dementia have been excluded from diagnostic consideration. Alzheimer's dementia is the most common and accounts for 60–80 percent of all cases of dementia.

Senile plaques, also referred to as amyloid plaques, are much more indicative of Alzheimer's disease, although they are also present in Down's syndrome and, to some extent, in normal aging. Senile plaques are composed of a particular protein β/A4, astrocytes, dystrophic neuronal processes, and microglia. The number and the density of senile plaques present in postmortem brains have been correlated with severity of the disease.

The course of the dementia varies from a steady progression commonly seen with dementia of the Alzheimer's type, to an incrementally worsening dementia seen in vascular dementia, to the stable dementia seen in dementia of head trauma.

DIAGNOSTIC CRITERIA FOR DEMENTIA IN ALZHEIMER'S DISEASE (DSM-IV)

A1. The disturbance is not better accounted for by another Axis I Psychiatric disorder (e.g. major depressive disorder, schizophrenia).

A2. The deficits do not occur exclusively during the course of a delirium.

A3. The cognitive deficits in criteria A1 and A2 are not due to any of the following:

1. Other central nervous system conditions that cause progressive deficits in memory and cognition (e.g. cerebrovascular disease, Parkinson's disease, Huntington's disease, subdural hematoma, normal-pressure hydrocephalus, brain tumour).
2. Systemic conditions that are known to cause dementia (e.g. hypothyroidism.
   Vitamin B12 or folic acid deficiency, niacin deficiency, hypercalcemia, neurosyphilis, HIV infection, etc.
3. Substance-induced conditions/ disorders.

A4. The course is characterized by gradual onset and continuing cognitive decline.

A5. The cognitive deficits in criteria A1 and A2 each cause significant impairment in social or occupational functioning and represent a significant decline from a previous level of functioning.

A6. The development of multiple cognitive deficits as follows:

1. Memory impairment (impaired ability to learn new information or to recall previously learned information).
2. One (or more) of the following cognitive disturbances:
   a. Aphasia (language disturbance)
   b. Apraxia (impaired ability to carry out motor activities despite intactmotor function)
   c. Agnosia (failure to recognize or identity objects despite intact sensory function)
   d. Disturbance in executive functioning (i.e. planning, organizing, sequencing, abstracting, etc.)

Classic course is with onset in the patient's 50s or 60s, with gradual deterioration over 5 to 10 years, leading eventually to death. Once dementia is diagnosed, the patient must undergo a complete medical and neurological check-up.

Although the symptoms of the early phase of dementia are subtle, the symptoms become conspicuous as the dementia progresses, and family members may then bring the patient to a physician's attention. Demented patients may be sensitive to the use of benzodiazepines or alcohol, which may precipitate agitated, aggressive, or psychotic behavior. In the terminal stages of dementia, patients become empty shells of their former selves, profoundly disoriented, incoherent, amnesic (grossly forgetful), and incontinent of urine and faeces.

Recent memory is lost before remote memory in most cases of dementia; many patients are highly distressed because they can clearly recall how they used to function while observing their obvious deterioration. At the most fundamental level, the self is a product of brain functioning. Hence, the patients' identities fade as the illness progresses, and patients can recall less and less of their past. Emotional disturbances ranging from depression to severe anxiety to catastrophic terror can stem from the realization that the sense of self is disappearing before one's eyes.

The clinician can assist patients in finding ways to deal with the defective ego functions, such as keeping calendars for orientation problems, making schedules to help structured activities, and taking notes for memory problems.

Loved ones who take care of the patient struggle with feelings of guilt, grief, anger, and exhaustion as they watch the family member gradually deteriorate.

VASCULAR DEMENTIA (DSM-IV)

The general symptoms of vascular dementia are the same as those for dementia of the Alzheimer's type, but the diagnosis of vascular dementia requires the presence of either clinical or laboratory evidence supportive of a vascular cause of the dementia.

1. The cognitive deficits in criteria A1 and A2 (as in Alzheimer's disease) each cause significant impairment in social or occupational functioning and represent a significant decline from a previous level of functioning.
2. The development of multiple cognitive deficits manifested by both:
   i. Memory impairment (impaired ability to learn new information or to recall previously learned information)
   ii. One (or more) of the following cognitive disturbances:
      a. Aphasia (language disturbance)
      b. Apraxia (Impaired ability to carry out motor activities despite intact motor function)
      c. Agnosia (failure to recognize or identify objects despite intact sensory function)

   d. Disturbance in executive functioning (i.e. planning, organizing, sequencing of and abstracting).
3. Focal neurological signs and symptoms (e.g. exaggeration of deep tendon reflexes, extensor plantar response, pseudobulbar palsy, gait abnormalities, weakness of an extremity) or laboratory evidence indicative of cerebrovascular disease (e.g. multiple infarctions involving cortex and underlying white matter) that are judged to be etiologically related to the disturbance).
4. The deficits do not occur exclusively during the course of a delirium.

Dementia of Medical Conditions

DSM-IV lists six specific causes of dementia that can be coded directly: HIV disease, head trauma, Parkinson's disease, Huntington's disease, Pick's disease, and Creutzfeldt-Jakob disease. A seventh category allows the clinician to specify other non-psychiatric medical conditions associated with dementia.

- The development of multiple cognitive deficits manifested by both:
  1. Memory impairment (impaired ability to learn new information or to recall previously learned information).
  2. One (or more) of the following cognitive disturbances:
     a. Aphasia (language disturbance)
     b. Apraxia (impaired ability to carry out motor activities despite intact motor function)
     c. Agnosia (failure to recognize or identify objects despite intact sensory function).
     d. Disturbance in executive functioning (i.e. planning organizing sequencing abstracting.
- The cognitive deficits in criteria A1 and A2 (as in Alzheimer's disease) each cause significant impairment in social or occupational functioning and represent a significant decline from a previous level of functioning.
- There is evidence from the history, physical examination, or laboratory findings that the disturbance is the direct physiological consequence of one of the general medical conditions listed above.
- The deficits do not occur exclusively during the course of a delirium.

Transient Ischemic Attacks

Transient ischemic attacks are brief episodes of focal neurological dysfunction lasting less than 24 hours (usually 5 to 15 minutes). The episodes are mostly the result of microembolization from a proximal intracranial arterial lesion that produces transient brain ischemia. The episodes usually resolve without significant pathological alteration of the brain parenchyma.

CASE LAW

Kamla Devi *vs* Kishori Lal AIR 1962 Punj 196, p 200

Case Law: The testator's age, disease and mental weakness are important considerations. Debility, physical or mental, militates strongly against the voluntary character of the Will.

Ram Nath Das *vs* Ram Nigina Chaubey AIR 1962 Pat 481, p 483

Mere old age of the testator, 90 years in the instant case, does not lead to an inference that the testator had no capacity to execute the Will, in the absence of medical evidence to the effect.

Krishna Kumar Sinha *vs* Kayastha pathshala, Allahabad AIR 1966 All 570 (1965) ILR 1 All 483

Testamentary capacity has to be judged not by an absolute standard but as relative to a particular testamentary act.

(1883) 8 PD 171

Pereira *vs* Pereira (1901) AC 354 followed in De Souza *vs* De Souza AIR 1956 Madh Bha 227; Re Amulya Kumar Bose 42 Cal WN 649; Gorandas *vs* Bai Suraj AIR 1921 Bom 193, 23 Bom LR 1068; Venkata *vs* Beggiamal 23 Mad LJ 54; Rajendra *vs* Brojendra 14 MIA 67; Suradindunath *vs* Sudhir 50 Cal 100; Woolmer *vs* Daly 1 Lah 173

The decision in Parker *vs* Felgate was to the effect that if a testator has given instructions to a solicitor at a time when he was able to appreciate what he was doing in all its relevant bearings and if the solicitor prepares the Will in accordance with these instructions, the Will shall stand good though at the time of execution of the Will, the testator is capable of only understanding that he is executing the Will which he has instructed but is no longer capable of understanding the instructions themselves or the clauses in the Will which give effect to them.

(1883) 8 PD 171

The principle enunciated in Parker *vs* Felgate should be applied with greatest caution and reserve when the testator does not himself give instructions to the solicitor who draws the Will, but to a lay intermediary who repeats them to a solicitor.

Battan Singh *vs* Amirchand AIR 1948 PC 200, (1948) 1 Mad LJ 232 (PC)

The opportunities for error in transmission and of misunderstanding and of deception in such a situation are obvious, and the court ought to be strictly satisfied that there is no ground for suspicion and that the instructions given to the intermediary were unambiguous and clearly understood, faithfully reported by him and rightly apprehended by the solicitor, before making any presumption in favour of validity.

Eussof Ahmad *vs* Ismail Ahmed AIR 1938 Rang 322

Wills are frequently made by the sick and the dying; the degree of understanding, therefore, which the law requires is such as may reasonably be expected from persons in that condition. It is not enough that a testator is able to answer familiar and usual questions. He must be able to exercise a competent understanding as to the general nature of the property, the state of his family, and the general condition and claims of the objects of his bounty, the nature of the instrument which he executes, and the general nature and general objects and the provisions which it contains; if he can do that, though he may be very feeble and debilitated in understanding and be at the point of death, it is enough to make the Will valid.

Makhan Mal *vs* Pritam Devi AIR 1961 Punj 411 p, 414

Where the testator lived for nearly three years after the execution of the Will and the attesting witnesses deposed that he was of sound mind when the Will was executed, the fact that the testator was almost blind and the persons to whom the property was bequeathed were living with him for a long time would not be sufficient to justify a finding of undue influence or lack of a proper dispositive mind.

Ajit Chandra *vs* Akhil Chandra AIR 1960 Cal 551, 64 Cal WN 576

All that can be said is that the conscience of the court must be satisfied on the evidence that the testator had sufficient mental capacity at the time of making the Will.

Carapiet *vs* Derderian AIR 1961 Cal 359

The court may zealously examine and carefully scrutinize evidence to remove the suspicion of the court when the propounder happens to be the biggest beneficiary under the Will.

Chapter

13

Substance-induced Dementia

The specific substances that (DSM-IV) can cause dementia are alcohol; inhalants; sedatives, hypnotics and anxiolytic substances.

DIAGNOSTIC CRITERIA FOR SUBSTANCE-INDUCED DEMENTIA (DSM-IV)

In addition to the general criteria for the diagnosis of other types of dementia,

- There is evidence from the history, physical examination or laboratory findings that the deficits are etiologically related to the persisting effects of substance used (e.g. a drug of abuse, a medication).

The diagnosis of dementia is based on a clinical examination of the patient, including a mental status examination, and on information from the patient's family, friends, and employers.

At the initial stages of dementia, the patient shows difficulty in sustaining mental performance, fatigue, and a tendency to fail when a task is novel or complex or requires a shift in problem-solving strategy. The severely demented patient requires constant supervision and help in order to perform even the most basic tasks of daily living. The major defects involve orientation, memory, perception, intellectual functioning, and reasoning. Affective and behavioral changes like defective control of impulses and lability of mood are frequent, as are accentuations and alterations of premorbid personality traits.

Changes in a demented person's personality are the most disturbing features for the families of affected patients. Pre-existing personality traits are accentuated during the development of a dementia. Patients with dementia also become introverted. Patients with frontal and temporal involvement have marked personality changes and may be irritable and explosive.

Patients with dementia may also exhibit pathological laughter or crying and extremes of emotions without apparent provocation.

Primitive (release) reflexes may be evident on neurological examination, and myoclonic jerks are seen in 5 to 10 percent of patients.

The patient has difficulty in generalizing from a single instance, in forming concepts, and in grasping similarities and differences among concepts. Lack of judgment and poor impulse control are found when the frontal lobes are involved. Examples of those impairments include coarse language, inappropriate jokes, the neglect of personal appearance and hygiene, and a general disregard for the conventional rules of social conduct.

The use of Single-photon emission computed tomography (SPECT) images may help in the differential diagnosis of dementing illnesses.

Delirium

Delirium is distinguished by rapid onset, brief duration, and fluctuation of cognitive impairment during the course of the day, nocturnal exacerbation of symptoms, marked disturbance of the sleep-wake cycle, and prominent disturbances in attention and perception.

Some patients with depression manifest cognitive impairment that can be difficult to distinguish from symptoms of dementia. The clinical picture is sometimes referred to as *pseudodementia*.

Factitious Disorder (Malingering)

Persons who attempt to simulate memory loss, as in factitious disorder, do so in an erratic and inconsistent manner. In true dementia, memory for time and place is lost before memory for person, and recent memory is lost before remote memory.

Aging

Aging is not always associated with any significant cognitive decline. Minor memory problems can occur with normal aging, referred as *benign senescent forgetfulness*.

Amnesia

The amnestic disorders primarily present a memory disorder with significant impairment in social or occupational functioning.

Amnesia is commonly found in alcohol disorders and head injury.

Diagnosis (DSM-IV)

- The development of memory impairment as manifested by impairment in the ability to learn new information or the inability to recall previously learned information.
- The memory disturbance causes significant impairment in social or occupational functioning and represents a significant decline from a previous level of functioning.
- The memory disturbance does not occur exclusively during the course of a delirium or a dementia.
- There is evidence from the history, physical examination, or laboratory findings that the disturbance is the direct physiological consequence of a general medical condition (including physical trauma or substance abuse).

DIAGNOSTIC CRITERIA FOR SUBSTANCE-INDUCED PERSISTING AMNESIA (DSM-IV)

- The development of memory impairment as manifested by impairment in the ability to learn new information or the inability to recall previously learned information.
- The memory disturbance causes significant impairment in social or occupational functioning and represents a significant decline from a previous level of functioning.
- The memory disturbance does not occur exclusively during the course of a delirium or a dementia and persists beyond the usual duration of substance intoxication or withdrawal.
- There is evidence from the history, physical examination or laboratory findings that the memory disturbance is etiologically related to the persisting effects of substance use (e.g. drug of abuse, a medication).

CLINICAL FEATURES AND ASSOCIATED CONDITIONS

The central symptom of amnestic disorders is the development of a memory disorder characterized by impairment in the ability to learn new information (*anterograde amnesia*) and the inability to recall previously remembered knowledge (*retrograde amnesia*). The symptom must result in significant problems for patients in their social or occupational functioning. The period of time for which a patient is amnesic may begin directly at the point of trauma or may include a period before the trauma. Memory for the time during the physical insult (for example, during a cerebrovascular event) may also be lost.

Patients cannot remember what they had for breakfast or lunch, the name of the hospital, or their doctor. In some patients the amnesia is so profound that the patients cannot orient themselves to city and time, although orientation to person is very rarely lost in amnestic disorders.

The onset of symptoms is sudden in trauma, cerebrovascular events, and neurotoxin chemical assaults or gradual in nutritional deficiency and cerebral tumours.

Cerebrovascular diseases: Cerebrovascular diseases affecting the hippocampus involve the posterior cerebral and basilar arteries and their branches. Infarctions are rarely limited to the hippocampus; they often involve the occipital or parietal lobes. Cerebrovascular diseases affecting the bilateral medial thalami, particularly the anterior portions, are often associated with symptoms of amnesia.

In cases of multiple sclerosis when plaques develop in the temporal lobe and the diencephalic regions, symptoms of memory impairment occur.

Korsakoff's syndrome is an amnestic syndrome caused by thiamine deficiency associated with the poor nutritional habits of chronic alcohol abusers. Korsakoff's syndrome is often preceded by Wernicke's encephalopathy, which is the associated syndrome of confusion, ataxia and ophthalmoplegia. In patients with thiamine deficiency-related symptoms, the neuropathological findings include hyperplasia of the small blood vessels with occasional haemorrhages, hypertrophy of astrocytes, and changes in neuronal axons. Recent memory tends to be affected more than remote memory; however, that feature is variable. Confabulation, apathy and passivity are prominent symptoms in the syndrome. With treatment, patients may remain amnestic for up to three months and then gradually improve over the next year. The administration of thiamine may prevent the development of additional amnestic symptoms, but rarely is the treatment able to reverse the severe amnestic symptoms, once they are established. About a third to a quarter of all patients recover completely, and about a quarter of all patients have no improvement of their symptoms.

Head injury

The severity of the brain injury is correlated with the duration and the severity of the amnestic syndrome, but the best correlate of eventual improvement is the degree of clinical improvement of the amnesia during the first week.

Transient Global Amnesia

Transient Global Amnesia is characterized by a lack of insight regarding the problem, a clear sensorium, some mild degree of confusion, and sometimes the ability to perform some well learned complex tasks. Episodes last from 6 to 24 hours.

Alcoholic Blackouts

An acute impairment in memory may be associated with alcohol intoxication. In some persons with severe alcohol abuse, the syndrome commonly referred to as an alcoholic blackout may occur. The alcoholic person awakens in the morning with a conscious awareness of being unable to remember a period of time the night before, while intoxicated. Sometimes specific behaviors like hiding money in a secret place and provoking fights are associated with a person's blackouts. That memory can be retrieved in some persons during the next stage of intoxication, which is termed 'State-dependant Learning'.

As the realization of the injury sets in, the patients may become angry and feel victimized by the malevolent hand of fate. The patient may view others, including the clinician, as bad or destructive, and the clinician must handle those projections without becoming punitive or retaliatory. As the patient accepts what happened, the clinician can help the patient form a new identity by connecting current experience of the self with past experiences of the self. Thus the clinician plays the role of the patient's missing ego.

Chapter

14

Schizophrenia

INTRODUCTION

Schizophrenia is a major mental disorder with an onset usually in the late adolescence and early adulthood. Early-onset schizophrenia (EOS: Onset between the ages, 13 and 18 years), although relatively rare, is associated with a proportion of offending and violent crime.

DIAGNOSIS

Schizophrenia is characterized by a 'fundamental distortion of thinking and perception, and by inappropriate affect or blunted affect. Clear consciousness and intellectual function are usually maintained' (WHO 1992). The essential features of schizophrenia are the psychotic symptoms.

1. Thought echo, thought insertion or withdrawal, and thought broadcasting
2. Delusions of control or of persecution, influence or passivity, etc.
3. Hallucinatory voices giving a running commentary on the patient's behavior, or discussing the patient amongst themselves.
4. Persistent delusions which are culturally inappropriate, bizarre or impossible
5. Persistent hallucinations with half-formed, non-affective delusions
6. Thought disorder with resultant incoherent speech or irrelevant speech and neologisms
7. Catatonic behavior
8. Negative symptoms of apathy, paucity of speech, social withdrawal, etc.
9. A significant and consistent change in personal behavior: Loss of interest, aimlessness, etc.

For a diagnosis there must be one clear or two less clear-cut symptoms from 1–4, and at least two symptoms from 5–8.

GENETIC FACTORS

The aetiology of adolescent or early-onset schizophrenia is multifactorial. Evidence of a genetic component to the liability to schizophrenia is from family, twin and adoption studies. Inheritance pattern, across the age range, is compatible with an oligogenetic disorder (Risch 1990)—that is, transmission by a few but not many genes. Early-onset schizophrenia may be a more severe form of the disorder or perhaps phenotypically different from adult-onset cases, with D3 receptor heterogeneity.

While the general population life time prevalence is about 1%, relatives of schizophrenic probands have a higher risk of schizophrenia and related disorders. The risk of developing schizophrenia in family members increases with the degree of biological relatedness to the patient—greater risks are associated with higher levels of shared genes

(Gottesman, 1991). For example, third-degree relatives (e.g. first cousins) share about 12.5% of their genes, and show a risk of 2% for developing schizophrenia. Second-degree relatives (e.g. half-siblings) share about 25% of their genes and show a risk of 6%. Most first-degree relatives (e.g. siblings, dizygotic (DZ) twins) share about 50% of their genes and show a risk of about 9%. Monozygotic (MZ) twins share 100% of their genes, and show risks near 50%. (Ming T. Tsuang, 2001)

ENVIRONMENTAL FACTORS

Environmental factors implicated in the genesis of schizophrenia include an excess of pregnancy and obstetric complications (Geddes and Lawrie 1995; Cannon et al. 2002a) which, it is estimated, doubles the lifetime risk to 2%. Gillberg et al (1986) found an excess of perinatal events in teenage psychotics. Some controversy remains over the finding, from several studies, of an excess of winter births and exposure to maternal influenza between the fifth and seventh month of gestation (Sham et al 1992). Crow and Done (1992), using direct maternal reports, found no such excess.

In the adolescent age range, the family environment is crucial. The importance of abnormal family communication ('communication deviance') and affective style was demonstrated in a 15-year prospective study of families of non-psychotic adolescent clinic attenders (Goldstein 1987).

There are psychosocial risk factors operative at the societal level, which include race or cultural factors. There is, for instance, a six times higher rate of schizophrenia in Afro-Caribbean second-generation people aged 16–25 (Harrison et al 1988). Social isolation in ethnic minorities also appears an important factor in the development of schizophrenia (Boydell et al 2001).

PRODROME

The prodromal phase of non-psychotic behavioral disturbance (NPBD) occurs in about half of early—onset schizophrenia (55%) and can last between one and seven years.

Acute presentations are more common in adolescence, but an insidious onset with predominantly negative symptoms-affective blunting, apathy, etc.—occurs, and heralds a poor prognosis.

PATHOGENESIS

In early-onset schizophrenia there is accumulating evidence of neurodevelopmental abnormalities (Murray et al 1992; Weinberger 1987) resulting in abnormal brain structures such as ventricular enlargement, smaller brain size (Frazier et al 1996) and loss of normal brain symmetry. Pre-schizophrenia boys are more hostile and anxious by the age of 7 years, while pre-schizophrenic girls demonstrate higher rates of withdrawal and under-reaction by age 11.

Violent schizophrenic subjects have been found on MRI to have smaller hippocampi bilaterally, and greater right-to-left asymmetry of the amygdale volumes.

GENERAL ISSUES

Data on forensic aspects of early-onset schizophrenia are limited, so some reliance is put upon studies of adult-onset schizophrenia. There are clearly problems with this: Adolescence represents a unique developmental phase with issues of increasing autonomy and independence and changes in relation to family, peers, school and occupation.

The early-onset group is more often characterized by histories of parental substance abuse, early school failure, conduct disorder and later antisocial personality functioning. They appear generally more deviant, committing more crimes including violent crimes, and displaying greater rates of substance abuse.

The prodromal phase of non-psychotic behavioral disturbances occurs in just over half of cases and can last on average six years. About half of these are externalizing behaviors—conduct disorder and attention-deficit disorder. As shown in the seminal studies of Farrington and West, of non-mentally ill boys, these behaviors, in conjunction with poverty, school failure, adverse parenting, and so on, represent risk factors for later offending behavior. The importance of this lies in the finding that one of the strongest predictors of offending behavior during a schizophrenic illness is pre-illness offending (Wessely and Taylor 1991).

Violent episodes are most likely to occur in the month prior to admission. Violence was more likely with an acute onset of schizophrenia.

Assaultive behavior is associated with hearing voices, manic excitement and going on a spending spree (Volavka et al 1997). Amongst adult psychotic prisoners, 20% are driven to offend by their symptoms; and alarmingly, 8% of those charged with homicide have schizophrenia—a high rate indeed (Taylor 1985).

Violent behavior was confined to the month prior to admission and the period of initial hospitalization and as in adult studies, even though severe, did not result in criminal proceedings. The violent episodes were in response to delusional, paranoid beliefs or hallucinatory experiences. Whilst the criminal behavior amongst the psychiatric controls was mundane (traffic and drug offences), that amongst the schizophrenic group was either serious (arson, stabbing, threatening behavior with a shotgun) or bizarre (being arrested for stealing £1 and causing a public nuisance by sitting cross-legged on a telephone kiosk). All were the direct result of delusional experiences.

DIFFERENTIAL DIAGNOSIS

The diagnosis of schizophrenia is often complex, requiring detailed phenomenological enquiry and longitudinal observation. The following clinical disorders need exclusion.

Mood Disorders

Bipolar disorder with psychotic symptoms is misdiagnosed as schizophrenia in up to 50% of cases.

Organic Disorders

All patients presenting with a psychotic illness should receive a through medical examination including blood tests, urine analysis and an MRI scan. The range of organic pathologies to be screened include:

- Delirium
- Central nervous system lesions—seizure disorders, brain tumours, congenital malformations, head injury
- Neurodegenerative disorders—Huntington's chorea, lipid storage disorder
- Metabolic disorders—Wilson's disease, endocrinopathies
- Infections-meningitis, encephalitis, human immunodeficiency virus-related syndromes
- Toxic encephalopathies—corticosteroids, illegal drugs (cannabis, amphetamines, LSD, cocaine, ecstasy, etc.)

The rate of illegal drug usage amongst first presentations of schizophrenia is high—up to 50% in some studies. In order to distinguish a drug-induced psychosis, a period of verified detoxification is necessary.

Pervasive Developmental Disorders

Although there are often developmental delays in cases of schizophrenia, including language, in autism and Asperger syndrome there is a lifelong history of aberrant social relatedness and characteristic speech abnormalities. The absence or transient nature of positive psychotic symptoms and the absence of a normal period of development help distinguish the conditions.

Personality Disorders and Dissociative States

The transient nature of the psychotic experiences in this disorder and the lack of delusions and thought disorder combined with the chaotic, demanding and dependent social relationships contrast with the schizoid, socially isolated and awkward relationships of the pre-schizophrenic adolescent.

Obsessive-compulsive Disorder

Severe obsessive-compulsive symptoms, such as intrusive thoughts or fears of contamination, without the patient being able to recognize these ideas as his or her own, can lead to diagnostic difficulty.

ASSESSMENT

The forensic assessment of schizophrenia can be divided into two interrelated parts: clinical assessment and risk assessment.

1. ***Clinical assessment***: The assessment of schizophrenia can be a complex task, broadly consisting of two areas.
   a. *History:* Acute presentations occur in about half of the cases; in others, there is an insidious onset with gradual withdrawal and isolation, loss of interest in activities—even those previously enjoyed—and a decline in sociability. The crucial factor is a change in personality functioning.
   b. *Observation:* If the patient is severely ill, at risk of self-harm or being violent or behaviorally disturbed, admission to hospital is indicated. Clear accounts of the patient's behavior are extremely useful. It should be possible to judge the patient's:
      - Response to abnormal experiences and his/her ability to resist these
      - Sociability and the potential to form relationships
      - Interaction with family and other significant figures
      - Level of general functioning
      - Likely response to treatment
2. ***Risk assessment:*** The risk assessment should be specific and address the following.
   a. *Historic risk behaviors*
      - When?
      - In what situation?
      - With whom or to whom were these behaviors directed?
      - Precipitating, aggravating and ameliorating factors?
      - What was the associated mental state?
      - Usage of illicit drugs or alcohol?

      Past behavior is one of the best or strongest predictors of future behavior.
   b. *Current risk behaviors:* Have there been changes in:
      - External circumstances or situation?
      - Mental state?
      - Usage of illicit drugs or alcohol?
      - Social support network, including psychiatric and social services?
   c. Mental state examination: This should cover:
      - *Subjective feelings of tension or* 'explosiveness'—ideas or feelings of violence
      - Persecutory ideation—especially delusions, paying particular attention to whether those currently around the patient are incorporated into the delusional system

- *Passivity phenomena*—note the important association of—threat/control-override' symptoms with violence (Link and Stueve 1994)
- *Hallucinations*—their nature and quality whether the source is benevolent or malevolent; also the omnipotence of the source (e.g. what are the consequences of not complying with any commands, why comply with some and not others?)
- *Depression*—for example 'I wish I was dead, there's nothing to live for, I might as well kill her and myself too'.
- *Jealousy of morbid intensity*— nature and detail, and importantly who is targeted
- *Insight*—not only into any psychiatric disorder but also previous violent or aggressive behavior (insight, however, may have poor predictive value for future violent episodes: Yen et al, 2002).
- The great majority of those who are mentally ill present no increased risk to others.
- The best predictors of future offending among mentally disordered people are the same as for the whole population: Previous offending, criminality within the family, poor parenting, etc.
- People suffering from severe mental illness such as schizophrenia may present an increased risk to others when they have active symptoms.
- People suffering from severe mental illness who have active symptoms and also abuse drugs or alcohol present a seriously increased risk to others.

Preliminary evidence suggests that those more likely to act on a delusion do the following; identify evidence, especially in the last week, to support their delusional beliefs; seek evidence to confirm their beliefs; feel frightened as a result of delusional beliefs; and have no insight.

TREATMENT

General Issues

The treatment of schizophrenia can be divided broadly into two parts: Specific treatment of the psychotic symptomatology, and general treatment of the psychological, social and educational needs.

Specific Treatment

Antipsychotics form the sheet anchor of treatment of schizophrenia. Older (typical) antipsychotics are less expensive but can cause more adverse effects such as sedation, weight gain, extrapyramidal symptoms, postural hypotension, etc. Patients on atypical antipsychotics—risperidone, olanzapine, quetiapine, amisulpride and clozapine—experience fewer side-effects, but many do gain significant weight (Barnes and McPhillips 1999). There is evidence of improvement in cognitive functioning with atypicals such as qutiapine (Herold et al 2002). Overall, patients on these medications may have a higher quality of life (Franz et al 1997). Clozapine may offer particular benefit in a forensic population as it is suggested that it reduces aggression because of its central serotonergic effects (Meltzer H.Y., 1992). However, as it is associated with a greater risk of inducing agranulocytosis, its use is restricted to only the treatment of refractory patients.

For severely disturbed patients, intramuscular preparations of antipsychotics such as haloperidol, olanzapine, zuclopenthixol acetate are effective. In some cases, oral or intramuscular benzodiazepines such as

Lorazepam and clonazepam are used to augment antipsychotics and achieve sedation (McAllister-Williams 2001). While experience is being gained with the use of intramuscular forms of the newer atypical antipsychotics, the older neuroleptics are found to be often associated with disturbing adverse effects. The adverse effects can however be tackled with appropriate doses of anticholinergics such as trihexyphenidyl, or with anti-histaminics such as promethazine.

The Individual

Cognitive-behavioral therapy.

The Family

A psycho-educational approach with the family is essential and has been shown, in combination with other interventions such as long-term drug prophylaxis, to reduce relapse rates by up to 50% (Falloon and Brooker 1992). Last few decades of research has shown that family interventions aimed at reducing the expressed emotions (such as hostile or critical comments and over involvement) in the family members is effective in reducing relapses in schizophrenia.

Social Functioning

Active rehabilitation

Management

It is a fundamental principle that the patient should be treated in the least restrictive setting appropriate to that person's needs.

DISCHARGE

Requires

- An assessment of need, including an assessment of risk.
- An agreed package of care.
- A nominated key-worker.
- Regular reviews and monitoring.

OUTCOME

There is no systematic cure for schizophrenia. A small percentage of 10–17% (Cawthron et al 1994; Werry et al 1991; Hollis 2000) appear to recover after the first episode, while the majority continue to experience symptoms, with some disintegration of the personality and social handicap.

The major deterioration occurs within the first few years of the onset, with a levelling off or plateauing thereafter (Bleuler 1978). Two broad patterns are seen: a relapsing course and a continuous illness.

The suicide rate, up to 15% in one study (Werry et al 1991), is greatest within the first six years (Westermeyer et al 1991) and is often associated with a depressive illness and feelings of hopelessness surrounding the illness itself. Continued social support and active treatment may mitigate this. In particular, there is evidence that the atypical antipsychotics olanzapine and risperidone have antidepressant effects and clozapine reduces the suicide rate (Meltzer 1995).

CONCLUSIONS AND FUTURE DIRECTIONS

Research

The first requirement is an accurately defined incidence and prevalence study on a defined population of DSM-IV or ICD-10 diagnosed early-onset schizophrenia. Prospective population studies would give greater understanding of the patterns of development and mechanisms of offending, and those factors specifically associated with persistence and remission of the violence and dangerous behavior.

Alongside the systematic application of research-based risk assessments of dangerousness, the development of a measure of the 'burden of care' for the family and professionals is needed to help plan service delivery on a more rational basis.

CASE LAW

Times of India, 2 December 1936

In the case of Katrak *vs* Khorshedbai before the High Court of Bombay, the Will of a Parsi was contested on the following grounds:

i. That the deceased was suffering from a delusion that his brother and sister had been instrumental in causing his son's death with a view to inherit his property. This delusion so operated on his mind that he had lost his testamentary capacity.
ii. That the deceased was not in a sound mind as he moved about in dirty clothes, kept food in cupboards for days and then ate the same in that condition, took away sandalwood offered at the agiary (fire temple) and sold the same for his benefit and sold sacred water of the sea to non-Zoroastrians and so on.

Dealing with the alleged delusion, it was stated that the evidence led in the case did not justify this conclusion. Even if there was this delusion, it did not prevent the deceased from making a valid Will, inasmuch as it had not influenced him in not considering the claims of his relatives. The other allegations only showed that the deceased was a miser and did not at all prove that he had lost his testamentary capacity or was of unsound mind.

Having regard to the life led by the deceased and the fact that he had ceased to live with his brother and sister for over 30 years, it was observed that there was nothing unusual in his leaving his whole fortune amassed by leading a very frugal life, to the agiary, to which he devoted his whole life. The evidence of the alleged delusion and unsoundness of mind was meagre, unsatisfactory and unreliable and was unjustified. It was concluded that he was not incapable of making a testamentary disposition. His habits of life might be eccentric, but the deceased was able to look after his affairs and showed clear-headedness. The Will having been proved to have been properly executed by the deceased, the plaintiffs were granted probate and the caveat was dismissed making the defendants pay their own costs.

1997 CR LJ 1461

In Khuraijam Somoi Singh *vs* State of Manipur, the accused was alleged to have killed the deceased, his step father, by an axe, but no ill will or animosity was shown to exist; rather, the witnesses' evidence showed that the accused was a lunatic and was living with the deceased for treatment. Medical evidence showed that the accused was suffering from a schizophrenic form of psychosis. The Guwahati High Court extending the benefit of Sec. 84 of the Indian Penal Code 1860 set aside the conviction of the trial court.

Ansar Ahmad Through Zaki Ahmed *vs* State, 34 (1988) D.L.T

Magistrate cannot Issue Arrest Warrant Against a Person Whose Trial has been Postponed on the Basis of Mental Unsoundness

The appellant, Ansar Ahamed, had schizophrenia and was accused of criminal charges under Secs. 506/323 of the Indian Penal Code. Zaki Ahmed, who was his next friend and surety, had asked for the proceeding to be conducted under Sec. 329 of the Code of Criminal Procedure, while placing on record a medical certificate affirming the unsoundness of the mind of the accused. The magistrate of the lower court had suddenly dropped the proceedings under Sec. 329 and issued a non-bailable warrant against the accused along with a warrant of attachment against the surety.

The High Court set aside the order of the magistrate and held that the mandate of the law is that if an accused is incapable of defending himself, the proceeding ought to be postponed till his capacities to make his defence are restored. It further held that the Magistrate has no jurisdiction to issue a warrant of arrest against a person of unsound mind. Also if the person is of unsound mind, the High Court said there is no question of proceedings against the surety.

Chandrashekar *vs* State of Karnataka, 1998 Cr. L.J. 2237 (Knt)(D.B.); Sanna Eranna *vs* State of Karnataka, 1983 Cr. L.J. 619: 1983 1 Knt L.J. 115 (Knt) (D.B.)

Opinion of Expert

The opinion of the expert as to the mental disease is relevant. Where reliable medical evidence shows that the accused was of unsound mind, when the offence was committed, the accused cannot be convicted and detained in prison, but has to be admitted in mental hospital.

Raghu Pradhan *vs* State of Orissa, 1993 910 Crimes 430: 1993 Cr. L.J. 1159 (Orissa)

Defence of Insanity—Accepted

Where the accused without any reason committed murder of two ladies, on earlier occasions had also suffered attacks of mental disorder, the plea of insanity under Sec. 84 of the Indian Penal Code was accepted.

Ajaya Mahakund *vs* State 1993 Cr.L.J. 1201 (Ori) (D.B.)

Where the accused pushed a four year child into fire resulting in its death, the act was without deliberation or preparedness, the accused was acquitted.

Ram Swarup Thakur *vs* State of Bihar, 2000 Cr. L.J. 26 (Pat) (D.B.)

Accused father killing his 3 years old minor child, for no apparent reason, accused remained in mental hospital for about 2 years, plea of unsoundness mind accepted, accused acquitted.

Pundalik Laxman Chavan *vs* State of Maharashtra, 199493) Crimes 298 (Bom)

Insanity—According to the medical certificate, the accused has improved and thereafter discharged. The record from mental hospital Ratangiri showed that the appellant was suffering from serious mental trouble, and the medical officer has deposed that the accused was admitted in the hospital on 14/12/1985, that he was running away from the home and suffering from insomnia. He was talking irrelevantly and drinking excessively. It was observed that the appellant was dishevelled and unkempt, muttering to self, talking irrelevantly, dull and was apathetic. He was diagnosed as a case of schizophrenia and treated up to 16/12/1985 when he was discharged.

In case of paranoid schizophrenia, it has been mentioned that the main characteristics of this illness are bizarre delusions with an intelligence that is otherwise well preserved, the patient gets very irritative and excited owing to these painful and disagreeable hallucinations and delusions. The totality of the cumulative effect of all the evidence and the circumstances brought on record duly considered carefully lead to the irresistible inference that at the crucial moment the state of mind of the appellant was such that he was not able to know or understand that what he was doing was wrong or contrary to the law due to unsoundness of mind. Therefore, his killing does not amount to an offence.

Inder Bir Singh *vs* Avneet Kaur, 1990 Marriage L J 560 (P & H)

Insanity: Wife suffering from schizophrenia even at the first wedding night. Parties lived together for three days after the marriage—what is required to be established is that the spouse was suffering from mental disorder and this fact was concealed?

Four varieties of schizophrenia were noticed by the court in Rameshwari Gupta *vs*

Ramnarain Gupta, 1987 (1) DMC 263 (All): In the first variety, i.e. simple schizophrenia, the patient loses interest in his best friends and has conflicts about sex. In the second variety, i.e. hebephrenia, disordered thinking is the outstanding characteristic. In this view of the matter, the wife held to have suffered from schizophrenia. According to the husband, he tried to consummate the marriage but there was no response. At the time of the intercourse her eyes became stable and she had a fixed gaze and her face was horrible —in the circumstances, the Hon'ble Court held, that the marriage was liable to be annulled.

(**Note:** The other two varieties of schizophrenia are the catatonic and the paranoid.)

State of H.P. *vs* Gian Chand, 2001 (3) SC 565.

Schizophrenia: Schizophrenia is one of a group of severe emotional disorders, usually characterized by misinterpretation and retreat from reality, delusions, hallucinations, ambivalence, inappropriate affect, and withdrawn, bizarre or regressive behaviors; popularly but erroneously called split personality. Accused suffering from schizophrenia cannot be held as suffering from unsoundness of mind and that too of a nature which would have rendered him incapable of knowing the nature of the act which he was doing or incapable of distinguishing between wrong or right as per law. Such an accused, therefore, cannot be granted benefit of Sec. 84, IPC.

Chapter

15

Suicidal Behavior and Attempts at Suicide

- Introduction
- Methods and incidence
- Religious attitude
- Psychological attitude
- Legal attitude
- Law of attempt at suicide
- Some cases

INTRODUCTION

Suicidal attempts and suicide are associated with depressive disorders, and those suicidal phenomena particularly in adolescence, constitute an important medicolegal problem. Suicidal tendencies and behavior are detectable or visible in many instances.

METHODS AND INCIDENCE

Completed suicide is rarely carried out as a realistic suicide plan. The decision to engage in suicidal behavior may be impulsive, without a great deal of forethought, or it may be the culmination of prolonged rumination. The method of the suicide attempt influences the morbidity and the completion rate independent of the severity of the intent to die at the time of the suicidal behavior. Thus, the common methods of completed suicide in children and adolescents are by using poisoning or self-immolation which account for about two thirds of all suicides in boys and almost half the suicides in girls. The second most common method of suicide in boys, occurring in about a fourth of all cases, is by hanging, in girls about a fourth commit suicide through the ingestion of toxic substances. Carbon monoxide poisoning is the next most common method for suicide in boys but occurs in less than 10 percent; suicide by hanging and carbon monoxide poisoning are equally frequent among girls, accounting for about 10 percent each. In the Nellore and Kadapa districts of Andhra Pradesh state in India, Supervasmol-33 (hair dye) liquid (50–200 ml)consumption is becoming a popular method of attempting suicide.

Suicide is among the ten leading causes of death in the west. In the United States, 30,000 suicides occur each year. In addition to completed suicides, more than 2,00,000 people attempt suicide each year and that nearly 3% of Americans have made a suicide attempt at some time in their lives. Hungary has an annual incidence of 44.9 per 1,00,000. India has second position after Hungary with 37.8 per 1,00,000 persons. Other countries with high rate, i.e. 20 per 1,00,000 or higher include-Switzerland, Finland, Austria, Sweden, Denmark and Germany. Countries with low rate (less than 9 per 1,00,000) include Egypt, Greece, Italy, Israel, Spain, Mexico and Ireland. According to National Crime Record Bureau of India, in 2006–07, 5857 young men committed suicide which is 16 per 1,00,000 whereas average of world suicide rate is 14.5 per 1,00,000.

There has been a steady increase in suicide rate. The increased suicide rates are thought to reflect changes in the social environment, growing stresses of life, and the increasing availability of the means to commit suicide.

The rates for suicide depend on age, and they increase significantly after puberty. Whereas less than one completed suicide per 100,000 occurs under 14 years of age, about 10 per 100,000 completed suicides occur in adolescents between 15 and 19 years of age. Under 14 years of age, suicide attempts are at least 50 times more common than suicide completions. While between 15 and 19 years, however, the rate of suicide attempts is about 15 times greater than suicide completions. The number of adolescent suicides over the past several decades has shown three to four-fold increase.

Suicidal adolescents are unable to synthesize solutions to problems and lack mature coping strategies to deal with immediate stressors, commit or attempt suicides. A narrow view of the options available to deal with recurrent family discord, rejection, or failure contributes to a decision to commit suicide.

GENETIC FACTORS

Evidence for a genetic contribution to suicidal behavior is based on family suicide risk studies and the higher concordance for suicide among monozygotic twins compared with dizygotic twins. The risk for suicide is high in persons with mental disorders—like schizophrenia, major depressive disorder, and bipolar disorders. The risk for suicide is much higher in the relatives of those with mood disorders than in the relatives of persons with schizophrenia.

OTHER BIOLOGICAL FACTORS

The mechanism linking decreased serotonin function and aggressive or suicidal behavior is unknown, and low serotonin may turn out to be a marker, rather than a cause, of aggression and suicidal propensity.

SOCIAL FACTORS

Children and adolescents are vulnerable to overwhelmingly chaotic, abusive, and neglectful environments. A wide range of psychopathological symptoms may occur owing to exposure to violent and abusive homes. Aggressive, self-destructive, and suicidal behaviors seem to occur with greatest frequency in persons who have endured chronically stressful family lives.

DIAGNOSIS AND CLINICAL FEATURES

Direct questioning of children and adolescents about suicidal thoughts is necessary, because studies have consistently shown that parents are frequently unaware of such ideas in their children. Suicidal thoughts (e.g. children's talk about wanting to harm themselves) and suicidal threats (that is, children's statements that they want to jump in front of a car) are more common than suicide completion.

Adolescents who attempt suicide and those who complete suicide are similar in conduct and behavior and about one third of those who complete suicide made prior attempts. Mental disorders present in some suicide attempters and completers include major depressive disorder and psychotic disorders. Adolescents with mood disorders in combination with substance abuse and a history of aggressive behavior are particularly at higher-risk. Those who are violent, aggressive, and impulsive are prone to suicide during family or peer conflicts. High levels of hopelessness, poor problem-solving skills, and a history of aggressive behavior predict suicide. Depression alone is a more serious risk factor for suicide in girls than in boys, but boys who commit suicide often have more severe psychopathology than the girls. An adolescent who commits suicide is occasionally one of high achievement and perfectionist character traits; such an adolescent may have recently felt humiliated for a perceived failure, such as diminished academic performance.

Psychiatrically disturbed and vulnerable adolescents attempt suicide. The precipitating factors include conflicts and arguments with family members and boyfriends or girlfriends. Alcohol and other substances also predispose vulnerable adolescents to suicidal behavior. In other cases, an adolescent attempts suicide in anticipation of punishment after being caught by the police or other authority figures for a forbidden behavior.

About 40 percent of youthful suicide completers had previous psychiatric treatment, and about 40 percent made a previous suicide attempt. The precipitating factors include loss of face with peers, a broken romance, school difficulties, unemployment, bereavement, separation, and rejection.

Cluster suicides among adolescents who know one another and go to the same school are reported. Suicidal behavior may precipitate similar attempts within a peer group through identification—so called copycat suicides. Some studies have found an increase in adolescent suicide after television programs were shown whose main theme was the suicide of a teenager. Many other factors are also involved, including a necessary substrate of psychopathology.

The tendency of disturbed young persons to imitate highly publicized suicides has been called the Werther syndrome, after the protagonist in Johann Wolfgang von Goethe's novel. *The Sorrows of Young Werther*. The novel, in which the hero kills himself, was banned in some European countries after its publication more than 200 years ago because of a rush of suicides by young men who had read it; some, when they killed themselves, dressed like Werther or left the book open to the passage describing his death. In general, although imitation may play a role in the timing of suicide attempts by vulnerable adolescents, the overall suicide rate does not seem to increase when media exposure increases.

Suicide has been a disputed phenomenon from ancient times the world over. In ancient Greece, the attempted suicide was punished by maiming the person. Classical Greeks believed indignity in death and people who were extremely ill could get permission from the state to commit suicide. Officials of State gave out Hemlock (a specific poison) to those who received such permission.

Christians believe that their lives are given by God and that everyone has an important role to play in society. They do not believe that one owns his individual life and therefore one should not choose to end it deliberately.

Suicide is forbidden in Islam. It is haraam and regarded as one amongst the major sins. The person who commits suicide is never allowed in Jannat. At numerous places in Quran, life is described by Allah as a favour on human beings, out of all the bounties Allah bestowed upon human beings, the most precious is the gift of life. Each one of us should remember that life, Allah has granted us, is not our personal possession or our personal property. In fact, it is a trust from Allah, making us merely trustees. Because we are trustees, we should utilise each and every moment of our lives in the paths that please Allah. A muslim should work and behave in his life in accordance with the path shown by the prophet Muhammad (let peace be on him). In this way he can attain Jannat after his death. As to the disparity and irony of life is concerned, Allah tests men by blessing them with countless bounties to see if the servant appreciates what he has been blessed with by Allah and he shows gratitude towards Allah for blessing him with these bounties. At times Allah in his infinite wisdom, puts a person in intense grief to see if the servant turns to Allah and seeks guidance and help or disbelieves in him.

There are specific sanctions expressed in Quranagainst suicide. The prophet Muhammad (let peace be on him) assigns suicide to the lower levels of Hell (Dojakh). Allah says explicitly in Quraan—"And do not kill yourself. Surely, Allah is most merciful to you"—(Surah An—Nisa Verse 29). In another verse of Quran, Allah says—"And do not throw yourself in destruction" (Surah A1-Baqarah Verse 195). Prophet Muhammad said, "whoever commits suicide with a piece of iron, he will be punished with the same piece of iron in the Hell—fire" and "He who commits suicide by throttling shall keep on throttling himself in the Hell fire forever. Moreover "He who commits suicide by stabbing himself he shall keep stabbing himself in the Hell fire forever".

Parasar IV-1-2 provides that if a man or a woman commits suicide out of extreme pride, or love or anger, or on account of fear, he or she falls into hell for sixty thousand years. Yama 20–21 provides, if a person tries to commit suicide but survives should be punished with a fine of two hundred panas, and he should undergo penance. If the person dies the body should be smeared with an impure substance.

The commentators on Manu hold the view that a man may undertake the Mahaprasthhaana (great departure) or on a journey which ends in death when he is incurably diseased or meets with a great misfortune and that because it is taught in the Sastras, it is not opposed to the Vedic rules which forbid suicide. But this form of suicide was allowed only for hermits, sages and to some extent for those leading Vanaprastha and Sanyas Ashrams. It was never allowed for common people. The general law was that suicide was prohibited for common people.

The eminent sociologist of the 19th century in his masterpiece "Le Suicide" Emile Durkheim considered suicide to be a social fact and social forces to be responsible for it. Suicide waves are formed in society and these waves are formulated by specific social circumstances. He defined suicide as, "Every case of death which results directly or indirectly from a positive or negative act of the victim himself which he knows will produce this result".

Durkheim mentions four types of suicides:

1. Egoistic suicide
2. Altruistic suicide
3. Anomic suicide
4. Fatalistic suicide

1. ***Egoistic suicide:*** The main cause of egoistic suicide is excessive individualism. A man fulfils the purpose and his desires in society. If we have affection with society we will be more involved in social activities. Segregation brings distance from society and here one feels doubts about oneself. He finds a hollowness in his life, feels rejected and dejected and becomes neutral to society and ultimately commits suicide.

2. ***Altruistic suicide:*** Society gobbles up the personality of individuals, and encourages or requires the individual to sacrifice his life. In the modern times this happens in armies. In some countries, suicide bombs are also a type of altruistic suicide.

   During World War II many villagers in Japan committed suicide when forced with imminent capture by Allied Forces. The soldiers of Denmark in their old age jumped from a hill and committed suicide. Buddhists commit suicide by self-immolation or self-destruction. Jains do so by hunger strikes. Durkheim says that in this type of suicide one has a specific objective to achieve but that lies beyond this life and present life is a hindrance in achieving that goal.

3. ***Anomic suicide:*** It is man's nature to be eternally dissatisfied and to have unlimited

desires. An anomic suicide happens when a sudden change occurs and society has no ideals before it. It often happens in economic crisis as well as in breakdown of conjugal relations in the society. It occurs due to the society's insufficient presence in the individual's life.

4. ***Fatalistic suicide:*** It is the result of excessive social regulation of persons with future pitilessly blocked and passions violently choked by oppressive discipline. The suicide of slaves and of those who were subject to excessive physical and moral despotism is an example. Psychological studies point out that mostly (about 90%) suicides happen due to depression which is the result of severe mood disorders. In mood disorders extreme variations either low or high are the predominant features. We all experience such variations at mild to moderate levels in the natural course of life but when grief and agony increases so high that the means to tackle are lessened then the feeling of suicide overbears the mind.

   More than 90% who commit suicide are suffering from stress. Constant stress leads to acute depression. Besides this, painful negative events such as severe bodily injury, any type of major failure, emotional shock, being victim of severe crime, extreme anger, severe financial reverses, unemployment, loss of social status, sense of hopelessness, escape from self, loss of love, one's imprisonment or interpersonal crisis are chiefly responsible for depression. These events lead to the loss of a sense of meaning to life and hopelessness about the future which can both produce independently or in combination a mental state that looks to suicide as a possible way out.

   In unipolar depression, the person experiences a range of affective, cognitive and emotional symptoms including persistent sadness, negative thoughts about self and the future, and lack of energy or initiative to engage in formerly pleasurable activities. Basic biological functioning is often also altered, i.e. the sleep pattern may be dramatically altered or the person may become uninterested in food and eating. In bipolar disorder, the person experiences episodes of both depression and hypomania or mania. During manic or hypomanic episodes the symptoms are essentially the opposite of those during a depressive episode, viz. elated mood, over talkativeness, grandiosity and later on aggressive behavior. For bipolar disorders biological causal factors play a very strong role.

   Biochemical imbalances and abnormalities of the hypothalamic-pituitary-adrenal-axis are also often implicated.

MANAGEMENT

Those who fall into high-risk groups should be hospitalized until the suicidality is no longer present, e.g. those who have made an attempt with a lethal method, such as a gun or a toxic ingested substance; those with major depressive disorder characterized by social withdrawal, hopelessness, and a lack of energy; girls who have run away from home, (or) pregnant. A child or an adolescent with suicidal ideation must be hospitalized, if the clinician has any doubts about the family's ability to supervise the child or cooperate with treatment in an outpatient setting.

Psychotherapy, pharmacotherapy, and family therapy are administered as indicated. A written contract with the adolescent, outlining the adolescent's agreement not to engage in suicidal behavior and providing an alternative, if suicidal ideation re-occurs, should be in place. In addition, a follow-up outpatient appointment should be made before the discharge, and a telephone number of a hotline should be provided to the adolescent and to the family in case suicidal ideation reappears any time before the next review date.

In criminal law, Secs. 305, 306 and 309 of IPC deal with the offence of suicide. Sections 305 and 306 provide punishment for abetment to suicide while Sec. 309 deals with the attempt to commit suicide. The main penal provision, Sec. 309 is as follows.

Section 309: Attempt to commit suicide. "Whoever attempts suicide and does any act towards the commission of such offence, shall be punished with simple imprisonment for a term which may extend to one year (or with fine or with both)".

Justice Amareshwari speaking for the Division Bench held that courts have sufficient power to see that unwarranted harsh treatment or prejudice is not meted out to those who need care and attention.

In P. Rathinam's case, the Double Bench of R.M. Sahai and B.L. Hansaria held Sec. 309, IPC as archaic law which deserves to be effaced from the statute book to humanize our penal laws. The Raisond' êtrethat it is a cruel and irrational provision resulting in punishing a person again (doubly) who has suffered agony and would be undergoing ignominy because of his failure to commit suicide.

In 1996, a Constitution Bench of the Supreme Court comprising Chief Justice J.S. Verma, G.N. Ray (JJ), N.P. Singh, Faizannuddin and G T Nanavati in the case of Gian Kaur held that Sec. 309 is not violative of Art. 21 or 14 of Constitution. When a person commits suicide he has to undertake certain positive overt acts and the genesis of those acts cannot be traced to or be included within the protection of the 'right to life' under Art. 21. The significant aspect of sanctity of life is also not to be overlooked. Art. 21 is a prohibition guaranteeing protection of life and personal liberty and by no stretch of imagination can extinction of life be read to be included in 'protection of life'.

The 'right to die' if any is inherently inconsistent with the right to life. The Court opined that the 'right to life' including the right to live with human dignity would mean the existence of such a right upto the end of natural life. This also includes the right to a dignified life up to the point of death including a dignified procedure of death. In other words, this may include the right of a dying man to also die with dignity when his life is ebbing out. The 'right to die' with dignity at the end of life is not to be confused or equated with the 'right to die' an unnatural death curtailing the natural span of life.

Proviso: Provided "an attempt by a person under delirium or acute depression shall not be punishable under this section".

- Suicidal attempts and successful suicides are medicolegal issues of importance
- There are different types and methods related to the above issues.
- Law should consider suicidal attempt as a medical problem and not as a crime (the Indian scenario).

First punishment he has already undergone when he goes through depression being the cause of suicide and second one the legal order which is ready to entrust on him. The best effort to reconcile the victim with the world will be that he is referred to a psychiatrist.

Chapter

16 Adjustment Disorders

Adjustment disorders cause significant impairment in a person's social, vocational, or academic functioning. The disorder is common in adolescents but may occur at any age.

The ratio of females to males is about 2:1. Single women are generally overly represented as being more at risk. Among adolescents of either sex, common precipitating factors are school problems, parental rejection, parental divorce, and substance abuse. Among adults, marital problems, divorce, moving to a new environment, and financial problems lead to adjustment disorders.

CAUSES

The stressor severity is a complex function of degree, quantity, duration, reversibility, environment, and personal context. For example, the loss of a parent is different for a 10 year old and a 40 year old. Personality organization, cultural or group norms and values contribute to the disproportionate responses.

Stressors may be single, such as a divorce or the loss of a job, or multiple, such as the death of an important person occurring at the same time as one's own physical illness and loss of a job. Stressors may be recurrent, such as seasonal business difficulties, or continuous, such as chronic illness or living in poverty. A discordant intra-familial relationship may produce adjustment disorder that affects the whole family system. Or the disorder may be limited to the patient, as when the patient is the victim of a crime or has a physical illness. Sometimes adjustment disorder occurs in a group or community setting, and the stressor affects several people, as in a natural disaster or in racial, social, or religious persecution. Specific developmental stages—such as like beginning school, leaving home, getting married, becoming a parent, failing to achieve occupational goals, having one's last child leave home, and retiring—are often associated with adjustment disorder.

PSYCHOANALYTIC FACTORS

Stresses of ordinary life produce illness in some and not in others. Why an illness takes a particular form, and why some experiences and not others predispose a person to psychopathology? Constitutional factors interact with a person's life experiences to produce fixation.

PSYCHODYNAMIC FACTORS

Pivotal to the understanding of adjustment disorder is an understanding of three factors: (1) The nature of the stressor, (2) The conscious and unconscious meanings of the stressor, and (3) The patient's pre-existing vulnerability.

DIAGNOSTIC CRITERIA FOR ADJUSTMENT DISORDERS (DSM-IV)

- The development of emotional or behavioral symptoms in response to an identifiable stressor occurring within 3 months of the onset of the stressor.
  1. Marked distress that is in excess of what would be expected from exposure to the stressor.
  2. Significant impairment in social or occupational (academic) functioning.

Specify if:

Acute: If the disturbance lasts less than 6 months.
Chronic: If the disturbance lasts for 6 months or longer.

Adjustment disorders are coded based on the subtype, which is selected according to the predominant symptoms. The specific stressor(s) can be specified on Axis IV.

With depressed mood
With anxiety
With mixed anxiety and depressed mood
With disturbance of conduct
With mixed disturbance of emotions and conduct

Adjustment Disorder with Anxiety

Palpitations, jitteriness, and agitation are present in adjustment disorder with anxiety which must be differentiated from anxiety disorders.

Adjustment Disorder with Depressed Mood

Depressed mood, tearfulness, and hopelessness: This type must be distinguished from major depressive disorder and uncomplicated bereavement.

Adjustment Disorder with Disturbance of Conduct

The predominant manifestation involves conduct in which the rights of others are violated or age-appropriate societal norms and rules are disregarded. Examples of behavior are truancy, vandalism, reckless driving, and fighting.

Posttraumatic Stress Disorder

The symptoms develop after a psychologically traumatizing event or events outside the range of normal human experience. Rape or assault, military combat, mass catastrophes, floods, airplane crashes, atomic bombings, and death-camps constitute psychological component, and a concomitant physical component may directly damage the nervous system.

Treatment—Psychotherapy

Psychotherapy is the treatment of choice for adjustment disorder. Group therapy can be particularly useful for patients who have undergone similar stresses.

Crisis Intervention: Crisis intervention, a brief type of therapy, is aimed at helping the person with adjustment disorder to resolve the situation quickly by supportive techniques, suggestion, reassurance, environmental modification, and even hospitalization,

Pharmacotherapy: A patient may respond to an antianxiety agent or to an antidepressant, depending on the type of adjustment disorder.

Chapter

17

Relational Problems

Relationships are the sources of comfort, connection, and happiness for people; they are also the sources of obligation, responsibility, and friction. Psychological problems affect the way people function in a variety of relationships. The lack of relationships or the loss of relationships can lead to feelings of isolation and depression.

RELATIONAL PROBLEM RELATED TO A MENTAL DISORDER OR GENERAL MEDICAL CONDITION

According to DSM-IV, this category should be used when the focus of clinical attention is a pattern of impaired interaction associated with a mental disorder or a general medical condition in a family member.

A problem that is now receiving attention is the abuse of the elderly parents by some caretaking children. The problem is most likely to occur when the abusing offspring have substance abuse problems, are under economic stress, and have no relief from their caretaking duties and when the elderly parent is bedridden or has a chronic illness that requires constant nursing attention. More elderly women are abused than are elderly men, and most abuse occurs in the elderly over age 75.

It requires adaptation on the part of the sick person and other family members. The sick person frequently deals with some loss of autonomy, an increased sense of vulnerability, and sometimes a taxing medical regimen. Other family members also experience the loss of the person as he or she was before the illness and usually have substantial caretaking responsibility especially in debilitating neurological diseases, including dementia of the Alzheimer's type, and with such diseases as acquired immune deficiency syndrome (AIDS) and cancer. In those cases the whole family has to deal with the stress of both prospective death and the current illness.

Chronic illness frequently causes depression in family members and may cause them to withdraw from one another or to attack one another. The burden of caring for ill family members falls disproportionately on the women in a family—mother, wife, daughters-in-law, and daughters.

PARENT-CHILD RELATIONAL PROBLEM

A family in which the parents are divorced presents parent-child problems. The remarriage of a divorced or widowed parent can also lead to aparent-child problem. The birth of a child can also be troublesome if the parents had already adopted a child in the belief that they were infertile.

Other situations causing a parent-child problem are the development, in either a parent or a child, of a fatal, crippling, or chronic illness–such as leukaemia, epilepsy, sickle cell anaemia, or a spinal cord injury —or the birth of a child with serious congenital defects like, cerebral palsy, blindness, or deafness. Although those situations are rare, they challenge the emotional resources of the people involved. The parents and the child have to face present and potential loss and must adjust their day-to-day lives physically, economically, and emotionally. Those situations can try the healthiest families and produce parent-child problems, not just with the sick child but also with the unaffected siblings. Those siblings may be resented, preferred, or neglected because the ill child requires so much time and attention.

PARTNER RELATIONAL PROBLEMS

According to DSM-IV, this category should be used when the focus of clinical attention is a pattern of interaction between the spouses or the partners characterized by negative communication (e.g. criticisms), distorted communication (e.g. unrealistic expectations), or non-communication (e.g. withdrawal) associated with clinically significant impairment in individual or family functioning or symptoms in one or both partners.

Demands of Marriage

Adjustment to marital roles can be a problem, if the partners are of different backgrounds and have been raised with different value systems. Members of low socioeconomic status groups perceive the wife as making most of the decisions regarding the family and accept physical punishment as a way to discipline children. Middle-class persons perceive the decisionmaking process as shared, the husband often being the final arbiter, and they prefer to discipline children by verbal chastisement.

Sibling Relational Problem

Improper interaction and rivalries among siblings can be associated with clinically significant impairment in individual or family functioning or symptoms in one or more of the siblings. Competition among children for the attention, affection, and esteem of their parents is a fact of family life. That rivalry can extend to others who are not siblings and remains a factor in normal and abnormal competitiveness throughout life. In good sibling relationships the pleasures of companionship and the bonds created by kinship and shared experiences outweigh feelings of rivalry.

Relational Problem Not Otherwise Specified

Difficulties with co-workers: Problems causing sufficient strain to bring a person into contact with the mental health care system may arise in relationships with romantic partners, co-workers, neighbours, teachers, students, friends, and social groups.

Chapter

18

Victims Turning Perpetrators

Young sex offenders, bullies and young perpetrators of violence have often been themselves the subject of abuse. The idea that abusing parents were themselves abused makes intuitive sense, and the histories of patients often support this notion.

Symptoms of depression and low self-esteem, anxiety, sadness, school and behavior problems and a sense of powerlessness are all associated with sexual abuse. Longer term sequelae include depression, low self-esteem, increased risk of further victimization, eating disorders, functional bowel disease, chronic pelvic pain, attempts at suicide and self-injury, interpersonal difficulties, drug abuse and criminality.

In Widom's (1989a) retrospective longitudinal study, early childhood victimization produced long-term consequences of delinquency, adult criminality and violent criminal behavior. Specifically, physical abuse and neglect were found to further increase the likelihood of later violent offending.

Factors exacerbating a propensity for crime include family criminality, large and poor broken families, low intelligence, school failure, and learning difficulties. 'Maltreatment' (physical, sexual, emotional abuse and neglect) of children increases their risk for both later alcohol and drug abuse (Dembo et al. 1992). Involvement in crime itself increases the risk of further victimization (Lauritsen et al. 1991).

Spitzer et al (1991), describing sadistic personality disorder in the patients of forensic psychiatrists, found that 90% had childhood backgrounds of emotional abuse. Parental figures had been hostile, demeaning or neglecting. The background of violent offenders often includes a history of neglect and/or abuse.

Childhood sexual abuse per se (compared to other types of child abuse and neglect), does not on its own increase an individual's risk for later delinquent or adult criminal behavior (Widom and Ames 1994). Experiences of other types of abuse have lifelong consequences for later criminal behaviors. Experiences of emotional abuse, neglect and loss are also strongly associated with later delinquency.

Loeber and Hay (1994) argued that the developmental pathways of aggression from pre-school age to young adulthood represent diverse youth groups:

- Young people who desist from aggression
- Young people where aggression is stable and continues at the same level
- Youths who escalate in the severity of their aggression and make the transition into violence
- Youths whose aggression stabilizes.

SPECIFIC THEORIES

There are a number of theories to explain the link between the experience of abuse and becoming an abuser.

- *Intergenerational transmission of violence* (Curtis 1963; Spinetta and Rigler 1972). This theory is close to Bandura's (1973) social learning theory. In this, the rationalization of aggression in families provides models of learning for children whereby aggression is seen as an appropriate means of goal realization.
- *Differential association-reinforcement* (Akers et al. 1979; Burgess and Akers (1966). This theory incorporates conditioning and modelling elements by bringing in the effects of peers and families.
- *Importance of the model* is that it highlights the traumatic effects of sexual abuse and places emphasis on the wider aspects of the relationship between the victim and the abuser, the type of abuse endured and the possible reactions to it.
- *Control theory* (Hirschi 1969). This proposes that poor parental supervision and harsh discipline disrupts parent-child bonding, leading to poor identification with the primary object, poor internal controls and eventual delinquency.
- *Criminal personality theory* (Yochelson and Samenow 1976, 1997). This emphasizes cognitive processes in the maintenance of criminal behavior.
- *Labelling theory* (Smith et al. 1980). This proposes that systems label the victims and the abusers, thereby serving to perpetuate their career paths. In fact, there is nothing new in this view, and in the nineteenth century 'pauper' children and their criminal activities were seen as resulting from their social class. There was a predominant view that institutionalization crushed the spirit of children who, if treated like adult criminals, became later criminals themselves (Pearson, 1975).
- *The diathesis-stressor paradigm model:* This model (Davison and Neale 1990) views normal behavior as the outcome between the **following personal vulnerability factors and external stressors**. It provides a simple interaction in a comprehensively expandable way of looking at abnormal behavior.
  - Genetic and constitutional factors
  - Home atmosphere and child-rearing factors
  - Developmental milestones
  - Personality factors
  - Social, biological and developmental stages
  - Current life circumstances
  - Socio-demographic variables
  - Personal variables (cognition, perceptions and motivation)
  - Behavioral analysis.

ASSESSMENT ISSUES

The specific issues of assessment that arise in victims who go on to perpetrate abuse are the same as in other clinical assessments. Young offenders often perceive courts as unfriendly places where truth might lead to punishment. Engaging and relating to disturbed children is an acquired skill; it requires a way of relating that is understandable to them and at the same time provides trust, safety and emotional containment and at times physical containment (by means of security).

TREATMENT APPROACHES

Extreme behaviors and psychological disturbances, of course, may or may not form part of recognized psychiatric syndromes or diagnoses. They are associated with mental disorder—aggression in the psychoses, self-injurious behavior in conduct disorder, enuresis in anxiety disorder, etc.

Perpetrators with past histories of victimization present particular difficulties. It is often difficult to decide whether a child perpetrator with a history of abuse should be treated in the light of the victimization he or she has suffered, or in terms of the criminal behavior displayed. A society which focuses on the punishment of offenders may attach little importance to the effects past abuse has on individuals and might decide to channel interventions on pragmatic approaches to extinguish criminal behavior. Whether it achieves so by punishment or by focusing on here-and-now interventions to deter from further offending is to be decoded from expert evidence.

Having established that some of the long-term consequences of abuse include adult criminal behavior, it would make sense to provide interventions that deal with the effects of past abuse as part of strategies to deal with young offenders.

APPENDIX: CASE STUDY

Z is a 16-year-old English Afro-Caribbean adolescent serving a sentence under Sec. 53(2) of the Children and Young Persons Act 1933.

She has a history of physical abuse and neglect from her mentally ill mother since birth. Her play in childhood made references to death and she ceremonially buried the pets she had killed. At the age of 9, and for about 3–4 years, she was the subject of multiple sexual abuses as she was the victim in a paedophile ring. She killed her first victim at the age of 12 by stabbing, and seriously wounded her second victim at the age of 14, also by stabbing. She had spent time in secure care from the age of 13 and had also spent time in psychiatric hospitals. She was affectionless, had disturbed sexual orientation, sexual excitement to violence, physical violence and a history of self-harm by cutting. She had diagnoses of conduct disorder (ICD-10) and sexual arousal disorder (Vizard et al. 1996). She was already serving a fixed sentence for her second stabbing and was expecting a life sentence for her recently discovered first offence. She made a full confession of her first murder to the police. The details of that confession are incorporated in her risk assessment which identified the vulnerability of small, white attractive females, issues of jealousy, revenge and quick disinhibition into violence which was at times instrumental.

At the age of 17, after she was found guilty of her first offence, she was transferred back to prison. Z required interventions to effectively deal with her past abuse experiences. They were prominent in her mind, manifested in her behaviors and had the characteristic intrusive nature associated with post-traumatic states. She also needed specific inputs to curb her physical violence. It was too traumatic for her to deal with her past abuse, and the level of containment she required to deal with her physical aggression had eventually incarcerated her.

Chapter

19

Psychiatric Emergencies

ADOLESCENT CRISES

Manifestations

- Suicidal attempts and ideation
- Substance abuse
- Truancy
- Trouble with law
- Pregnancy
- Running away from home
- Eating disorders
- Psychosis

Treatment

- Evaluation of suicidal potential, extent of substance abuse and family dynamics
- Crisis-oriented family therapy and individual therapy
- Hospitalization when required
- Consultation with appropriate authorities

AGOROPHOBIA

Manifestations

- Panic
- Depression

Treatment

- Alprazolam 0.25 mg SOS, antianxiety medication (Fluoxetine 20 mg/day for adults)

AGRANULOCYTOSIS (CLOZAPINE-INDUCED)

Manifestations

- High fever
- Sore throat (Pharyngitis)
- Oral and perianal ulcerations

Treatment

- Discontinue medication immediately
- Administer granulocyte colony stimulating factor

AKATHISIA

Manifestations

- Agitation
- Restlessness
- Muscle discomfort
- Dysphoria

Treatment

- Reduce antipsychotic dosage;
- Propranolol (30 to 120 mg a day)
- Benzodiazepines
- Diphenhydramine (Benadryl) orally or IV

ALCOHOL-RELATED EMERGENCIES: ALCOHOLIC DELIRIUM TREMENS

Manifestations

- Confusion with multimodal hallucinations, illusions, delusions and psychomotor agitation.

- Disorientation
- Fluctuating consciousness and perception
- Autonomic hyperactivity
- Sometime fatal

Treatment

- Hospitalization in a Medical ICU
- Chlordiazepoxide or Lorazepam in high doses
- Haloperidol or olanzepine for psychotic symptoms may be added if necessary
- Injection thiamine 100 mg IV/IM bid for five days.
- Manage medical complications, e.g. seizures, liver dysfunction, electrolyte imbalance, infection, etc.

ALCOHOLIC INTOXICATION

Manifestations

- Disinhibited behavior
- Sedation at high doses

Treatment

- Wait and Watch
- Maintain airway
- Prevent injuries by physical restraint

ALCOHOLIC PERSISTING AMNESTIC DISORDER

Manifestations

Confusion, loss of memory even for all personal identification data

Treatment

- Vitamin B supplements especially thiamine.
- Other organic pathology must be excluded, e.g. chronic subdural hematoma.

ALCOHOLIC PERSISTING DEMENTIA

Manifestations

- Forgetfulness
- Agitation
- Impulsivity

Treatment

- Rule out other causes for dementia;
- Vitamin B supplements
- Hospitalization may help
- Memory enhancers, e.g. choline esterase inhibitors
- Antipsychotics if psychotic symptoms are present

ALCOHOLIC PSYCHOTIC DISORDER WITH HALLUCINATIONS

Manifestations

- Vivid auditory (at times visual) hallucinations with affect appropriate to content (often fearful)
- Clear sensorium

Treatment

- Oral haloperidol for psychotic symptoms or other atypical antipsychotics such as olanzapine, risperidone, etc.

ALCOHOL WITHDRAWAL SEIZURES

Manifestations

- Grand mal seizures
- Rarely status epilepticus

Treatment

- Diazepam or lorazepam IV/IM
- Phenytoin IV/IM
- Preventable by using chlordiazepoxide for detoxification over 5–7 days

SIMPLE ALCOHOL WITHDRAWAL

Manifestations

- Irritability
- Nausea
- Vomiting
- Insomnia
- Malaise
- Autonomic hyperactivity
- Shakiness

Treatment

- Fluid and electrolytes maintained;
- Sedation with benzodiazepines
- Monitoring of vital signs
- Injection thiamine IM 100 mg bid for 5 days

IDIOSYNCRETIC ALCOHOL INTOXICATION

Manifestation

Marked aggressive or assaultive behavior

Treatment

- Protective environment
- Haloperidol/olanzapine injectable

KORSAKOFF'S PSYCHOSIS

Manifestations

- Alcohol stigmata
- Amnesia
- Confabulation

Treatment

- Injection thiamine 100 mg in bid for 5 days
- Institutionalization often needed
- Vitamin supplements
- Haloperidol/olanzapine SOS

WERNICKE'S ENCEPHALOPATHY

Manifestations

- Acute in nature
- Oculomotor disturbances, e.g. ophthalmoplegia
- Cerebellar ataxia
- Mental confusion

Treatment

- Thiamine 100 mg IV or IM bid with $MgSO_4$ given before glucose loading
- Haloperidol/olanzapine SOS

AMPHETAMINE INTOXICATION

Manifestations

- Delusions
- Paranoia
- Violence
- Depression (during withdrawal)
- Anxiety
- Delirium

Treatment

- Antipsychotics
- Restraints
- Hospitalization as per the need
- No need of gradual withdrawal from amphetamine.
- Antidepressants when necessary.

ANOREXIA NERVOSA

Manifestations

Loss of 25 percent of body weight of the normal for age and sex

Treatment

- Hospitalization
- Electrocardiogram (ECG)
- Fluids and electrolytes
- Neuroendocrine evaluation
- Symptomatic and supportive medical treatment
- Cognitive behavior therapy
- Oral fluoxetine or mirtazapine

ANTICHOLINERGIC INTOXICATION

Manifestations

- Psychotic symptoms
- Dry skin and mouth
- Hyperpyrexia
- Mydriasis
- Visual hallucinations

Treatment

- Discontinue drug,
- IV physostigmine, 0.5 to 2 mg
- Antipsychotics such as injection Haloperidol/Olanzapine, (for severe agitation)
- Benzodiazepines
- Antipyretics/cold sponging

ANTICONVULSANT INTOXICATION

Manifestations

- Psychosis
- Delirium

Treatment

- Gastric lavage
- Dosage of anticonvulsant is reduced and monitored
- Forced alkaline diuresis especially for phenobarbitone intoxication

BENZODIAZEPINE WITHDRAWAL

Manifestations

- Irritability
- Seizures

Treatment

- Must be differentiated from major anxiety disorder
- Benzodiazepines

BENZODIAZEPINE INTOXICATION

Manifestations

- Sedation
- Ataxia
- Somnolence, drowsiness and later stupor

Treatment

- Supportive measures
- Injection flumazenil, a benzodiazepine antagonist
- Should be used only by skilled personnel with resuscitative equipment availability

Brief Psychotic Disorder

Manifestations

- Emotional turmoil and agitation
- Acutely impaired reality testing often after obvious psychosocial stress

Treatment

- Hospitalization often necessary
- Antipsychotics

CAFFEINE INTOXICATION

Manifestations

- Severe anxiety resembling panic disorder
- Sleep disturbance
- Agitated depression
- Mania
- Delirium

Treatment

- Cessation of caffeine-containing substances
- Benzodiazepines

CANNABIS INTOXICATION

Manifestations

- Delusions
- Panic
- Dysphoria
- Cognitive impairment

Treatment

- Benzodiazepines and antipsychotics as needed
- Evaluation of suicidal or homicidal risk
- Symptoms usually abate with time and reassurance but, some of the patients may evolve into a chronic schizophrenia like psychosis.

CATATONIC SCHIZOPHRENIA

Manifestations

- Marked psychomotor disturbance (either excitement or stupor)
- Exhaustion
- Can be fatal due to starvation or suicide

Treatment

- Rapid tranquilization with antipsychotics
- Monitor vital signs
- Lorazepam IV/IM oral
- Electroconvulsive therapy (ECT) is the treatment of choice. Catatonia can "melt like ice" with ECT.

CLONIDINE WITHDRAWAL

Manifestations

- Irritability
- Psychosis
- Violence
- Seizures

Treatment

- In mild cases, symptoms abate with time
- Antipsychotics as per need
- Requires to be lowered carefully and gradually.
- Antihypertensive measures

COCAINE INTOXICATION AND WITHDRAWAL

Manifestations

- Paranoia and violence
- Severe anxiety
- Cocaine bugs (tactile hallucinations)
- Delirium
- Schizophreniform psychosis
- Tachycardia
- Hypertension
- Myocardial infarction
- Cerebrovascular disease
- Depression and suicidal ideation

Treatment

- Antipsychotics and benzodiazepines
- Antidepressants, depression if persistent
- Hospitalization

DELIRIUM

Manifestations

- Fluctuating sensorium
- Suicidal and homicidal risk
- Cognitive clouding
- Multimodal hallucinations—visual, tactile, auditory, etc. worse during nights,
- Paranoia
- Psychomotor agitation

Treatment

- Hospitalization in an ICU
- Evaluate all potential contributing medical or surgical causes and treat each accordingly
- Reassurance and structured clues to orientation
- Benzodiazepines
- High-potency antipsychotics

DELUSIONAL DISORDER

Manifestations

- Most often brought into emergency room involuntarily
- Threats directed toward others

Treatment

- Antipsychotics, if patient will comply (IM if necessary)
- Intensive family intervention
- Hospitalization, if necessary

DEMENTIA

Manifestations

- Forgetfulness
- Unable to care for self
- Violent outbursts
- Psychosis
- Depression and suicidal ideation
- Confusion

Treatment

- Memory enhancers, e.g. Donepezil, Memantine, etc.
- Small dosages of high-potency antipsychotics and anti-depressants
- Clues to orientation
- Organic evaluation including brain imaging and metabolic work up.
- Evaluation of medication use for potential adverse effects/interactions
- Family intervention.

DEPRESSIVE DISORDERS

Manifestations

- Suicidal ideation and attempts
- Self-neglect
- Substance abuse

Treatment

- Assessment of danger to self
- Hospitalization, if necessary
- Non-psychiatric causes of depression must be evaluated, e.g. Hypothyroidism, vascular dementia, etc.
- Antidepressant drugs along with cognitive behavior therapy
- ECT for severe depression

L-DOPA INTOXICATION

Manifestations

- Mania
- Depression
- Schizophreniform disorder

Treatment

- Atypical antipsychotics such as quetiapine or aripiprazole
- Lower the dosage or discontinue drug and switch to other anti-parkinsonian drugs.

ACUTE DYSTONIA

Manifestations

- Intense involuntary spasm of muscles of neck, tongue, face, jaw, eyes or trunk

Treatment

- Decrease dosage of antipsychotic
- Benztropine or diphenhydramine IM
- Injection Promethazine 25–50 mg IV/IM

HALLUCINOGEN PSYCHOTIC DISORDER

Manifestations

- Symptomatology is a result of interaction of the type of substance, dose taken, duration of action and user's premorbid personality.
- Panic
- Agitation
- Psychosis

Treatment

- Serum and urine screens to rule out underlying medical or mental disorder
- Benzodiazepines orally (Lorazepam) (2 to 20 mg)
- Reassurance and re-orientation
- Rapid tranquilization

HOMICIDAL AND ASSAULTIVE BEHAVIOR

Manifestations

- Marked agitation with verbal threats

Treatment

- Seclusion
- Restraints (judicious use of)
- Medication (antipsychotics)

HYPERTENSIVE CRISIS

Manifestations

- Life-threatening hypertensive reaction secondary to ingestion of tyramine containing foods in combination with MAOIs
- Headache
- Stiff neck
- Sweating
- Nausea
- Vomiting

Treatment

- Adrenergic blockers (e.g. phentolamine [Regitine]
- Nifedipine (procardia) 10 mg orally
- Chlorpromazine (Thorazine)
- Make sure symptoms are not secondary to hypotension (side effect of monoamine oxidase inhibitors [MAOIs] alone)

MALIGNANT HYPERTHERMIA

Manifestations

- Extreme excitement, confusion, or stupor or a combination of them
- Extremely elevated temperature
- Agitation

Treatment

- Attempt at identifying the underlying cause
- Hydrate and cool; look if it is a drug reaction, e.g. neuroleptic
- Discontinue any drug
- Rule out infection

HYPERVENTILATION

Manifestations

- Anxiety
- Terror
- Clouded consciousness
- Giddiness
- Faintness
- Paradoxical feeling of warmth

Treatment

- Rebreathing bag to treat hypocapnia
- IV fluids and rewarming
- Cardiac status must be carefully monitored
- Avoidance of alcohol

INCEST AND SEXUAL ABUSE OF A CHILD

Manifestations

- Suicidal behavior
- Adolescent crises
- Substance abuse

Treatment

- Corroboration of charge
- Protection of victim
- Contact social services
- Medical and psychiatric evaluation
- Crisis intervention

INSOMNIA

Manifestations

- Daytime somnolence
- Depression and irritability
- Early morning agitation
- Frightening dreams and fatigue

Treatment

- Sleep hygiene
- Treat any underlying psychiatric disorder
- Hypnotics only in short term, e.g. Zolpidem 5 to 10 mg at bedtime; Ramelteon 8 mg Hs

INTERMITTENT EXPLOSIVE DISORDER

Manifestations

- Brief outbursts of violence
- Periodic attempts of suicide

Treatment

- Glucose tolerance curve, electroencephalogram (EEG)
- Computed tomography (CT) scan
- Benzodiazepines or antipsychotics for short term

LITHIUM TOXICITY

Manifestations

- Vomiting
- Abdominal pain
- Oliguria or anuria
- Palpitations
- Severe tremor
- Ataxia
- Myoclonic jerks
- Seizures
- Confusion
- Dysarthria
- Focal neurological signs
- Coma

Treatment

- Lavage with wide-bore tube if within 4 hours
- Medical consultation
- May require ICU treatment for cardiac arrhythmias
- Renal dialysis

MAJOR DEPRESSIVE EPISODE WITH PSYCHOTIC FEATURES

Manifestations

- Depressive symptoms
- Agitation, severe guilt
- Delusions (of nihilism, hypochondriasis or guilt)
- Suicide risk

Treatment

- Antipsychotics plus antidepressants
- Evaluation of suicide and homicide risk
- ECT
- Hospitalization, if necessary

MANIC EPISODE

Manifestations

- Pressured speech and aggressive behavior
- Decreased need for sleep and food
- Indiscriminate spending or disinhibited sexual behavior
- Grandiose delusions
- Substance abuse

Treatment

- Stop antidepressant drugs, if any
- Hospitalization for serious patients
- Judicious use of restraints, if necessary
- Rapid tranquilization with antipsychotics and/or clonazepam mouth dissolving tablets.
- Mood stabilizers such as lithium or valproate.
- ECT in some cases who do not respond to medication.

MIGRAINE

Manifestation

Throbbing unilateral headache

Treatment

Sumatriptan 6 mg as subcutaneous injection

NEUROLEPTIC MALIGNANT SYNDROME

Manifestations

- Hyperthermia
- Muscle rigidity
- Autonomic instability
- Stupor
- Neurological signs
- Elevated creatine phosphokinase
- 10 to 30 percent fatality

Treatment

- Discontinue antipsychotic
- Hydration and cooling
- Monitor CPK levels
- Benzodiazepines, e.g. Lorazepam
- IV dantrolene (Dantrium)
- Bromocriptine (parlodel) orally

OPIOID INTOXICATION AND WITHDRAWAL

Manifestations

- Intoxication can lead to coma and death
- Withdrawal is not life threatening

Treatment

- Urine and serum screens
- Psychiatric and medical illnesses (e.g. AIDS) may complicate picture and need attention
- IV naloxone, narcotic antagonist for intoxication
- NSAIDs for muscle aches of withdrawal from opioids
- Clonidine in divided doses while monitoring BP

PANIC DISORDER

Manifestations

- Episodes of intense anxiety and a feeling of impending doom
- Symptoms of sympathetic nervous system over-activity, e.g. palpitations
- Acute onset, lasts for about ten minutes and usually subsides spontaneously

Treatment

- Must differentiate from other anxiety-producing disorders, both medical and psychiatric
- ECG to rule out mitral valve prolapse
- Propranolol (10 to 30 mg); SOS
- Clonazepam (0.25 to 0.5 mg) SOS
- Long-term management includes anti-anxiety agents, e.g. Fluoxetine

PARANOID SCHIZOPHRENIA

Manifestations

- Third person auditory hallucinations
- Delusions of threat to others or themselves

Treatment

- Rapid tranquilization with anti-psychotics, e.g. haloperidol, olanzapine, etc.
- Threatened person must be notified and protected
- Hospitalization
- ECT
- Long-acting depot medication

DRUG INDUCED PARKINSONISM

Manifestations

- Secondary to antipsychotic medication
- Stiffness
- Tremor
- Bradykinesia
- Flattened affect
- Shuffling gait
- Salivation

Treatment

- Oral anti-parkinsonian drug for four weeks to three months or longer
- Decrease dosage of the antipsychotic or change to atypicals such as Quetiapine or Aripiprazole.

PHENCYCLIDINE INTOXICATION

Manifestations

- Violent behavior,
- Nystagmus,
- Tachycardia, hypertension,
- Anesthesia, and analgesia
- Can lead to death

Treatment

- Serum and urine assay
- Benzodiazepines for patients without psychosis
- Medical monitoring and hospitalization for severe intoxication
- Antipsychotics (such as haloperidol or olanzapine)

PHOBIAS

Manifestations

- Anxiety
- Fear
- Avoidance behavior

Treatment

- Pharmacological treatment same as for panic disorder
- Behavior therapy useful in the hands of clinical psychologists or psychiatrists

PHOTOSENSITIVITY

Manifestations

Easy sun burning secondary to use of antipsychotic medication (chlorpromazine).

Treatment

- Patient should avoid strong sunlight and use high-level sunscreens
- Change over to atypical antipsychotics

POSTPARTUM PSYCHOSIS

Manifestations

- Childbirth can precipitate psychosis
- Depression
- Reactive psychoses
- Mania
- Depression
- Suicide risk is reduced during pregnancy but increases in the postpartum period.

Treatment

- Danger to self and others (including infant) must be evaluated and proper precautions taken for their safety.
- Medical illness presenting with behavioral aberrations included in the differential diagnosis and must be sought and treated.
- Antipsychotics
- Mood stabilizers
- Nursing the baby is not permitted

POSTTRAUMATIC STRESS DISORDER

Manifestations

- Panic and terror
- Depression and insomnia
- Flashbacks
- Heightened arousal state with startles
- Suicidal ideation

Treatment

- Reassurance
- Encouragement of return to responsibilities
- Avoid hospitalization, if possible, to prevent chronic invalidism
- Monitor suicidal ideation
- Antidepressants such as escitalopram, mirtazepine, etc.

PRIAPISM

Manifestations

Persistent penile erection accompanied by severe pain

Treatment

- Intra-corporeal epinephrine
- Mechanical or surgical drainage

RAPE

Manifestations

Not all sexual violations are reported. Silent rape reaction is characterized by:

- Loss of appetite
- Sleep disturbance and startle reactions
- Anxiety, and sometimes agoraphobia
- Long periods of silence and social withdrawal
- Mounting anxiety, stuttering, and physical symptoms during the interview when the sexual history is taken
- Fear of violence and death
- Fear of contracting a sexually transmitted disease or being pregnant

Treatment

- Rape is a major psychiatric emergency
- Victim may have enduring patterns of sexual dysfunction
- Crisis-oriented therapy
- Social support
- Ventilation
- Reinforcement of healthy traits and encouragement to return to the previous level of functioning as rapidly as possible
- Legal counsel
- Thorough medical examination and tests to identify the assailant (e.g. obtaining samples of pubic hairs with a pubic hair comb, vaginal smear to identify blood antigens in semen)
- In a woman, methoxyprogesterone or diethylstilbestrol orally for five days to prevent unwanted pregnancy
- If menstruation does not commence within one week of cessation of the estrogen, all alternatives to stop the pregnancy including abortion should be offered.
- If the victim has contracted a venereal disease, appropriate antibiotics; victim's

written permission is required for the physician to examine, photograph, collect specimens and release information to the authorities.

- Obtain consent; record the history in the patient's own words, obtain required tests, record the results of the examination; save all clothing; defer diagnosis and provide protection against disease, psychic trauma, and pregnancy.
- Men's and women's responses to rape are reported similarly although men are more hesitant to talk about the assault particularly, if it was homosexual for fear that they will be assumed to have consented.

SCHIZOPHRENIA IN EXACERBATION

Manifestations

- Social and emotional withdrawal, or
- Agitation
- Suicidal and homicidal risk

Treatment

- Suicide and homicide evaluation
- Screen for medical illness
- Restraints and rapid tranquilization
- Hospitalization, if necessary
- Re-evaluation of medication regimen

SEDATIVE, HYPNOTIC, OR ANXIOLYTIC INTOXICATION AND WITHDRAWAL

Manifestations

- Alterations in mood, behavior, thought or delirium
- Intoxication can progressively cause drowsiness, stupor or coma
- Derealisation and depersonalization
- Untreated, can be fatal
- Withdrawal can cause seizures

Treatment

- Naloxone to differentiate from opioid intoxication
- Slow withdrawal with phenobarbital or sodium thiopental or benzodiazepine
- Hospitalization

COMPLEX PARTIAL SEIZURES

Manifestations

- Anxiety
- Feelings of impending doom
- Gustatory or olfactory hallucinations
- Confusion
- Derealisation and depersonalization
- Fugue-like state

Treatment

- Rule out pseudo seizures by careful history and clinical observation
- Immediate EEG
- Admission, sleep-deprived and 24-hour EEG
- Anticonvulsants.

PSYCHOTROPIC MEDICATION WITHDRAWAL

Manifestations

- Abdominal pain
- Insomnia or drowsiness
- Delirium
- Seizures
- Eruption of manic or schizophrenic symptoms

Treatment

- Symptoms of psychotropic drug withdrawal may spontaneously disappear with time or with the reinstitution of the substance
- Symptoms of antidepressant withdrawal can be successfully treated with anticholinergic agents, such as atropine
- Gradual withdrawal of psychotropic substances over two to four weeks generally obviates development of symptoms

SUICIDE

Manifestations

- Feelings of helplessness and hopelessness
- Suicidal ideation

Treatment

- Hospitalization
- Remove all dangerous objects, e.g. knife, fire-arms, etc.
- Antidepressants prescribed for short durations
- ECT
- Not to leave the person unattended even for a minute till the suicidal risk has abated.

TARDIVE DYSKINESIA

Manifestations

- Dyskinesia of mouth, tongue, face, neck, and trunk
- Choreoathetoid movements of extremities
- Usually but not always appearing after long-term treatment with antipsychotics, especially after a reduction in dosage
- Incidence highest in the elderly and brain damaged
- Symptoms are intensified by antiparkinsonian drugs and masked, but not cured by increased dosages of antipsychotic

Treatment

- No effective treatment reported
- May be prevented by prescribing the least amount of drug possible for as little time as is clinically feasible and using drug-free holidays for patients who need long-term medication.
- Decrease or discontinue drug on the first sign of dyskinetic movements
- Benzodiazepines
- Switch over to clozapine

Conservative measures may be adequate. In some instances drugs such as thiothixene and haloperidol, 5 mg every half hour to an hour up to a maximum dose of 20 mg in 24 hours are needed until a patient is stabilized. Benzodiazepines are used instead of or in addition to antipsychotics (to reduce the antipsychotic dosage).

MANAGEMENT OF A VIOLENT PATIENT

Violent, struggling patients are most effectively subdued with an appropriate sedative or antipsychotic. Diazepam (Valium), 5 to 10 mg, or lorazepam (Ativan), 1 mg, may be given IM or slowly intravenously (IV) over two minutes. The clinician must give the IV medication with great care to prevent respiratory arrest. Patients who required IM medication can be sedated with haloperidol 5 mg IM, or with chlorpromazine 50 mg IM. If the furore is due to alcohol or is part of a post seizure psychomotor disturbance, the sleep produced by a relatively small amount of an IV medication may go on for hours. On awakening, the patients are often entirely alert and rational and typically have a complete amnesia for the violent episode.

If the furore is part of an ongoing psychotic process and returns as soon as the IV medication wears off, continuous medication may be given. It is sometimes better to use small IM or oral doses at half-hour to one-hour intervals—e.g. haloperidol 2–5 mg, up to a maximum dosage of 20 mg in 24 hours or diazepam 5 mg, up to a maximum of 20 mg—until the patient is controlled, rather than to use large dosages initially and end up with an overmedicated patient. As the patient's disturbed behavior is brought under control, successively smaller and less frequent doses should be used. During the preliminary treatment, the patient's blood pressure and other vital signs should be monitored.

RAPID TRANQUILIZATION

Antipsychotic medication can be given rapidly at 30 to 60 minutes intervals to achieve a therapeutic result as quickly as possible. The procedure is useful in agitated patients and those in excited states. The drugs of choice for rapid tranquilization are haloperidol and other high-potency antipsychotics. In adults 5 mg of haloperidol can be given orally or IM and repeated every 20 to 30 minutes up to a maximum dose of 20 mg in 24 hours until the patient becomes calm. Some patients may experience mild extrapyramidal symptoms or acute dystonic reaction within the first 24 hours after rapid tranquilization; although the side effects are rare, the psychiatrist should not overlook them. In general, most patients respond before a total dose of 20 mg is given. The goal is not to produce sedation or somnolence; rather, the patient should be able to cooperate in the assessment process and, ideally, be able to provide some explanation of the agitated behavior. Agitated or panic-stricken patients can be treated with small doses of lorazepam, 1 mg IV or IM, which can be repeated if necessary in 20 to 30 minutes until the patient has quietened down.

The extrapyramidal emergencies respond well to Inj Promethazine 25–50 mg IV/IM, benztropine (Cogentin), 2 mg orally or IM, or diphenhydramine 50 mg IM or IV. Some patients respond to diazepam 5 to 10 mg orally or IV.

RESTRAINTS

Restraints are used when patients are so dangerous (to themselves or to others) that they pose a severe threat that cannot be controlled in any other way. Patients may be restrained temporarily to receive medication or for long periods if medication cannot be used. Most often, patients in restraints quieten down after some time has elapsed. On a psychodynamic level, such patients may even welcome the control of their impulses that restraints provide.

Chapter

20

Antisocial Behavior and Crime

- Introduction
- Early interventions
- Interventions targeting youth
- Restorative justice

INTRODUCTION

Antisocial behavior (ASB) includes littering, vandalism, kerb crawling, reckless driving, and shoplifting, among others. In the United States, where much research on ASB is conducted, the concept refers to a cluster of related behaviors, including disobedience, aggression, temper tantrums, stealing, and violence, which can be strong predictors of future delinquent and criminal activity.

The British Crime Survey 2003/4, reports that 76% of people perceive one or more types of antisocial behavior to be a problem (Wood, 2004).

ASB is "behavior by one household or individual that threatens the physical or mental health, safety or security of other households and individuals".

The concept of ASB in USA refers to "a cluster of related behaviors, including disobedience, aggression, temper tantrums, lying, stealing, and violence" (Eddy and Reid, 2002) while ASB is seen as a conduct disorder (thus emphasizing its psychological dimension), American scholarship recognizes that ASB in childhood and adolescence serves as "the strongest predictor of adjustment problems including criminal behavior, during adulthood" thus making the link between the psychological dimension and its social, legal and criminological ramifications.

EARLY INTERVENTIONS TO PREVENT THE ONSET OF ASB AND DELINQUENCY

Early interventions are critical to the prevention of crime and ASB because the presence of ASB and delinquent behavior in a child is one of the strongest predictors of an individual's future deviant or antisocial behavior (Greenwood et al, 1998). Moreover, longitudinal studies reveal that poverty (i.e. low income, dependency on welfare), parents' history of convictions and imprisonment, single parenthood, and youthfulness of parents are some of the factors most closely associated with the risk of ASB and delinquency in children's later life.

According to Farrington, antisocial personality in this context refers to a cluster of associated behaviors such as committing property crimes, drunkenness, repeated lying and conning and reckless driving. It also includes personality traits such as lack of remorse or guilt feelings, aggressiveness, low frustration tolerance, impulsiveness and selfishness.

INTERVENTIONS TARGETING AT-RISK YOUTH

Measures to prevent ASB and delinquency have also been developed targeting youths at risk of offending, and not exclusively those who have already committed an offence. A type of intervention for at-risk youths that has been rigorously evaluated is the educational incentive. Although it is not clear exactly what the relationship is between increased education and reduced crime, crime statistics in England and elsewhere appear to show that crime rates are lower in areas with higher levels of education, suggesting that education could have a potentially significant influence in reducing an individual's propensity to commit offences and ASB (Feinstein and Sabates, 2005).

While there is no methodologically sophisticated research evaluating the effectiveness of treatment of antisocial behavior offenders (ASBOs), the available evidence tends to show that ' coercive' sanctions (those designed as restrictive, regulatory or punitive) cannot be relied on to prevent, or even necessarily to reduce, re-offending particularly among young offenders (Prior and Paris, 2005).

Restorative justice is an innovative rehabilitative approach in dealing with offenders. The predominant view of restorative justice in the UK is that it consists of a "process whereby the parties with a stake in a particular offence come together to resolve collectively how to deal with the aftermath of the offence and its implications for the future".

The outcome of situational interventions can go beyond the reduction of crime and delinquency. Street lighting and clean spaces, for example, can contribute to perceptions of public safety and to increased use of public places by law-abiding citizens.

CONCLUSIONS

While it has been clear for many years that some person-centred interventions to tackle ASB and delinquency do in fact work, it is difficult to isolate the types of interventions that achieve the best results. Responding to the general and specific learning needs of the offender, i.e. interventions that focus on the offender's behavioral and skill needs, addressing specific issues in terms of gender, age, ethnicity and cultural identity is of good assistance.

- Early interventions are critical to the prevention of crime
- 'Coercive' sanctions cannot be relied on to prevent or to reduce, re-offending
- The outcome of situational interventions go beyond reduction of crime and delinquency.

Chapter

21

Personality Disorders

Personality can be defined as all emotional and behavioral traits that characterize the person in day-to-day living under ordinary conditions; it is relatively stable and predictable. Patients with personality disorders show deeply ingrained, inflexible, and maladaptive patterns of relating to and perceiving both the environment and themselves.

Cluster A personality disorders (paranoid, schizoid, and schizotypal) are more common in the biological relatives of schizophrenic patients. Cluster B personality disorders (antisocial, borderline, histrionic, and narcissistic) also have a genetic base. Antisocial personality disorder is associated with alcohol use disorders.

Temperamental factors: Temperamental factors identified in childhood may be associated with personality disorders in adulthood. Childhood central nervous system dysfunctions associated with soft neurological signs are most common in antisocial and borderline personality disorders. Children with minimal brain damage are at risk for personality disorders, particularly antisocial personality disorder. Some personality disorders arise from poor parental fit—a poor match between temperament and child-rearing practices. Cultures that encourage aggression unwittingly reinforce and contribute to paranoid and antisocial personality disorders.

NEUROTRANSMITTERS

Endorphins have effects similar to those of exogenous morphine, including analgesia and the suppression of arousal. High endogenous endorphin levels may be associated with a phlegmatic-passive person. Studies of personality traits and the dopaminergic and serotonergic systems indicate an arousal-activating function for those neurotransmitters. Levels of 5-hydroxy indole acetic acid (5-HIAA), a metabolite of serotonin, are low, in persons who attempt suicide and in patients who are impulsive and aggressive.

Serotonin reduces depression, impulsivity, and rumination in many persons and can produce a sense of general well-being. Increased dopamine in the central nervous system, produced by certain psycho stimulants (for example, amphetamines) can induce euphoria. The effects of neurotransmitters on personality traits have generated a great deal of interest and controversy about whether personality traits are inborn or acquired.

Fantasy: Many persons—especially eccentric, lonely, frightened persons who are often labelled schizoid—make extensive use of the defense of fantasy. They seek solace and satisfaction within themselves by creating imaginary lives, especially imaginary friends, within their minds.

UNCONSCIOUS EGO DEFENCE MECHANISMS

Dissociation

Dissociation consists of the replacement of unpleasant affects with pleasant ones. Frequent users of dissociation are often seen as dramatizing and as emotionally shallow; they may be labelled histrionic personalities. Their behavior is reminiscent of the stunts of anxious adolescents who carelessly expose themselves to exciting dangers (to erase anxiety). Accepting such patients as exuberant and seductive is to miss their anxiety; however, confronting them with their vulnerabilities and defects is to make them still more defensive.

Isolation

Isolation as characteristic of the orderly, controlled person, often labelled an obsessive-compulsive personality, who, unlike the histrionic personality, remembers the truth in detail but without affect. In a crisis the patient may show an intensification of self-restraint, overformal social behavior, and obstinacy. The patient's quest for control may be annoying or boring to the clinician. Such patients respond well to precise, systematic, and rational explanations.

Projection

In projection, the patients attribute their own unacknowledged feelings to others. Excessive fault finding of the therapist and sensitivity to criticism are common. These patients are hypervigilant and collect what they perceive to be injustices.

Splitting

In splitting, the patient divides ambivalently regarded people, both past and present, into good people and bad people. For example, in an inpatient setting, some staff members are idealized, and others are uniformly disparaged. The effect of that defensive behavior on a hospital ward can be highly disruptive; it ultimately provokes the staff to turn against the patient.

Passive Aggression

In passive-aggressive defenses, the anger is turned against the self; most often termed masochism. It includes failure, procrastination, silly or provocative behavior, selfdemeaning, clowning, and frankly self-destructive behavior. The hostility in such behavior is never entirely concealed; indeed, the mechanism, as in wrist cutting, engenders such anger in others that they feel that they themselves have been assaulted and view the patient as a sadist, not a masochist. Passive aggression is best dealt with by trying to get the patients to ventilate their anger.

Acting Out

In acting out, direct expression through action of an unconscious wish or conflict avoids being conscious of either the idea or the affect that accompanies it. Tantrums, apparently motiveless assaults, child abuse, and pleasureless promiscuity are common examples. The clinician must recognize: (1) that the patient has lost control, (2) that anything the interviewer says will probably be misheard and (3) that getting the patient's attention is of paramount importance.

Projective Identification

The defense mechanism of projective identification is used mainly in borderline personality disorder. It consists of three steps: (1) An aspect of the self is projected onto someone else, (2) The projector tries to coerce the other person to identify with what has been projected, and (3) The recipient of the projection and the projector feel a sense of oneness or union.

PARANOID PERSONALITY DISORDER

Persons with paranoid personality disorder show longstanding suspiciousness and mistrust of people. They refuse responsibility for their own feelings and assign responsibility to others. They are hostile, irritable, and angry. The bigot, the pathologically jealous spouse, and the litigious crank often have paranoid personality disorder.

Epidemiology

The disorder is more common in men than in women, and it does not appear to have a familial pattern. The incidence among homosexuals is no higher than usual.

Diagnosis

Muscular tension, an inability to relax and a need to scan the environment for clues may be evident. The patient's affect is often humourless and serious. Although some premises of their arguments may be false, their speech is goal-directed and logical. Their thought content shows evidence of projection, prejudice, and occasional ideas of reference.

Clinical Features

They pride themselves on being rational and objective, but that is not the case. They lack warmth and are impressed with and pay close attention to power and rank, expressing disdain for those who are seen as weak, sickly, impaired, or defective in some way. In social situations, persons with paranoid personality disorder appear business-like and efficient, but they often generate fear in others.

Course and Prognosis

Patients with paranoid personality disorder have lifelong problems working and living with others. Occupational and marital problems are common.

SCHIZOID PERSONALITY DISORDER

Schizoid personality disorder is diagnosed in patients who display a lifelong pattern of social withdrawal. Persons with schizoid personality disorder are often seen by others as isolated, or lonely.

SCHIZOTYPAL PERSONALITY DISORDER

Persons with schizotypal personality disorder are strikingly odd or strange, even to laypersons. Magical thinking, peculiar ideas, ideas of reference, illusions, and derealisation are seen.

Diagnosis

Schizotypal personality disorder is diagnosed based on the patients' peculiarities of thinking, behavior, and appearance. They show poor interpersonal relationships and may act inappropriately.

Course and Prognosis

Thomas McGlashan reported that 10 percent of persons with schizotypal personality disorder eventually committed suicide. Many patients maintain a stable schizotypal personality throughout their lives and marry and work in spite of their oddities.

Chapter

22

Women Offenders

Adult females suffer from mental disorders similar to those of men. There are some striking differences in the prevalence of specific disorders, and in their presentation and management. Some mental illnesses occur only in women. Women patients may have a different experience of treatment. There are particular issues unique for women patients in relation to childhood sexual abuse, rape and domestic violence.

Women seem to have more social contact problems and fewer legal difficulties but more problems with victimization and medical illness (Brunette and Drake, 1997).

Two crimes of violence associated with females are infanticide and physical abuse of children. When women kill, it is often assumed that they are mentally disturbed. In particular, the mysterious workings of the female body have long been blamed for women running riot and becoming violent. The creation by the law of the offence of infanticide was an important stage in this tradition. The offence applies only to women who kill their children under the age of 12 months when the balance of their mind is disturbed as a result of childbirth or lactation.

When offenders commit crimes, the law presumes they are sane until it is shown otherwise. Yet the infanticide provisions enshrine a virtual presumption that a certain class of offender is mentally disturbed. Further, it has to be shown only that the offender's imbalance of mind coincided with the criminal act, rather than having directly caused it. Of particular interest in adolescent females is the act of neonaticide (killing of an infant within 24 hours of birth) and undisclosed teenage pregnancy.

WOMEN AND FAMILIES

Women threatened with having their children taken into custodial care may distrust services and feel inhibited from seeking help. A significant proportion of women with a severe mental illness have children, but health professionals are only beginning to recognize the importance of these women's role as parents.

WOMEN AND ABUSE

Violence against women, in particular the effects of childhood sexual abuse, domestic violence and rape, has been found to be on the increase.

Childhood Sexual Abuse

Women who have experienced childhood sexual abuse are more likely to suffer social, interpersonal and sexual difficulties in adult life. Abuse may also correlate with an increased risk for a range of mental health problems (Mullen et al., 1994).

Domestic Violence

A high proportion of women attending accident and emergency departments report a history of domestic violence, and in this group there is a high level of mental health problems. A history of childhood abuse increases a women's risk of subsequent mental health problems, especially if she is also abused as an adult. In this double abuse group, there may also be an increased risk of substance abuse (Roberts et al. 1998).

Rape

Victims of completed rape are at increased risk of suicide attempts and of having a depressive illness. In addition, perceptions of life threat and actual injury increase the risk of post-traumatic stress disorder (Mezey and Stanko 1996).

ADOLESCENT FEMALE OFFENDERS

Statistics

All the evidence supports the conclusion that, compared with young males, young females commit fewer and different crimes and follow different offending careers. Although there has been evidence over the years that young females are treated differently by the criminal justice system (Morris 1987), this does not account for the overall difference in statistics with respect to young offenders; a real difference in behavior does exist. Known risk factors for delinquency do vary by sex, but this still does not offer a full explanation of gender differences in rates of juvenile crime and the associated evolution of severe antisocial behavior and parallel acts of violence through childhood and into adolescence.

In the case of individuals aged 21 years or more with at least ten convictions, 22% of males but only 13% of females were sentenced to immediate imprisonment. This differential processing of males and females should tend to lead to an increase in the sex ratio over time; in fact the opposite has taken place and the sex ratio has gradually but steadily diminished over the last 40 years. Crimes by females have been increasing at a faster rate than crimes by males. Consideration is now given to how gender, crime and violence are linked, how the small but significant rise in violent crimes carried out by adolescent females is understood, and the ways in which these issues are being addressed by the mental health services.

ASSESSMENT OF YOUNG FEMALES

Given the transitional nature of adolescent influences on mental health and young females, assessment involves not only the consideration of the presence or absence of illness or disorder, but also an evaluation of the various components of development, which must encompass personality, social and moral development, including empathy and ability to form relationships. Physical and intellectual development will have a considerable bearing on psychological development. Any judgement about the presence or absence of psychiatric disorder has to take into account different presentations at different stages through development. The interplay between assessment, development and presence or absence of disorder is highlighted in the assessment of adjustment to a trauma, or a series of negative life events.

Those coming to the attention of the adolescent forensic services have commonly started to repetitively self-harm and exercise control over their lives through an array of high-risk behaviors, such as fire setting and sustained repetitive, assaultive behavior, the latter not infrequently against their residential carers.

Psychiatric disorders in adolescence fall into three main developmental categories: continuing childhood disorder; mental illness typical of adulthood; and disorders which although not confined exclusively to adolescence, are characterized in the main by difficulties in surmounting this particular stage of development.

The early life experiences of adolescent females presenting with aggressive and violent behavior render such tasks at times not only alien but frequently impossible to achieve. This situation, in turn, acts as a strong reinforcer for escalating maladaptive coping strategies to survive for the moment, while young women are unable to plan or think about future.

Assessment of a high-risk female adolescent with a possible mental health problem can be beset with many difficulties. Not least of these is the viewing of the adolescent solely as a target for complaint, the still prevalent attitude of stigma attached to mental illness adding to discrimination against this already negatively labelled group of young female offenders.

In practice, assessment has to strike a balance between engagement, the need to elicit information, and formal mental state examination, whether the assessment is a stand-alone exercise for the purpose of a report to a court when the practice of least harm must be one of a set of competing priorities, or whether the assessment is but a prelude to long-term treatment for the young female facing the possibility of a life sentence for an act of extreme violence.

PSYCHIATRIC DISORDERS AND VIOLENCE: A GENDER PERSPECTIVE

There is an urgent need to explore the evolution of such personality types in young females. Key indicators include:

- *Family features*—parental antisocial personality disorder; witnessing violence, abuse, neglect or rejection
- *Personality features*—callous, unemotional, interpersonal style; evolution of violent and sadistic fantasy; people regarded as objects; morbid identity; paranoid ideation; hostile attribution.
- *Situational features*—history of repeated loss and rejection in relationships; threats to self-esteem; crescendos of hopelessness and helplessness; social disinhibition (group processes, substance misuse); changes in mental state over time.

Childhood onset of psychosis is, in itself rare in both males and females. It can be associated with violent behavior but the association is complex. Psychosis with onset in the teenage years has a tendency to go unrecognized, the psychotic behavior being attributed to the very process of adolescence. The risk of violence however is related less to the actual psychosis than to the previous history of antisocial behavior and unsupportive rearing. Nevertheless, it remains important, in any overall assessment of young females by multi-professional agencies, to consider the possibility of early-onset psychosis.

At-risk mental states associated with violence include perceptual changes, in ideas of reference, and paranoid delusions. Mental states in young females which should alert professionals to risk of imminent violence include subjective feelings of tension, ideas of violence, delusional systems that incorporate those currently close to the young female, persecutory delusions with fears of imminent attack, feelings of sustained anger and fear, passivity experiences, reduction of self-control, believing oneself to be controlled by others, and command hallucinations telling one what to do.

A critical protective factor against violent acts is a fear of their own potential for violence, not only against others but turned against themselves. Such severe self-harm includes cutting of breasts and genitals, and attempts at self-immolation.

UNDERSTANDING GENDER DIFFERENCES

General Issues

It is possible, that biological factors link with other factors predisposing to violence.

Antisocial girls are much more likely than other girls to become teenage unwed mothers. This may well expose such girls to a range of social difficulties and make it more likely that they will experience failure in parenting. As a consequence they may have a higher rate of interpersonal conflict, including violence with partners and children alike. On the other hand, their domestic commitments in late adolescence and early adult life may possibly make it more difficult for them to be part of a delinquent peer group and thus to engage in criminal activities, including violence outside the home (Maccoby 1998).

Widom and White (1997), in an important America prospective design cohort study, reported that among abused and neglected children, females but not males are at a significantly higher risk for substance misuse or dependence diagnosis and arrest for violent crimes in adulthood. The younger group of females, as compared with young males, have higher rates for re-offending than their male and female adult counterparts, Food Page et al. (2000).

THE DISADVANTAGE OF MALE OFFENDERS

Learning from the Adult Literature

In adult men with severe mental illness, addictions and affective illnesses are greatly over-represented in forensic populations when compared with the general population, whether in Court diversion schemes, remand, or sentenced prison populations (Kennedy 2001). The rising suicide rate among young men in small cities at a time when suicide rates for other groups are falling (Drever and Bunting 1997) underlines the same apparent failure in early case finding and early intervention for adolescent males.

Suicide and Deliberate Self-harm

The suicide rate for young males continues to rise (Fombonne 1998). The male:female ratio of deaths from suicide in 15 to 19 years olds is approximately 4:1, and the ratio for deliberate self-harm is approximately 1:6 (Cotgrave et al. 1995).

Stanway and Cotgrave (2001) summarize the main characteristic features which predispose to completed suicide in adolescence:

- Individual features of psychiatric disorder— depressive psychosis; substance misuse; conduct disorder; isolation; low self-esteem and chronic physical illness.
- Family and environmental factors—loss of a parent in childhood; family dysfunction; abuse and neglect; family history of psychiatric illness or suicide.

Deliberate self-harm may be a serious attempt to die or to escape from unbearable feelings or situations. It can be a dramatic action to change things the individual feels powerless about—a communication that includes a cry for help but so often involves hostility and anger directed at self or others. The act can release feelings of inner tension, or may reflect low self-worth or be a means of self-punishment. Estimates of those who go on to kill themselves vary, but at the extreme, Otto (1972) found that 4% of girls and 11% of boys had killed themselves at five-year follow-up.

CASE LAW

BMJ, 18 April 70, 186

Mrs. A.M., a sleepwalking shop lifter was acquitted on the evidence of a psychiatrist, as she was suffering from somnambulism. When the commission of an offence involves the doing of a certain definite act, it must be welled by the accused for being convicted according to law. However, an involuntary act or automatism is not liable to punishment.

AIR 1959 Mad 239

In another case, a recently delivered woman jumped into a well with her child at night and the child was drowned. She was charged of murder and attempt to commit suicide, and the plea of somnambulism was not sustained.

Chapter

23

Sexual Dysfunction

Seven major categories of sexual dysfunction are listed in DSM-IV: (1) Sexual desire disorders, (2) Sexual arousal disorders, (3) Orgasmic disorders, (4) Sexual pain disorders, (5) Sexual dysfunction due to a general medical condition, (6) Substance-induced sexual dysfunction, and (7) Sexual dysfunction not otherwise specified.

PHASES OF NORMAL HUMAN SEXUAL RESPONSE CYCLE AND ASSOCIATED SEXUAL DYSFUNCTIONS

1. Desire

Characteristics

This phase is distinct from any identified solely through physiology and reflects the patient's motivations, drives, and personality. The phase is characterized by sexual fantasies and the desire to have sex.

Dysfunction

Hypoactive sexual desire disorder, sexual aversion disorder, hypoactive sexual desire disorder due to a general medical condition (male or female) and substance induced sexual dysfunction with impaired desire.

2. Excitement

Characteristics

This phase consists of a subjective sense of sexual pleasure and accompanying physiological changes. All the physiological responses noted in Masters and Johnson's excitement and plateau phases are combined and occur in this phase.

Dysfunction

Female sexual arousal disorder; male erectile disorder (may also occur in stage 3 and in stage 4); male erectile disorder due to a general medical condition; dyspareunia due to a general medical condition (male or female); substance-induced sexual dysfunction with impaired arousal.

3. Orgasm

Characteristics

This phase consists of a peaking of sexual pleasure, with release of sexual tension and rhythmic contraction of the perineal muscles and pelvic reproductive organs.

Dysfunction

Female orgasmic disorder; male orgasmic disorder, premature ejaculation; other sexual dysfunction due to a general medical condition (male or female), substance-induced sexual dysfunction with impaired orgasm.

4. Resolution

Characteristics

This phase entails a sense of general relaxation, well-being, and muscle relaxation. During this phase male is refractory to orgasm for a period of time that progressively increases with age. Some women are capable of having multiple orgasms without a refractory period.

Dysfunction

Postcoital dysphoria, postcoital headache.

SEXUAL DYSFUNCTION—TYPES

1. **Primary:** This type of sexual dysfunction is present since the onset of sexual functioning.
2. **Secondary (Acquired):** This applies if the sexual dysfunction develops only after a period of normal functioning. One of the following subtypes may be used to indicate the context in which the sexual dysfunction occurs.
3. **Generalized type:** This applies if the sexual dysfunction is not limited to certain types of stimulation, situations or partners.
4. **Situational type:** This applies if the sexual dysfunction is limited to certain types of stimulation, situations, or partners. Although in most instances the dysfunctions occur during sexual activity with a partner, in some cases it may be appropriate to identify dysfunctions that occur during masturbation.

   One of the following subtypes may be used to indicate etiological factors associated with the sexual dysfunction:

Due to psychological factors: This applies when psychological factors are judged to have the major role in the onset, severity, exacerbation, or maintenance of the sexual dysfunction, and general medical conditions and substances play no role in the etiology of the sexual dysfunction.

Due to combined factors: This applies when: (1) Psychological factors are judged to have a role in the onset, severity, exacerbation or maintenance of the sexual dysfunction; and (2) A general medical condition or substance use is also judged to be contributory but is not sufficient to account for the sexual dysfunction. If a general medical condition or substance use (including medication side effects) is sufficient to account for the sexual dysfunction, sexual dysfunction due to a general medical condition and/or substance-induced sexual dysfunction is diagnosed.

SEXUAL AROUSAL DISORDERS

In the DSM-IV, sexual arousal disorders are divided into: (1) female sexual arousal disorder, characterized by the persistent or recurrent partial or complete failure to attain or maintain the lubrication-swelling response of sexual excitement until the completion of the sexual act, and (2) male erectile disorder, characterized by the recurrent and persistent partial or complete failure to attain or maintain an erection until the completion of the sex act.

Diagnosis of Female Sexual Arousal Disorder

- Persistent or recurrent inability to attain, or to maintain until completion of the sexual activity, an adequate lubrication swelling response of sexual excitement.
- The disturbance causes marked distress or interpersonal difficulty.
- The sexual dysfunction is not better accounted for by another Axis I disorder (except another sexual dysfunction) and is not exclusively due to the direct physiological effects of a substance (e.g. a drug of abuse or a medication) or a general medical condition.

Diagnosis of Male Erectile Dysfunction

- Persistent or recurrent inability to attain, or to maintain until completion of the sexual activity, an adequate erection.
- The disturbance causes marked distress or interpersonal difficulty.

- The erectile dysfunction is not better accounted for by another Axis I disorder (other than a sexual dysfunction) and is not exclusively due to the direct physiological effects of a substance (e.g. a drug of abuse or a medication) or a general medical condition.

Diagnosis of Female Orgasmic Disorder

- Persistent or recurrent delay in, or absence of, orgasm following a normal sexual excitement phase. Women exhibit wide variability in the type or intensity of stimulation that triggers orgasm. The diagnosis of female orgasmic disorder should be based on the clinician's judgment that the woman's orgasmic capacity is less than would be reasonable for her age, sexual experience, and the adequacy of sexual stimulation she receives.
- The disturbance causes marked distress or interpersonal difficulty.
- The orgasmic dysfunction is not better accounted for by another Axis I disorder (except another sexual dysfunction) and is not exclusively due to the direct physiological effects of a substance (e.g. a drug of abuse or a medication) or a general medical condition.

Diagnosis of Male Orgasmic Disorder

- Persistent or recurrent delay in, or absence of, orgasm following a normal sexual excitement phase during sexual activity that the clinician, taking into account the person's age, judges to be adequate in focus, intensity, and duration.
- The disturbance causes marked distress or interpersonal difficulty.
- The orgasmic dysfunction is not better accounted for by another Axis I Disorder (except another sexual dysfunction) and is not exclusively due to the direct physiological effects of a substance (e.g. a drug of abuse or a medication) or a general medical condition.

Diagnosis of Premature Ejaculation

- Persistent or recurrent ejaculation with minimal sexual stimulation before, on or shortly after penetration and before the person wishes it. The clinician must take into account factors that affect duration of the excitement phase, such as age, novelty of the sexual partner or situation, and recent frequency of sexual activity.
- The disturbance causes marked distress or interpersonal difficulty.
- The premature ejaculation is not due exclusively to the direct effects of a substance (e.g. withdrawal from opioids).

Diagnosis of Dyspareunia

- Recurrent or persistent genital pain associated with sexual intercourse in either a male or a female.
- The disturbance causes marked distress or interpersonal difficulty.
- The disturbance is not caused exclusively by vaginismus or lack of lubrication, is not better accounted for by another Axis I disorder (except another sexual dysfunction), and is not exclusively due to the direct physiological effects of a substance (e.g. a drug of abuse or a medication) or a general medical condition.

Diagnostic Criteria of Vaginismus

- Recurrent or persistent involuntary spasm of the musculature of the outer third of the vagina that interferes with sexual intercourse.
- The disturbance causes marked distress or interpersonal difficulty.
- The disturbance is not better accounted for by another Axis I disorder (e.g. somatization disorder) and is not exclusively due to the direct physiological effects of a general medical condition.

Diagnosis of Sexual Dysfunction due to a General Medical Condition

- Clinically significant sexual dysfunction that results in marked distress or interpersonal difficulty dominates the clinical picture.
- There is evidence from the history, physical examination, or laboratory findings that the sexual dysfunction is fully explained by the direct physiological effects of a general medical condition.
- The disturbance is not better accounted for by another mental disorder (e.g. major depressive disorder)

Diagnosis of Substance-Induced Sexual Dysfunction

- Clinically significant sexual dysfunction that results in marked distress or interpersonal difficulty dominates the clinical picture.
- There is evidence from the history, physical examination or laboratory findings that the sexual dysfunction is fully explained by substance use as manifested by either (1) or (2) of the following:
  1. The symptoms in criterion developed during, or within a month of, substance intoxication
  2. Medication use is etiologically related to the disturbance
- The disturbance is not better accounted for by a sexual dysfunction that is not substance induced; Evidence that the symptoms are better accounted for by a sexual dysfunction that is not substance induced might include the following: The symptoms precede the onset of the substance use or dependence (or medication use); The symptoms persist for a substantial period of time (e.g. over a month) after the cessation of intoxication, or are substantially in excess of what would be expected given the type or amount of the substance used or the duration of use; or there is other evidence that suggests the existence of an independent non substance-induced sexual dysfunction (e.g. a history of recurrent non-substance-related episodes).

Surgical treatment is rarely advocated, but improved penile prosthetic devices are available for men with inadequate erectile responses who are resistant to other treatment methods or who have deficiencies of organic origin. The placement of a penile prosthesis in a man who has lost the ability to ejaculate or have an orgasm because of organic causes will not enable him to recover those functions. Men with prosthetic devices have generally reported satisfaction with their subsequent sexual functioning. Their wives, however, report much less satisfaction than do the men. Pre-surgical counselling is strongly recommended so that the couple have a realistic expectation of what the prosthesis can do for their sex lives. Some physicians are attempting revascularization of the penis as a direct approach to treating erectile dysfunction caused by vascular disorders. In patients with corporal shunts that allow normally entrapped blood to leak from the corporal spaces, leading to inadequate erections (steal phenomenon), such surgical procedures are indicated. There are limited reports of prolonged success with the technique. Endarterectomy can be of benefit if aortoiliac occlusive disease is responsible for erectile dysfunction.

Surgical approaches to female sexual dysfunctions include hymenectomy in the case of dyspareunia in an unconsummated marriage, vaginoplasty in multiparous women who complain of reduced vaginal sensations, and the release of clitoral adhesions in women with sexual arousal disorder. Such surgical treatments have not been carefully studied and should be considered with great caution.

Injections of vasoactive materials into the corporal bodies of the penis produce erections for several hours; usually, a mixture of papaverine (Cerespan), prostaglandin E, and phentolamine (Regitine) is used. Usually, an urologist teaches the patient to inject himself in a series of training sessions. However, fibrosis and prolonged erections (lasting many hours) are occasional side effects of the approach. In addition, some patients become resistant to treating themselves. Vacuum pumps can also be used by patients without vascular disease to obtain erections but they are not very satisfactory.

Chapter

24

Sexually Abusive Behavior

- Introduction
- Five variables
- Seven categories
- Three categories of Juvenile offenders
- Assessment and treatment approaches

INTRODUCTION

Adult sexual offenders against children are now acknowledged to exist both inside and outside of family system and to pose a limited but recognizable threat to vulnerable children. Media coverage of sexually aggressive children and adolescents has brought awareness but not understanding of the problem and recent changes in the law relating to young offenders highlights the need for professional assessment of risk. (Soothill, 1997; Vizard 1999).

The concept of sexually aggressive and abusive is discussed in the light of research evidence that 30–50% of all sexual abuse of children is perpetrated by people under 21 years old (Vizard et al. 1995). The natural history of sexually abusive behavior by children towards other children is not fully understood. Work with adult and adolescent perpetrators of abuse suggests that some of these individuals have started patterns of abusive behavior even before puberty.

In 1971, Michael Rutter noted that 'psychosexual issues occupy a central place in child development'. Professional inter pretations of sexualized interactions between children vary between cultures and from time to time.

Five variables that predict sexual behavior problems among sexually abused children (Hall J et al. 1998) are:

1. Sexual arousal
2. Sadism during the child's sexual abuse
3. A history of physical abuse
4. A history of emotional abuse
5. Who the child blamed for that abuse.

Every culture follows rules and attitudes which protect children and help towards a healthy sexual fulfilment and development from childhood into adulthood rather than towards perverse, cruel, punishing or deviant behavior.

It has become apparent that even younger children, well below the age of criminal responsibility (<10 years old) are now involved in abusing other children.

Seven different categories of adolescent sexual abusers are:

1. Naive experimenter/abuser
2. Under-socialized child exploiter
3. Pseudo-socialized child exploiter
4. Sexual compulsive
5. Disturbed impulsive
6. Group-influenced
7. Miscellaneous (not coming under above categories)

Three categories of juvenile sexual offenders with distinct psychosocial profiles were identified (Graves, 1996). They are:

1. The paedophilic offender
2. The sexual-assault offender
3. The mixed-offence offender.

Bremer 1993 describes sexual behaviors as follows:

- Normative
- Inappropriate
- Hyper sexualized
- Orgasm-oriented
- Aggressive.

Many of these cognitive-behavioral concepts are used in the construction of treatment programmes for child and adolescent sexual abusers. The natural developmental processes push the child back towards a normative developmental trajectory when external corrupting influences are removed (e.g. the recovery of seriously abused children placed in safe alternative care).

WHY DO CHILDREN ABUSE?

There is no single-factor theory (e.g. being sexually abused) which can explain the origins of sex offending in adolescent life.

GIRLS WHO ABUSE

Many sexually aggressive girls are currently described as victimized or abuse reactive and therefore do not get referred for sexually abusive behavior.

Female adolescent sexual abuser girls are more likely than boys to be known to the victim, that they use persuasion rather than force with victims. They gain physical access to younger victims sooner, perhaps through baby sitting activities—which are seen as innocuous with girls whereas a boy may be viewed with more caution by parents. (Hunter et al, 1993).

HIGH-RISK INDICATORS

A typical high-risk sexually abusive adolescent: The adolescent is a developmentally delayed, mild learning disabled, abused and neglected boy with several placement changes in the past, few close friends, hobbies and interests centring on younger children, childhood-onset conduct disorder with evidence of sexual fantasies about younger children, and patterns of targeting, isolating and grooming victims becoming more evident with each known or suspected incident. Typically such a boy and his sexual proclivities are well known to agencies and this type of case is characterized by the 'fat file' syndrome where all the above features are meticulously recorded but little coherent multi-agency action is taken (Skuse et al. 1998).

SEXUAL HOMICIDE AND OTHER OFFENCES

Most children and adolescents with sexually aggressive or abusive behavior will hurt their victims through emotional blackmail and abuse, physical and sexual violence and betrayal of trust. A small number of more dangerous children abduct, rape and sometimes murder other children (Bailey, 1996).

APPROACHES TO ASSESSMENT AND TREATMENT

Specialist outpatient assessment of juvenile sexual offenders consists of three stages (Vizard 1996):

1. Clarification and rapport building.
2. Mapping the abuse: The fantasies, strategies and behaviors.
3. The future placement, treatment and personal change

The following do's and don'ts are recommended when interviewing high-risk youth including antisocial clients, adolescent sexual offenders, aggressive and passive-aggressive clients, clients who frequently lie and exploit and juvenile fire-setters' (Gray and Wallace, 1992):

- Do control the interview
- Do state immediately and clearly the nature of the interview.
- Do keep the focus on the client and swiftly and repeatedly bring the client back to task
- Do ask 'what' and 'how' questions. Not 'why'.
- Do track your feelings during the interview (if you are feeling exploited, validate this through changing course).
- Do respect the client as a whole individual, capable of change.
- Do not agree to keep secrets (obtain all necessary releases of information at the time of the initial interview).
- Do not relinquish interview control (do use control positively to reinforce the client when responsibility is taken for any personal behavior).
- Do not be diverted (do keep the focus firmly on the client, where you want it).
- Do not 'need' or 'want' something from the client (do care and detach).
- Do not isolate yourself (do seek colleague input and support, share concerns, ideas and feelings; attend trainings and network).

TREATMENT PROGRAMMES

The treatment approaches for young sexual abusers of other children is reviewed by Sirles et al. (1997), and a helpful summary of the programmes reviewed is laid out as a chart which includes the name of the program (SPARK, etc.), the ages served, the theories utilized and the treatment modalities offered. The review confirms that 'multiple theoretical approaches and treatment modalities have been found useful for intervening with sexually abusive or aggressive children' and that such complex, integrated interventions are preferable to a single-model approach.

Spark

The treatment is based on theories derived from post-traumatic stress disorder, addiction theory and the sexual abuse cycle as well as other concepts from within the victim and offender field of work.

Step

The STEP programme is cognitive-behavioral but uses a modified relapse prevention approach adapted to the developmental needs of the much younger perpetrator who may also be a victim.

- Offenders are found inside and outside family systems
- Even younger children are involved in abusing other children.
- There is no single factor that can explain the origin of sex offending in adult life
- Young sex offenders under watch do not try to repeat.

The strong clinical impression is that the young sex offender is very much less likely to try to re-offend if there is a watchful professional network in place to review his or her behavior.

Chapter

25

Paraphilias

Paraphilias are sexual disorders characterized by specialized sexual fantasies and intense sexual urges and practices that are usually repetitive and distressing to the person.

Classification: The major categories of paraphilias in the fourth edition of Diagnostic and Statistical Manual of Mental Disorders (DSM-IV) are exhibitionism, fetishism, frotteurism, pedophilia, sexual masochism, sexual sadism, voyeurism, transvestic fetishism, and paraphilias not otherwise specified (NOS)—for example, zoophilia. One person may suffer multiple paraphiliac disorders also.

Epidemiology: Repetitive nature of the disorders results in the high frequency of the commission of paraphiliac acts; and a large proportion of the population are victimized by paraphiliac persons.

Among legally identified cases of paraphilias, pedophilia is far more common than the others. Ten to twenty percent of all children have been molested by age 18. Because a child is the object, the act is taken more seriously, and greater effort is spent tracking down the culprit than in other paraphilias. Persons with exhibitionism, who publicly display themselves to young children, are also commonly apprehended. Those with voyeurism may be apprehended, but their risk is not great. Twenty percent of adult females have been the targets of persons with exhibitionism and voyeurism. Sexual masochism and sexual sadism are under represented in any prevalence estimates. Sexual sadism usually comes to attention only in sensational cases of rape, brutality, and lust murder.

Paraphilias are more male conditions. Fetishism almost always occurs in men.

Psychosocial factors: A person with paraphilia is supposed to have failed to complete the normal developmental process toward heterosexual adjustment;

Failure to resolve the oedipal complex by identifying with the father-aggressor (for boys) or mother-aggressor (for girls) results either in improper identification with the opposite-sex parent or in an improper choice of object for libido cathexis.

Trans-sexualism and transvestic fetishism are both disorders which involve identification with the opposite-sex parent, instead of the same-sex parent.

Exhibitionism and voyeurism are also seen as expressions of feminine identification, since persons with the paraphilias must constantly examine their own or others' genitals to calm their anxiety about castration.

The person with a shoe fetish unconsciously denies that women have lost their penises through castration by attaching libido to a phallic object, the shoe, which symbolizes the female penis. Persons with pedophilia and sexual sadism have a need to dominate and control their victims, as though to compensate for their feelings of powerlessness during the oedipal crisis. Persons with sexual masochism overcome their fear of injury and their sense of powerlessness by showing that they are impervious to harm.

Psycho-physiological tests are available to measure penile volumetric size in response to paraphiliac and non-paraphiliac stimuli. The procedures are of questionable diagnostic validity because some men are able to suppress their erectile responses.

Exhibitionism: Exhibitionism is the recurrent urge to expose one's genitals to a stranger or an unsuspecting person. Sexual excitement occurs in anticipation of the exposure, and orgasm is brought about by masturbation during or after the event.

The psychodynamics of the man with exhibitionism is to assert his masculinity by showing his penis and by watching the reaction of the victim—fright, surprise, disgust.

Fetishism: In fetishism the sexual focus is on objects (such as shoes, gloves, pantyhose, and stockings) that are intimately associated with the human body. The particular fetish is linked to someone closely involved with the patient during childhood and has some quality associated with that loved, needed, or even traumatizing person. The disorder begins by adolescence. Although the fetish may have been established in childhood, once established, the disorder is chronic. Sexual activity may be directed toward the fetish itself (for example masturbation with or into a shoe), or the fetish may be incorporated into sexual intercourse (for example, the demand that high-heeled shoes be worn). The disorder is almost exclusively found in males.

Frotteurism: Frotteurism is usually characterized by the male's rubbing his penis against the buttocks or other body part of a fully clothed woman to achieve orgasm. The person with frotteurism is extremely passive and isolated, and frottage is often his only source of sexual gratification.

Pedophilia: Pedophilia involves, over a period of at least six months, recurrent intense sexual urges toward or arousal by children 13 years of age or younger. The person with pedophilia is at least 16 years of age and at least five years older than the victim.

The vast majority of child molestations involve genital fondling or oral sex. Ninety-five percent of those with pedophilia are heterosexual, and 50 percent have consumed alcohol to excess at the time of the incident.

Sexual masochism: According to DSM-IV, persons with sexual masochism have a recurrent preoccupation with sexual urges and fantasies involving the act of being humiliated, beaten, bound, or otherwise made to suffer. Persons with sexual masochism may have had childhood experiences that convinced them that pain is a prerequisite for sexual pleasure.

Sexual sadism: Pleasure is derived from expressing the aggressive instinct. The disorder was named after the Marquis de Sade, an 18th-century French author, who was repeatedly imprisoned for his violent sexual acts against women. Sexual sadism is related to rape, although rape is more aptly considered a form of aggression. Some sadistic rapists, however, kill their victims after having sex (so-called lust murders). He lists five contributory causes of sexual sadism: hereditary predisposition, hormonal malfunctioning, pathological relationships, a history of sexual abuse, and the presence of other mental disorders.

Voyeurism: Voyeurism is the recurrent preoccupation with fantasies and acts that involve observing people who are naked or are engaged in grooming or in sexual activity.

Transvestic fetishism: Transvestic fetishism is marked by fantasies and sexual urges by heterosexual men to dress in female clothes for purposes of arousal and as an adjunct to masturbation or coitus. Transvestic fetishism typically begins in childhood or early adolescence. As years pass, some men with transvestic fetishism want to dress and live permanently as women.

Telephone scatologia: In telephone scatologia or obscene phone calling, tension and arousal begin in anticipation of phoning, an unsuspecting partner is involved. The recipient of the call listens while the paraphiliac (usually male) verbally exposes his preoccupations or induces her to talk about her sexual activity. The conversation is accompanied by masturbation, which is completed after the contact is interrupted. People use computer interactive networks to transmit obscene messages by electronic mail. Some use computer networks to transmit sexually explicit messages and video images. Some persons compulsively use these services.

Necrophilia: Necrophilia is obtaining sexual gratification from cadavers. Most persons with necrophilia find corpses for their exploitation from morgues. They may rob graves. Persons even murder to satisfy their sexual urges. Persons with necrophilia believe that they are inflicting the greatest conceivable humiliation on their lifeless victims.

Partialism: In partialism the person concentrates on one part of the body leaving other parts. Mouth-genital contact—such as **cunnilingus:** Oral contact with the external female genitals, **fellatio:** Oral contact with the penis, and **anilingus:** Oral contact with the anus–are considered a part of foreplay. Freud recognized the mucosal surfaces of the body as being erotogenic and capable of producing pleasurable sensation. When a person uses these activities as the sole source of sexual gratification and cannot have coitus or refuses to have coitus, it is a paraphilia. It is also known as **oralism**.

Zoophilia: Some predilection for animal contact is present in opportunistic zoophilia.

Urophilia: Urophilia is interest in sexual pleasure associated with the desire to urinate on a partner or to be urinated on; it is a form of urethral eroticism. It may be associated with masturbatory techniques involving the insertion of foreign objects into the urethra for sexual stimulation in both men and women.

Hypoxyphilia: Hypoxyphilia is the desire to achieve an altered state of consciousness secondary to hypoxia while experiencing orgasm. In the disorder the persons may use a drug (such as a volatile nitrite or nitrous oxide) that produces hypoxia. Autoerotic asphyxiation is also associated with hypoxic states but should be classified as a form of sexual masochism.

Unconsummated marriage: A couple involved in an unconsummated marriage has never had coitus and is typically uninformed and inhibited about sexuality. Couples present with the problem after having been married several months or several years. William Masters and Virginia Johnson reported a case of an unconsummated marriage of 17 years duration.

Causes of unconsummated marriage are varied: lack of sex education, sexual prohibitions, overly stressed by parents or society, problems of an oedipal nature, immaturity in both partners, over dependence on primary families, and problems in sexual identification. Many patients can be helped by simple education about genital anatomy and physiology, by suggestions for self-exploration, and by correct information from a physician.

Nymphomania: Nymphomania is an excessive or pathological desire for coitus in a woman. It can be a symptom of another psychiatric illness such as schizophrenia. These patients usually have one or more sexual disorders. They may also have a fear of loss of love.

Chapter

26

Decriminalization of Homosexuality

INTRODUCTION

Attitudes toward homosexuality and homosexual relations continue to be one of the more complex areas of public opinion in a country like India. The treatment of homosexuals can be linked to Indian traditional society, which tends to be deeply conservative and disapproving of sex outside of marriage. Family is an important part of Indian culture, and institution of marriage is seen as strengthening family values. As Indian society is very collective in its nature, it excludes the promotion of homosexual values. Indian society by and large not only disapproves of homosexuality but also justifies it being treated as criminal offence. And accordingly the criminal law of India (IPC) criminalizes homosexual behavior.

Though very little is known regarding the extent of homosexual crimes, there is no reference to the offence in Government of India's bulletin Crime in India. A perusal of the law reports suggests that cases on the subject are scant. However, it is a stark reality that homosexual behaviors have always existed in India, sometimes in forms, which are culturally sanctioned (such as the hijra) and at other times in invisibility and silence. The Government of India estimates the homosexuals number at around 25 lakhs.

In Western countries homosexuality is not a big issue. The contemporary trend is clearly towards greater tolerance of homosexuality. Since 1974, homosexuality ceased to be considered an abnormal behavior and was removed from the classification of mental disorder. It was also decriminalized in different countries. Since then various States across the globe enacted anti-discriminatory or equal opportunity laws and policies to protect the rights of homosexual persons. But homosexual relations are technically still a crime in India.

In recent past both due to liberal attitudes and need to control HIV/AIDS, several non-profit organisations demanded legalization or at least decriminalization of homosexuality and acceptance, tolerance and equality for homosexuals. The gays' rights activists argued that the criminalization of homosexuality among consenting adults in private cannot be justified because it does not cause any harm to anyone. Thus, regardless of one's personal view of morality, many feel that it should not be made a criminal offence; law has no business in the bedroom of consenting adults engaging in an activity that harms no one, though on the other hand, a significant group of the society as well as the Government took the other view. While the right to respect for private and family life is undisputed, interference by public authority in the interest of public safety and protection of morals is equally permissible. They argued that Criminal law should be used to sustain public morality and therefore, homosexuality should remain a crime, otherwise it may send a wrong message that law is encouraging and endorsing it as part of our mainstream way of life. It is in this back ground that Delhi High Court has given a land mark judgment, resolving certain complex legal issues which have led a lot of public debate in the legal community.

In Naz Foundation *vs* Government of NCT of Delhi a Division Bench of the Delhi High Court consisting of Chief Justice Ajit Prakash Shah and Justice S. Muralidhar dealt with the various aspects relating to homosexuality. The main issues agitated before the Court were whether (1) Public morality is a ground of a restriction of fundamental rights; (2) Section 377 of IPC violates constitutional guarantee of equality, privacy and dignity; (3) Decriminalization of consensual homosexuality would corrupt public morals and increase delinquent behavior; (4) State has a compelling interest of public health to interfere upon a fundamental right; (5) Criminalization of homosexuality is an impediment to public health and HIV/AIDS prevention.

BRIEF FACTS OF PETITION

In 2001, the Naz Foundation, a New Delhi-based NGO working on HIV/AIDS and sexual education and health filed a writ petition in the Delhi High Court, challenging the constitutional validity of Sec. 377 of IPC on account of it covering sexual acts between consenting adults in private, claiming that the impugned law was in violation of Arts. 14, 15, 19, and 21 of the Constitution of India. The writ petition was dismissed by the Delhi High Court in 2004 on the ground that there is no cause of action in favour of the petitioner and that such a petition cannot be entertained to explain the academic challenge to the constitutionality of the legislation. The Supreme Court set aside the said order of Delhi High Court observing that the matter does require consideration and is not of a nature which could be dismissed on the aforesaid ground. The Supreme Court directed the High Court to examine the matter, deeming it worthy of consideration.

THE PETITIONERS' MAIN GROUNDS OF CHALLENGE

1. Section 377 of IPC is based upon traditional Christian Moral Standard which conceives sex in purely functional terms, i.e. for the purpose procreation only. Any non-procreative sexual activity is thus viewed as being against the order of nature.
2. Section 377 is discriminatory because it criminalizes predominantly homosexual acts and imposes traditional gender stereotypes of "natural" sexual roles for men and women upon sexual minorities. In effect, Sec. 377 provides moral and legal sanction for the continued social discrimination of sexual minorities.
3. The law is a hurdle in the AIDS awareness campaigns run by the various AIDS welfare agencies as the laws restricts many men from coming forward to receive information on how to protect themselves from the disease.
4. Homosexuals are extremely vulnerable to AIDS infection. The AIDS preventive efforts were severally impaired by the discriminatory attitudes of the State agency towards homosexuality as the same is covered under Sec. 377 of IPC, as a result of which basic fundamental right of such groups stood denied and they were subject to abuse, harassment and assault from public as well as public authorities.
5. Section 377 leaves the homosexuals vulnerable to blackmail by the police. Police uses it arbitrarily and any arrest is rarely registered since they are merely out to make quick money from homosexuals

who are easy prey because of this Sec. Recent past execution of the provision shows that it has generally been employed in cases of child sexual assault and abuse and not on private consensual same sex conduct and thus criminalizing consensual oral and anal sex is outdated and served as the weapons for money and perpetuate negative and discriminative beliefs towards homosexual.

6. Section 377 to the extent of their application violates the Arts. 14, 15, 19(1)(a)(b)(c) and (d) and Art. 21 of the Constitution of India and thus consensual sexual intercourse between two willing adults in private is required to be saved and excepted from the penal provision contained in Sec. 377 of IPC.

THE RESPONDENT'S MAIN GROUNDS IN FAVOUR OF SECTION 377

1. The criminal law should represent the wishes of majority of the population and homosexuality should be a crime as a majority of Indian is intolerant towards it. Section 377 was enacted in response to prevailing morals in Indian society and public condemnation of homosexuality remains strong enough today to justify its criminalization.
2. State should criminalize homosexuality "to preserve public order and decency" and protect citizens from what is offensive or injurious. Decriminalizing homosexuality would corrupt public morals and encourage delinquent behavior.
3. Section 377 has been generally invoked in cases of allegation of child sexual abuse and for complementing lacunae in the rape laws and not mere homosexuality. It has been used particularly in cases of assault where bodily harm is intended and/or caused.
4. Anything which is illegal cannot be legalized by the consent of the party who is party to such illegality.
5. There is no fundamental right to engage in the same sex activities. In our country, homosexuality is abhorrent and can be criminalized by imposing proportional limits on the citizens' right to privacy and equality. Right to privacy is not absolute and can be restricted for compelling State interest. Article 19(2) expressly permits imposition of restrictions in the interest of decency and morality.
6. Spread of AIDS is curtailed by Sec. 377, IPC and decriminalization of consensual same sex acts between adults would cause a decline in public health across society generally since it would foster the spread of AIDS.
7. The subject is relating to policy of law rather than the legality. In parliamentary secular democracy the legal conception of crime depends upon political as well as moral consideration. Notwithstanding, overlap existing between legal and moral factors.

RATIONALE OF THE DECISION

The Delhi High Court has extensively dealt with the above issues and also other related issues, with the help of variety of sources, both domestic and international. The response of the High Court can better be understood if certain areas which have been emphasized be categorized into following rubrics.

RIGHT TO LIFE, PRIVACY AND DIGNITY UNDER ARTICLE 21

The Court conducted its analysis of Sec. 377 in light of the right to life and liberty. Indian Constitution conforms on every person the fundamental right to life and personal liberty which has become an inexhaustible source for many other rights. These rights are as much available to citizen as to a foreigner. In the instant case, the court has extensively discussed the nature of the right to life, privacy as well as dignity in general and that of homosexuals in particular. The development of the Supreme Court's interpretation of Art. 21 is summarized by the court.

Until the decision of the Supreme Court in Maneka Gandhi *vs* Union of India, AIR 1978 SC 597 a rather narrow and constricted meaning was given to the guarantee embodied in Art. 21. But in Maneka Gandhi, it was held that the expression "personal liberty" in Art. 21 is of the widest amplitude and it covers a variety of rights which go to constitute the personal liberty of man and some of them have been raised to the status of distinct fundamental rights and give additional protection under Art. 19. Any law interfering with personal liberty of a person must satisfy a triple test: (i) It must prescribe a procedure; (ii) The procedure must withstand a test of one or more of the fundamental rights conferred under Art. 19 which may be applicable in a given situation; and (iii) It must also be liable to be tested with reference to Art. 14. The Court thus expanded the scope and ambit of the right to life and personal liberty enshrined in Art. 21 and sowed the seed for future development of the law enlarging this most fundamental of the fundamental rights. This decision in Maneka Gandhi became the starting point for a very significant evolution of the law culminating in the plethora of decisions.

The Court referred to evolution of the right to privacy as a fundamental right emanating from right to life and personal liberty under Art. 21 of the Constitution of India in Kharak Singh *vs* State of U.P., Gobind *vs* State of M.P., R. Raja Gopal *vs* State of Tamil Nadu, PUCL *vs* Union of India, and Sharda *vs* Dharampal; and finally endorsed, which was just an affirmation what has been held earlier by the Apex Court in a number of judgments:

In India, our Constitution does not contain a specific provision as to privacy but the right to privacy has, as we shall presently show, been spelt out by our Supreme Court from the provisions of Art. 19(1) (a) dealing with freedom of speech and expression, Art. 19(1)(d) dealing with right to freedom of movement and from Art. 21, which deals with right to life and liberty.

The Court also referred cases from foreign jurisdiction, Art. 12 of UDHR, Art. 17 of ICCPR, Art. 8 of the European Convention on Human Rights. The Court reviewed the development of privacy jurisprudence and concluded.

The sphere of privacy allows to develop human relations without interference from the outside community or from the State, "and that this" exercise of autonomy enables an individual to attain fulfilment, grow in self-esteem, build relationships of his or her choice and fulfill all legitimate goals that he or she may set.

Moreover, sexual identity intersects with the privacy and is thus implicated in the Constitution's protection of personal autonomy. The Court opined:

Privacy deals with persons and not places, "and that for" every individual, whether homosexual or not, the sense of gender and sexual orientation of the person are so embedded... that the individual carries this aspect of his or her identity wherever he or she goes.

The courts have linked the issue with dignity and peak of judicial concern was reached when it was held that the right to privacy is derived from, and intimately related to, the right of each person to dignity. The constitutional protection of dignity requires us to acknowledge the value and worth of all individuals as members of our society. It recognizes a person as a free being who develops his or her body and mind as he or she sees fit. At the root of the dignity is the autonomy of the private will and a person's freedom of choice and of action. Human dignity rests on recognition of the physical and spiritual integrity of the human being, his or her humanity, and his value as a person, irrespective of the utility he can provide to others. The expression "dignity of the individual" finds specific mention in the Preamble to the Constitution of India.

While discussing Sec. 377 of IPC, the Court made it clear that it affects dignity of a man as it exposes a person of his sexual orientation and also punishes him and sends him to prison which violates his right to live a dignified life. The Court in its own style opined:

The criminalization of homosexuality condemns in perpetuity a sizeable section of society and forces them to live their lives in the shadow of harassment, exploitation, and humiliation, cruel and degrading treatment at the hands of the law enforcement machinery. The Government of India estimates the MSM (males who have sex with males) number at around 25 lacs. The number of lesbians and transgender is said to be several lacs as well. This vast majority (borrowing the language of the South African Constitutional Court) is denied "moral full citizenship". Section 377, IPC grossly violates their right to privacy and liberty embodied in Art. 21 insofar as it criminalizes consensual sexual acts between adults in private.

Thus having established the right to privacy as both zonal and decisional, the Court provides a new strength of right to privacy. In so doing, the High Court articulates a unique non-spatial and portable understanding of privacy. By its innovative interpretation to locate the notion of dignity into preamble of the Constitution it provides both a firmer base as well as constitutional value to the right to privacy. Recognition of autonomy as a root of dignity is another innovative approach which will open up many new directions.

COMPELLING STATE INTEREST

The Court then disposed of claims that this invasion of privacy was justified within the exception to Art. 21. The State may only infringe upon a fundamental right protected under Art. 21, if it has a compelling interest in doing so. If such an interest exists, the interference must be rationally related to a legitimate State end and must be proportional to achieving that end. Regarding contention of public morality and an obligation to protect young people from sexual exploitation, the Court referred to the report of Wolfendon Committee of England and 172 report of the Law Commission of India. While considering protection of public morality as compelling interest, Court rightly observed:

While it could be "a compelling State interest" to regulate by law, the area for the protection of children and others incapable of giving a valid consent or the area of non-consensual sex, enforcement of public morality does not amount to a "compelling State interest" to justify invasion of the zone of privacy of adult homosexuals engaged in consensual sex in private without intending to cause harm to each other or others.

The Court was of the opinion that the popular morality or public disapproval for certain acts is not a valid justification for restriction of the fundamental rights under Art. 21. Popular morality, as distinct from a constitutional morality derived from constitutional values, is based on shifting and subjective notions of right and wrong. If there is any type of "morality" that can pass the test of compelling state interest, it must be "constitutional" morality and not public morality.

The Court further examined the issue of public health as compelling interest. There is almost unanimous medical and psychiatric opinion that homosexuality is not a disease or mental illness that needs to be, or can be, 'cured' or 'altered', it is just another expression of human sexuality. Safeguarding public health may indeed be a compelling state interest that can justify reasonable limitation on the right to privacy. However, the Court reasons, such an interest would in far compel the state to decriminalize homosexuality, because it demonstrably hampers HIV prevention efforts. The Court dismissed State's arguments in following manner:

That Sec. 377 is an impediment to successful public health and the submission of ASG that Sec. 377 IPC helps in putting a break in the spread of AIDS and if consensual same-sex acts between adults were to be decriminalized, it would erode the effect of public health services by fostering the spread of AIDS, is completely unfounded since it is based on incorrect and wrong notions. It held that Sexual transmission is only one of the several factors for the spread of HIV and the disease spreads through both homosexual as well as heterosexual conduct. There is no scientific study or research work by any recognized scientific or medical body, or for that matter any other material, to show any causal connection existing between decriminalization of homosexuality and the spread of HIV/AIDS. The argument, in fact, runs counter to the policy followed by the Ministry of Health and Family Welfare in combating the spread of this disease.

Thus the Court rightly found that there is no compelling State interest at all to intervene in the private lives of consenting adult homosexuals. The Court while acknowledging devastating impact of criminalization of homosexuality placed much emphasis on scientific findings, leading decisions and scholarship from foreign jurisdictions and made its firm approach to Sec. 377 absolutely clear in the above observation. Constitution is a live document to serve for all times, which enacts principles to be interpreted in tune with the times. The perception of public morality at a given time may be a relevant factor to interpret a constitutional principle in tune with the times so that no gap is seen between them.

RIGHT TO EQUALITY UNDER ARTICLES 14 AND 15

The Court considered deeply Art. 14's guarantee of 'equality before the law or the equal protection of the laws'. The Court emphasized that the essence of Art. 14 is that it "eschews arbitrariness in any form" and thus" any action that is arbitrary must necessarily involve negation of equality" and must be held unconstitutional. Though Art. 14 forbids class legislation, it does not forbid reasonable classification for the purpose of legislation. A permissible classification must meet two conditions: (1) It must be founded on an intelligible differentia which distinguishes persons or things that are grouped together from those that are left out and (2) The differentia must have a rational relation to the objective sought to be achieved by the statute in question. However, while considering Sec. 377's mode of classification, the Court found that Sec. 377 targets homosexuals as a class and creates an arbitrary and unreasonable classification between penile-vaginal and penile-nonvaginal sexual acts. The Court expressed its view saying that although the provision is neutral and pertains only to acts, because these acts are closely associated with homosexuals, it unfairly targeted them as a class and had " the effect of viewing all gay men as criminals. The Court substantiated its argument in the following fashion.

It makes no distinction between adults and minors, between consensual and nonconsensual acts, between harmful and harmless acts, or between acts done in the public sphere versus those done in private. Public animus and disgust towards a particular social group or vulnerable minority is not a valid ground for classification under Art. 14. Section 377 targets the homosexual community as a class and is motivated by an animus towards this vulnerable class of people.

The Court makes an impressive survey of contemporary jurisprudence, including verdicts from different countries. The Universal Declaration of Human Rights, the International Covenant on Civil and Political Rights, the European Convention on Human Rights; these principles recognize that "human beings of all sexual orientation and gender identities are entitled to the full enjoyment of all human rights".

Art. 15 prohibits discrimination on grounds such as religion, race, caste and sex. Until recently, it had remained a largely sterile provision, subsumed entirely by the general guarantee of equality under Art. 14. In the instant case the Court made a progressive reinterpretation in Art. 15 and held that personal autonomy is inherent in the grounds mentioned in Art. 15. It is autonomy that allows us to form relationships and pursue the projects that give our lives meaning. Systematic discrimination diminishes the quality of all our lives by denying us access to an adequate range of valuable options, in all the things that matter most in our lives: Housing, jobs and partners.

The Court substantiated its view by referring a similar approach, both of which have been adopted by the Courts of other countries as well as have been recognized by the various international instruments that gender and sexual orientation are an intrinsic and inalienable part of every human being; they are constituents of a person's identity and declared:

We hold that sexual orientation is a ground analogous to sex and that discrimination on the basis of sexual orientation is not permitted by Art. 15.

Furthermore, the Court added that Art. 15 provides protection from discrimination perpetrated not only by the State ('vertical' protection) but also by a private individuals ('horizontal' protection). In other words, it even prohibits discrimination of one citizen by another in matters of access to public spaces.

The Court then addressed the proper standard of review to be applied to discrimination on the ground of sex. The Court, having noticed the concepts of strict scrutiny used in Anuj Garj *vs* Hotel Association of India and Ashok Kumar Thakur *vs* Union of India as the standard of review, read seemingly conflicting Supreme Court precedents harmoniously, and held that personal autonomy is inherent in the grounds enumerated in Art. 15, and that "grounds that are not specified therein, will be those which have the potential to impair the personal autonomy of an individual". The Court then held:

The impugned provision in Sec. 377, IPC criminalizes the acts of sexual minorities particularly men who have sex with men. It disproportionately impacts them solely on the basis of their sexual orientation. The provision runs counter to the constitutional values and the notion of human dignity which is considered to be the cornerstone of our Constitution. Section 377, IPC in its application to sexual acts of consenting adults in privacy discriminates a section of people solely on the ground of their sexual orientation which is analogous to prohibited ground of sex. A provision of law branding one section of people as criminal, based wholly on the State's moral disapproval of that class goes counter to the equality guaranteed under Arts. 14 and 15 under any standard of review.

It is submitted that above revolutionary reinterpretation of Art. 15 is a real contribution to the Jurisprudence. By drawing upon the notion of analogous ground of discrimination the Court is to keep the door open to other grounds which might suffer discrimination availing the protection of Art. 15. The Court's conclusion to horizontal application of the Art. 15 is another progressive interpretation which will create a powerful way to deal with State's inaction with societal harassment and discrimination. Though incorporation of US Supreme Court's application of strict scrutiny as the appropriate standard of review instead of twin-tests of a classification based on an intelligible differentia and a 'reasonable' nexus of such differentia with the object of the classification is needless because it serves no purpose and its rejection has been affirmed by the Apex Court.

THE RULING

The Court went on to hold that the Indian Constitution does not permit the statutory criminal law to be held captive by the popular misconception of who the LGBTs (lesbian gay bisexual transgender) are. It cannot be forgotten that discrimination is antithesis of equality and that it is the recognition of equality which will foster dignity of every individual. It observed that the inclusiveness that the Indian society traditionally displayed in every aspect of life manifested in recognizing a role in society for everyone. "Those perceived by the majority as deviants or different are not on that score excluded or ostracized". The Court delivered operative part of its order in following words:

We declare that Sec. 377 IPC, insofar it criminalizes consensual sexual acts of adults in private, is violative of Arts. 21, 14 and 15 of the Constitution. The provisions of Sec. 377, IPC will continue to govern non-consensual penile non-vaginal sex in adults, and penile non-vaginal sex involving minors. By 'adult' we mean everyone who is 18 years of age and above. A person below 18 would be presumed not to be able to consent to a sexual act.

CONCLUSION

The foregoing analysis and discussion makes it clear that the Delhi High Court has delivered a judgment of far reaching consequences. This is a welcome step, particularly because it dispels many misconceptions about the sexual orientation, homosexuality, public morality and fundamental rights. While the decision was technically only to decriminalize consenting homosexuality in private, arguments around equality, privacy, dignity and morality have meant a far wider impact in jurisprudence on liberty, diversity and pluralism in India. It inaugurates intersectional jurisprudence that examines questions of constitutionalism in relational terms that underscore inclusiveness. Further, it strengthens minority rights by making it clear that public morality and majoritarian opinion has to be subservient to constitutional morality and protection of fundamental rights. The Court's interpretation of 'privacy' to refer to a broad notion of autonomy and personhood has tremendous potential in other spheres as well. That is why this judgment has been rightly hailed as an affirmation of the equal rights of sexuality minorities.

However, to remove some doubts it may not be out of place to mention here that the Court did not declare Sec. 377 of IPC unconstitutional but rather clarified that its ambit does not include sexual activities between consenting adults in private. In addition to it, this ruling does not mean that homosexual act in India is legal, but that it is not criminal. So for the appreciation of the spirit of judgment it will be important to make this distinction in the judgment between decriminalizing the act and legalizing the act. Apart from it, decriminalization of homosexuality in private does not mean law endorses or approves of it. This will keep the police away and will serve the need against the grievance that police is abusing Sec. 377 for extortion. It will also enable prevention of AIDS. The scourge of the spread of HIV/AIDS is threatening to become pandemic, and India is in its grip. The Union Health Ministry and National AIDS Control Organization (NACO) have given statistics to prove that it is necessary to bring out of the closet homosexuals infected with the HIV/AIDS to aid the national programme for combating the spread of HIV/AIDS; and it is necessary to decriminalize consensual homosexuality in privacy to bring them out of the closet to treat them, and to arrest the spread of infection through them. This factual reality is significant for the decision of the limited issue before the Court. One another circulated misconception against the judgment is, it allows gay marriage which is totally baseless and judgment does not change the definition of marriage in the country and it continues to use bride and groom meaning that they are only between a man and a woman.

Apart from it, we have to understand that law is not merely the solution to all problems existing in our society as well as law is not always the best tool to change entrenched moral values and social attitudes. That is why legality is in no way social acceptance, in India homosexuality among consenting adults will legally no longer be a deviant behavior but may continue to be looked upon so. The judgment is simply an endeavour of the Court to appreciate the global trend towards decriminalizing consenting homosexuality and granting protection for the rights of homosexuals. The seed was sown by the Court and now it is high time for the society as well as legislatures that this judicial innovation be nurtured in the right perspective.

Chapter

27

Criminal Responsibility—Children

INTRODUCTION

The wisdom of protecting young children against the full rigour of the criminal law is beyond argument. The difficulty lies in determining when and under what circumstances that protection should be removed. [R (a child) *vs* Whitty (1993) 66 A Crim R 462]

Courts have always had to deal with the dilemma presented by the criminal behavior of children. On the one hand, breach of criminal laws made children liable to punishment. On the other hand, the Courts recognized the immaturity of children, and their need for nurture and protection.

Maturity of young adolescents, as of children in all age groups, is not only subject to biological and familial influence, but also cultural influence (Offer et al. 1996). Actual and perceived differences in their ability to take on adult roles and responsibilities may be enormous. Against this background the criminal process struggles with the very real task of managing the risk of adolescent crime (Rutter et al. 1998).

The doli incapax presumption provided a framework of considering individual maturity of child offenders when evaluating their capacity to be criminally responsible. The current approach to adolescent crime in the UK takes into account only the chronological age of the offender in determining his or her capacity to be criminally responsible. No consideration is given to the individual capacities of a young adolescent to shoulder the responsibility for personal behavior.

In the context of criminal law, if a defendant is considered responsible, then the finding of guilt will make him or her liable to the full punishment that law may dispense (Hart 1968). Attributing full responsibility to children would make them as liable for their crimes as adults.

'Doli incapax' means 'incapable of crime'. A Court applying this doctrine presumes that individuals who are in the 'intermediate stage' between the criminal incapacity of a child and full criminal capacity of an adult are incapable of committing crime. The 'intermediate stage' to which the presumption applies is between the ages of 10 and 14 years. This presumption of incapacity can be rebutted by the prosecution adducing evidence which proves the criminal capacity of the child defendant beyond reasonable doubt (Williams 1961). To prove the criminal capacity of the defendant the prosecution must show that the child knew at the time of the offence that his or her actions were 'seriously wrong' and not 'merely naughty or mischievous'. If it were established that the child knew this difference, the prosecution could then proceed to prove the necessary mental and physical elements of the crime.

By the law, the capacity of doing ill, or contracting guilt, is not so much measured by years and days, as by the strength of the delinquent's understanding and judgment. For one lad of eleven years old may have as much cunning as another of fourteen.

The courts have constantly struggled with the meaning of 'seriously wrong' and merely naughty or mischievous'. In C (A Minor) *vs* DPP (H.L.(E) [1995] 2 W.L.R. 383) the House of Lords cited authorities which propose that wrong means gravely wrong, seriously wrong, evil or morally wrong';and that 'wrong' refers to moral wrong as opposed to legal wrong. Another authority proposed that wrong means 'wrong' according to the principles of ordinary people (Field and SA *vs* Gent (1996) 87 A. Crim. R 225, at 230).

As early as age 2 years children have a basic understanding of rights and wrongs. They are sensitive to adult standards and attempt to uphold these (Kagan 1981).

Delinquents, may not have the benefit of family relationships for the development of moral understanding. Emotional development may be compromised in them.

Delinquents may have a reduced capacity for emotional awareness of right and wrong. They may not understand, or be concerned with, the emotional effect of their behavior on the victim. They may not be able to experience or acknowledge feelings of guilt or shame. Angry adolescents who appear indifferent to the consequences of their behavior can fall into this category.

Chapter

28

Delinquent and Criminal Behavior

- Antisocial behavior may be a part of growing up or beginning of a long-term criminal activity.
- Juvenile crime and delinquency are on the rise.
- Prevention of recurrent crime is possible through restorative justice.
- Juvenile delinquency groups may be concentrated around parks.
- Restorative justice is possible through reconciliation between offender and victim.

INTRODUCTION

Antisocial behavior may be a normal part of growing up or the beginning of a long-term pattern of criminal activity. The United Nations Guidelines for the prevention of Juvenile Delinquency (the Riyadh Guidelines) assert that "youthful behavior or conduct that does not conform to overall social norms and values is often part of the maturation and growth process and tends to disappear spontaneously in most individuals with the transition to adulthood"; a great majority of young people commit some kind of petty offence at some point during their adolescence without this turning into a criminal career in the long term. While delinquency is a common characteristic of the period and process of becoming an adult, it is very important to note that juveniles often create stable criminal groups with a corresponding subculture and start to engage in the activities of adult criminal groups, in effect choosing delinquent careers.

Young people who are at risk of becoming delinquent often live in difficult circumstances. Children who for various reasons—including parental alcoholism, poverty, breakdown of the family, overcrowding, abusive conditions in the home, the growing HIV/AIDS scourge, or the death of parents during armed conflicts—are orphans or unaccompanied and are without the means of subsistence, housing and other basic necessities, are at greater risk of falling into juvenile delinquency. The number of children in especially difficult circumstances is estimated to have increased from 80 million to 150 million between 1992 and 2000, and even much more by now.

Available data shows that delinquency and crime have strong gender associations. Police records indicate that the crime rates of male juvenile and male young adult offenders are more than double those of young females, and conviction rates are six or seven times higher. The number of male juvenile suspects for every 100,000 members of the designated age group is more than six times the corresponding figure for females; for those in the youth category the male-female suspect ratio is even higher, at 12.5 to 1.

CULTURAL FACTORS AND URBANIZATION

Delinquent behavior often occurs in social settings in which the norms for acceptable behavior have broken down.

Geographical analysis suggests that countries with more urbanized populations have higher registered crime rates than do those with strong rural lifestyles and communities. Rural groupings rely mainly on family and community control as a means of dealing with antisocial behavior and exhibit markedly lower crime rates. Urban industrialized societies tend to resort to formal legal and judicial measures, an impersonal approach that appears to be linked to higher crime rates.

When young people are exposed to the influence of adult offenders they have the opportunity to study delinquent behavior, and the possibility of their engaging in adult crime becomes more real. The "criminalization" of the family also has an impact on the choice of delinquent trajectories. A study carried out in prisons in the United States reveals that families involved in criminal activities tend to push their younger members towards violating the law. More than two-thirds of those interviewed had relatives who were incarcerated; for 25 percent it was a father and for another 25 percent a brother or a sister. The American Psychological Association upon review found that violence shown on television accounts for 10 percent of aggressive behavior of children.

PEER INFLUENCE

Membership in a delinquent gang, like membership in any other natural grouping, can be part of the process of becoming an adult. Through such primary associations, an individual acquires a sense of safety and security, develops knowledge of social interaction, and can demonstrate such qualities as loyalty or leadership. In "adult" society, factors such as social status, private welfare, race and ethnicity are of great value; however, all members of adolescent groups are essentially in an equal position and have similar opportunities for advancement in the hierarchical structure. In these groups well-being depends wholly on personal qualities such as strength, will and discipline. Quite often delinquent groups can counterbalance or compensate for the imperfections of family and school. A number of studies have shown that juvenile gang members consider their group a family. For adolescents constantly facing violence, belonging to a gang can provide protection within the neighbourhood. In some areas those who are not involved in gangs continually face the threat of assault, oppression, harassment or extortion on the street or at school. As one juvenile from the Russian Federation said, "I became involved in a gang when I was in the eighth (about 13 years old), but I joined it only when I was in the tenth (at 15 years of age). I had a girlfriend and I feared for her, and the gang was able to provide for her safety". The three types of adolescent victims identified are, accidental victims, people inclined to become victims and inborn victims.

SOME REGIONAL ASPECTS OF DELINQUENCY

Juvenile crime and delinquency are on the rise, a trend also linked to the rapid and dramatic social, political and economic changes that have taken place in Africa in recent decades. The principal offences committed by young people are theft, robbery, smuggling, prostitution, the abuse of narcotic substances, and drug trafficking.

Some countries are facing great difficulty because they are located near or within the "Golden Crescent" or the "Golden Triangle", two major narcotics-producing areas of Asia. Traffickers actively involve adolescents and youth in serving this industry, and many of them become addicted to drugs because of their low prices and easy availability. Another major problem is human trafficking: Unemployment is undeniably a major contributory factor.

PREVENTING JUVENILE DELINQUENCY

Violence against children endangers their fundamental human rights. It is therefore imperative to convince individuals and institutions to commit the time, money, expertise and other resources needed to address this global problem. A number of United Nations instruments reflect a preference for social rather than judicial approaches to control juvenile delinquency. The Riyadh Guidelines assert that the prevention of juvenile delinquency is an essential part of overall crime prevention in society, and the United Nations Standard Minimum Rules for the Administration of Juvenile Justice (the Beijing Rules) recommend instituting positive measures to strengthen a juvenile's overall well-being and reduce the need for State intervention.

Often it is possible to reduce the level of juvenile delinquency by changing an urban environment, altering the physical features through architectural and landscape planning and providing opportunities to engage young people's interests. A research study conducted in a town in the United States revealed that most of the activities of juvenile delinquent groups were concentrated around the town's only park. The layout of the park was redesigned to create many more leisure and recreational alternatives for juveniles and their parents. The number of positive afternoon activities held in schools and parks was also increased. All of these measures led to a considerable reduction in juvenile delinquency; in the United States juvenile crime, including violent offences, peaks at around 3 pm, generally right after school lets out.

Special programmes are needed to tackle the problem of unaccompanied and homeless children, including rehabilitation schemes that take children off the streets. The United Nations Convention on the Rights of the Child provides a framework for improving the living conditions of children, focusing on the following four broad areas:

- **Survival rights.** Articles 6.1, 6.2 and 24.1 deal with the basic needs that must be met for children to enjoy good health for adequate growth, including medical care, nutrition, shelter and clothing. For street children, most of these needs are not satisfied.
- **Development rights.** Articles 6, 26 and 28 relate to the opportunities and means for providing children with access to education, skills training, recreation and rest, information, parental care and social security.
- **Protective rights.** Articles 2, 19.1, 19.2, 32.1, 33, 34, 36 and 37 focus on the legal and social provisions that must be made by each country to protect children from exploitation, drug abuse, sexual abuse, cruelty, separation from family, discrimination, and the effects of all types of man-made or natural disasters.
- **Participation rights.** Articles 12, 13, 14 and 17 focus on the opportunities and means provided to children to enable them to express opinions on matters affecting their lives, including freedom of worship, access to information about oneself, and freedom to give evidence (where applicable). Children are knowledgeable about their situations and can devise innovative solutions to their problems if consulted. Street children, in particular, have already learned to make important decisions regarding their daily lives without the assistance of adults.

Prevention of recurrent crime is best achieved through "**restorative justice**", which is usually carried out by non-governmental remedial organizations and local communities. Restorative justice is regarded as an alternative mode of criminal justice. It involves a process whereby all the parties with a stake in a specific offence come together and collectively determine how best to deal with the aftermath of the offence and its implications for the future. The offender, through interaction with the victim, must understand the seriousness of the incident and together with the victim and social workers develop a series of steps towards reconciliation, arranging reparations for damages and providing whatever remedial assistance the victim might require. If successful resolution occurs, the juvenile is not placed in a correctional facility or labelled a delinquent, thereby avoiding the influence of an environment (jail) that can reinforce delinquent behavior.

One of the key elements of restorative justice is reconciliation between the offender and the victim, a process necessary not only for the correction of the offender, but also for the restoration of justice for the victim. The protection and support of victims and witnesses is recognized as an important basic element of overall crime prevention and crime control strategies. Support measures reduce the impact of crime on those most directly affected and are essential for preserving and protecting the role of victims and witnesses in the criminal justice process. It also helps the investigation and prosecution of crime by facilitating cooperation between victims, witnesses and law enforcement and prosecution agencies.

A crime prevention system will be effective only if: the contents and framework of prevention efforts are clearly defined and the functional opportunities of all agencies included in that system are appropriately utilized; all of the subjects and targets of prevention work (including adolescents themselves and their relations in different spheres of society) are covered and the specific characteristics of each are taken into consideration; and the mechanisms of administration, control and coordination for this type of prevention work have been developed.

If delinquency policies are to be truly effective, higher priority must be given to marginalized, vulnerable and disadvantaged young people in society, and issues relating to youth in conflict with the law should be a central focus of national youth policies. The administration of juvenile justice should be decentralized in order to encourage local authorities to become actively involved in preventing youth crime and reintegrating young offenders into society through support projects, with the ultimate aim of fostering responsible citizenship.

- Young people becoming delinquent often live in difficult circumstances.
- Juvenile delinquency is six times more common in males than in females.
- Families involved in criminal activities tend to push their juveniles and children towards violations of law.
- Special programs can tackle the problem of street children and orphans.
- Protection and support of victims and witnesses helps in overall prevention of crimes and criminal conduct.

Chapter

29

Child Sexual Behavior

- Child victims of sexual abuse display sexualized behavior.
- It is normal for children to indulge in sex play.
- There are four groups of observed sexual behavior in children.

INTRODUCTION

Sexual behavior in children has become increasingly relevant in recent years due to the attention paid to the problematic area of child sexual abuse.

Studies in Sweden have indicated that children in their homes and, in preschools demonstrate a number of different behaviors which can be linked to the body, sexual identity and sexuality but that more explicit sexual behavior which imitates adult sexuality is uncommon. Children who are found to have been the victims of sexual abuse on the other hand can display "sexualized" behavior.

Besides the behavior in itself, it is important to look at the child's entire situation: level of development, anxiety, shame, guilt, pain, relationships with adults and friends, the environment in which the child lives and is growing up, the total family situation, etc. What is considered to be sexualized behavior, with an explicit sexual content, may be due to the child having been the victim of abuse, but it is important to be aware that similar behavior can also have other causes.

Expressions of sexual desire, curiosity and behavior in children have aroused many feelings in adults. Since Freud, almost a century ago, we have accepted to a certain extent, that children are sexual beings from birth.

PURPOSE, METHODOLOGY AND TERMINOLOGY

The term "sexual behavior" refers to behavior which concerns the body, touching, sexual identity, exploring one's own body and that of others, sexual language, masturbation and games and interaction which can have sexual connotations. The term "child" is here primarily used to refer to the period up to puberty.

BASIC ASSUMPTIONS ON CHILDREN, SEXUALITY AND GENDER

The basic theory is that children are born with sexual energy and are initially entirely controlled on their seeking sexual experiences. Development then progresses through various stages, which at the same time involves adapting to the surrounding world and controlling sexual impulses. If something goes wrong during the various stages, the child's sexuality can stagnate, resulting in deviations in adult sexuality.
Gender socialization addresses how biological gender gradually becomes social and

psychological gender, i.e. how our thinking and behavior is shaped on the basis of the expectations for our gender. A child is not only a child but also a boy or a girl.

The social system and the economic, religious, medical as well as the cultural spheres determine the position held by and the nature of sexuality.

Our assumptions on sexuality and gender also form the basis for the way in which we address children's sexual behavior and their socialization in becoming women and men which is consciously or unconsciously part of our child-rearing.

NORMAL AND DEVIANT BEHAVIORS

The conceptual apparatus surrounding what is meant by "normal" or "deviant" sexual behavior is somewhat unclear. The term "normal" tends to be used most by researchers and practitioners in the field with links to the worlds of psychology, medicine or education. Normal sexual behavior is a result of natural human biological and psychological development process. The terms "pathological" or "abnormal" are used to describe behavior which indicates that something has happened to disrupt or change expected sexual behavior or the natural development process. When sexual behavior is defined in sociocultural terms, the term "normative" is used to indicate what is considered to be the norm in a given society, culture or group. The latter term is primarily used by sociologists, social work professionals and those connected with the legal system. Researchers and practitioners in these fields tend to use terms such as "deviant" or "criminal acts" more frequently to describe sexual behavior outside social norms or legislation (Araji, 1997).

Sexual behavior can be seen as normal and not typical but still healthy or, on the other hand, a behavior may occur often and still not be accepted or seen as healthy. Normality therefore does not exist as an absolute or a fact, instead it is about how we see each other and ourselves. What is seen as "normal" in one generation can be labelled "problematic" in the next. Normality is also culturally bound. What is seen as normal in one culture can be seen as deviant, bizarre or even as abuse in another (Rosenfeld and Wasserman, 1993; Larsson, 1994, Soderauist, 1995).

The same sexual behavior can, confusingly enough, be labelled normal, abnormal or pathological by taking a developmental view but described as normative, deviant or criminal by those who prefer an anthropological or sociological approach.

Behaviors imitating adult sexuality, like attempted intercourse or imitation of sex with another child or dolls/soft toys; attempts to insert objects in the child's own anus or vagina or the anus or vagina of another child; oral-genital contact and demanding that others take part in specific sexual activities with the child, are very uncommon in observations of normal groups of children but are more common among children who have been the victims of abuse.

Friedrich et al found a link between the incidence of domestic violence, which was manifested in aggression, and sexual behavior on the part of the child. Friedrich claims that this is because the sexual development of the child may be disrupted as a result of the family dysfunction evinced by the violence.

The most uncommon behaviors (seen in less than 5% of the children) were touching the sexual organs of another adult woman, attempting to get an adult to touch the child's genitals, attempting to undress other children, imitating sex play with dolls and soft toys and initiating sex play with other children. No parent stated that their child had attempted to touch the sexual organs of a man outside the family. On the other hand, children were curious about their father's penis on individual occasions (59%) and 23% had at some point touched their father's sexual organ. It was uncommon for this interest to be maintained in the long term.

Majority of the young people (74%) also thought it as normal for children to indulge in sex play, e.g. hugging and kissing games, playing doctors and nurses, looking at pictures of sexual acts, touching the sexual organs and masturbating. The vast majority considered it to be abnormal for children to take part in vaginal and anal intercourse or insert objects in the anus or vagina. Most stated that they had obtained their knowledge of sex primarily from friends and television but a majority also stated that their parents are the source of information. A comparative study between the US, Ireland, Sweden and the Netherlands (Cavanagh Johnson et al,) showed considerable cultural differences. The first two countries have the lowest figures, 57% and 59% respectively for young people who considered sexual activities among children to be normal. Figures for the Netherlands are around the same level as Sweden.

Sexual Behavior as a Symptom

Several studies show that there is a link between what we often call sexualised behavior in children and their having been the victim of sexual abuse (Friedrich et al, 1992, 1993; Kendall-Tackett, 1993; Cosentino et al, 1995). "Sexualised behavior" usually refers to sexual behavior in the child which is expressed, often recurring, takes over other activities and becomes a central aspect of the child's everyday life, involves the child screening him or herself off or attempting to involve other children in sexual activities and to which the children and/or adults surrounding the child react with concern. This may involve a specific behavior, e.g. masturbation, which the child constantly repeats, or consists of a number of different behaviors (and vocabulary) of a sexual nature. On the basis of the above studies sexualised behavior can be seen as the best indicator that a child may have been the victim of sexual abuse.

Post-traumatic Stress and Sexualised Behavior

Kendall-Tackett, Williams and Finkelhor (1993) have carried out a wide ranging summary and analysis of 45 studies of sexual abuse and found that children who have been the victims of abuse showed more symptoms of varied nature than children who had not been exposed to abuse. However, there was no single symptom which characterised the majority of the children who had been abused. *One in three of the children who had been the victims of abuse showed no symptoms at all.* It is also an observed sexualised behavior, which often involved excessive or public masturbation, sexualised games with dolls, seductive behavior, inserting objects in the anus or vagina, sexual knowledge not commensurate with the child's age and a desire for sexual stimulation from adults or other children.

In children aged 0 to 4, sexualised behaviors are touching one's own body from time to time, looking at others, interest in the toilet situation and playing doctors and nurses and mummies and daddies.

Children at ages 5 to 7 increased contact with friends, take part in experimentation with other children and have developed inhibitions in certain situations. The behavior consists of specific touching of the child's own body, questions about the body and bodily functions, curiosity about and distancing from the opposite sex, sexual vocabulary, role-playing, playing mummies and daddies and kissing and hugging games.

Children aged 8 to 12. The behavior may involve touching one's own sexual organs, exhibitionist behavior, asking out someone of the opposite sex, crushes, kisses, petting, touching the sexual organs of other children, imitating intercourse with clothes on and also proper intercourse.

On the basis of Sgroi et al (1988), who developed social criteria to determine sexually abusive behavior in young people, Gil proposes the following list to be used for children up to the age of 12 (Araji, 1997):

1. Age difference—more than three years' difference between the persons involved should give cause for concern.
2. Developmental age difference—children will vary greatly, with some having developmental delays or severe immaturity. These children may become targets of abuse.
3. Size difference—if children are the same age but there is a substantial difference in height, weight or strength, this should be seen as a variable which may cause problems.
4. Difference in status—when a child has the status, e.g. of a babysitter, this gives a special position which involves authority or power, which potentially can be used to coerce other children.
5. Type of sexual activity—one way of judging the appropriateness of the behavior is to see it on the basis of a developmental continuum, which is why data on normative sexual behavior in children is required.
6. Behavioral dynamics—Gil E (1993) thinks that the dynamics of age-appropriate sex play are completely different to those of "problematic behaviors". Sex play tends to be spontaneous and involves joy, laughter, embarrassment and varying levels of inhibition or uninhibitedness/openness. Problematic sexual behavior, on the other hand, involves dominance, force, threats and violence. Children who take part in this type of behavior show anxiety, hostility, anger or tension. They display higher levels of arousal. Their sexual behavior can be habitual and become compulsive in nature. Nor are they receptive to guidance from parents or other adults, nor to attempts to distract the child.

Cavangh Johnson and Feldmeth classified such children into four groups:

I. Normal sexual exploration
II. Sexually reactive
III. Extensive mutual sexual behaviors
IV. Children who molest

Group I

Normal sexual behavior is seen as healthy exploration or as sex play in which children of about the same age and size explore each other's bodies by touching or looking. Children in this group feel no shame or guilt about their behavior.

- Takes place as part of an information-gathering process or an act of curiosity.
- The children are of a similar age, size and developmental status.
- Both (or all) the children take part on a voluntary basis.
- Sex play takes place between children who have an ongoing mutually enjoyable play and/or school friendship over and above the sexual interaction.
- The sexual behaviors are limited in type and frequency and occur in several periods of a child's life.
- If the children are discovered and instructed to stop the activity, they do so, at least when in sight of adults. When they are discovered by adults they may be embarrassed or show feelings of guilt but normally they express no deep feelings of anger, anxiety, guilt or shame.
- The children's sexuality is generally light-hearted and spontaneous.

Group II

The **sexually reactive:** The children in group II do not use threats or violence against other children. When they are asked to cease the activity, they usually do as they are told. Intervention or treatment is generally received positively in this group.

Group III

Extensive mutual sexual behavior: Most children in group III have been the victims of sexual abuse, all have experienced some type of abuse—emotional, physical or sexual or all three. They come from dysfunctional environments and are found in all groups of children who are maltreated.

In some cases the children in group III use sex as a means of winning friends and for dealing with feelings of loss, abandonment, fear and loneliness. For these children the sexual behavior has become a way of dealing with their existence, a coping mechanism. They have organized their reactions around sex as a way of handling their life stresses. They seek out other children with similar conflicts and problems who might be thought to want to take part in mutual sex play. For children in group III sexual arousal and enjoyment are rarely the primary driving force behind taking part in sexual activities although some pre-pubertal children may experience physical feelings of desire. Many children in this group have been chronically wounded, abandoned and often have no success either in school or socially among classmates. They generally distrust adults and appear less receptive to treatment than children in group II.

Group IV

Children who molest manifest abusive behavior. They show an impulsive, compulsive and aggressive component in their sexual behavior. They use social and emotional threats to prevent the victim from telling anyone about the abuse. They show lack of empathy for victim. Children in this category have often been the victims of sexual abuse, like some children in groups II and III. The sexual behaviors of children in group IV continue and increase over time and represent a pattern. They linked feelings of loneliness, anger and fear with sex, which in turn is linked to aggression. Like the children in group III they tend to be found in dysfunctional environments. The group IV are the most difficult to treat. Require intensive and specialised therapy.

KEY LEARNING POINTS

- What is considered normal sexual behavior in children can vary from one period to another.
- The absence of knowledge about one's own body and its physical and emotional sensations may help to make the child more vulnerable and encourage secrecy should a child be the victim of some form of abuse.

Chapter

30

Learning Disability, Autism and Aggressive Criminal Behavior

INTRODUCTION

The adolescent with learning disability or autism faces the same challenges and tasks like young people. He does not share the general intellectual and social skills required for resolving complex matters. Without the ability to understand, communicate and consider their situation, antisocial and disturbed behavior is common in these people. Let us consider the factors which predispose adolescents with learning disability and autism to commit crime and the extent to which criminal behavior shows a distinct profile.

FACTORS RELATED TO CRIMINIAL BEHAVIOR IN ADOLESCENTS WITH LEARNING DISABILITY

- General issues
- Severity of learning disability
- Relevance of the cause/aetiology of learning disability
- Impact of the nature of an individual's learning disability/cognitive profile
- Importance of super-added psychiatric disorder among learning disabled adolescents
- Role of life experiences and personal history

PSYCHIATRIC DISORDER AND LEARNING DISABILITY

As we consider the impact of intervening variables on the occurrence of offending among adolescents with learning disability, psychiatric disorder proves to be of key importance. Psychiatric disorder is very common among adolescents with learning disability. One major epidemiological Swedish survey of 16 to 19 year olds with learning disability found rates as high as 64% in moderately to severely learning disabled young people (1Q < 50), and 57% in the mildly learning-disabled (1Q 51–70) (Gillberg et al 1986).

The phenomenon of prevalence rate of psychopathology 'peaking' in adolescence among people with learning disability is well recognized. The psychiatric problem which constitutes this is autism. Given the extent and social impact of this disorder, and the suggestion that the young person with learning disability who also has autism, such a child may particularly be at high risk of offending behavior.

The other common psychiatric disorders which constitute the high rate of psychopathology among these young people notably include attention deficit disorder with hyperactivity (ADHD).

Given the propensity for disruptive, antisocial and offending behavior which is seen in these disorders, these high prevalences are of considerable relevance to consideration of the offending behavior of young people with learning disability.

Conditions associated with high prevalence of antisocial and offending behavior:

- Autistic spectrum disorder is the most frequent diagnosis, followed by attention-deficit disorder with hyperactivity.
- Both autism and hyperactivity are increasingly more common in more severely learning disabled individuals.
- Schizophreniform psychosis is more common among the non-intellectually disabled population, and is more often non-specific or poorly-differentiated in type.
- Psychiatric disorder of this extent and nature has major implications for both understanding and management of learning—disabled adolescent offenders.

PERSONAL HISTORY

Aggression may have been learnt through the experience of being a victim of aggression, or may be some other reflection of an abusive or otherwise adverse early life experience. Indeed, it is now accepted that children and adolescents with learning disabilities, particularly those with more severe disabilities who are dependent on the care of others, may be more at risk of sexual and other physical abuse (O' Brien 1996, Holland 1997). Also, what seems at first sight to be a trait of serious and goal-directed aggression may reflect some long standing aspect of individual development, where previous aggressive acts were in some sense 'rewarded', and therefore have continued, or even worsened. Such a set of circumstances commonly presents in a learning disabled adolescent who has, virtually by a process of trial and error, learned that aggression can serve to remove him/herself from some undesirable situation.

In many cases, it is not possible to identify the mechanisms of specific early-life adverse experiences, and how these have predisposed to offending. More often, general indicators of adverse early-life experiences are identified, such as early admission in remand homes (usually due to deficient or otherwise inappropriate parenting) and severe emotional deprivation.

WHAT IS AUTISM?

The pervasive developmental disorders (including the autistic spectrum disorders) present with a number of clinical pictures, while sharing three core features:

- Impaired social reciprocity
- Impaired communication
- Restricted, repetitive repertoire of interests or behaviors.

As developmental disorders they will manifest differently according to the individual's developmental stage and chronological age. For example, autism commonly occurs in individuals with learning disability, but, most importantly, the triad of impairments must be of a greater magnitude than one would expect in the context of the given degree of intellectual disability.

Example, one young man with autism regularly flooded his mother's bathroom while indulging in his fascination for water.If prevented from carrying out this habitual behavior, he would typically resort to extremes of violence. On one he smashed holes in the bath with a brick. This man repeatedly set fire to the family home. By the age of 8 years he had repeatedly assaulted his mother, with fists, by biting and with any object to hand.

Violence, aggression or socially proscribed behaviors are common in autism. The autists are less likely to use drugs or alcohol, and substance misuse is not implicated in their offending. They committed offences during daylight hours, while others had offended both by day and night.

Howlin (1997) proposed that offending and aggression in autists might arise by four means:

1. Autists, because of their social naiveté, may be led into criminal acts by others (e.g. Rain Man card counting in the casino).
2. Aggressive behaviors may arise from a disruption of routines or changes in daily circumstances.
3. Antisocial behaviors are related to a lack of understanding or misinterpretation of social cues. This is not uncommonly seen particularly in Asperger syndrome, where the young man wishes to make friends but his attempts are often awkward and clumsy and can escalate to violence when rebuffed.
4. Antisocial or criminal behaviors can arise from obsessions. One man had a lifelong interest in cars, and this obsession led to his having in excess of twenty convictions for taking cars without consent.
   Example. A young man has an obsession with women's hair. He will become obsessed with and follow a woman with a particular hair type. This usually results in him stalking the woman. He misinterprets any discouragement apart from very concrete instructions to desist. As a result he becomes very angry towards the woman and the risk of assault is high.

   A group of men committed serious sexual assaults or homicide. They repeatedly fantasized about the acts that they eventually committed. When fantasy alone was not enough they carried out the initial stages of their fantasy, such as approaching their preferred victim type, collecting or carrying their preferred weapon, and so on, before escalating to the complete act. In Asperger's syndrome and high-functioning autists, one area of expertise may be present such as rote memory (being able to recite the telephone directory from memory) or mathematics. Some individuals with autism have heightened sensitivity to sounds (e.g. vacuum cleaners, aeroplanes, etc.) and exhibit extreme reactions in response to these stimuli-including severe aggressive behavior.

Aggression and autism: Three categories of aggression are:

- Inter-specific aggression—predatory type
- Intra-specific aggression—seen in social interactions
- Indiscriminate or reactive aggression—larsgely defensive or in response to fear.

Autists who have difficulty understanding social rules and interaction show abnormal aggressive behaviors.

Conclusion and Pointers to Diagnosis

A diagnosis of autistic spectrum disorder especially should be routsinely considered (even if it is rapidly discounted) where an offence or assault is characterized by:

- Bizarre nature
- A degree and nature of aggression which is 'unaccountable'
- A repeated and very stereotypic pattern of offending.

SOTOS SYNDROME

This is a sporadic, non-familial condition, and is sometimes called cerebral gigantism. The prevalence is unknown, because the features are so variable in expression. Individuals typically present with large body size, accelerated growth, advanced bone age, and a characteristic facial appearance with high forehead, prominent jaw, premature eruption of teeth and sparseness of hair, in addition to other eye and nasal features. The main behavioral problems are of aggressive behavior and emotional immaturity. These assume even greater importance, given the large stature and appearance of sufferers of the syndrome.

TUBEROUS SCLEROSIS

The condition has a classic triad of epilepsy, learning disability and certain skin problems —notably the so-called 'adenoma sebaceum' rash. The severity of learning disability of the condition varies enormously, according to the brain involvement of blood vessel malformations, which are essentially the same as those which appear on the face. As these are progressive, so is deterioration in intelligence. Prominent psychological findings are of generally disturbed, distractible and disinhibited behavior, often amounting to an autistic/ hyperactive constellation which may worsen in late adolescence and early adulthood (Hunt and Dennis 1987).

- Offending among adolescents with learning disability psychiatric disorder is of key importance.
- Autism is common among people with learning diasibility
- Violence and aggression are common in autism.

KEY LEARNING POINTS

- Persons with learning disabilities or autism face challenges and tasks.
- Autists may be lead to criminal acts by others.
- There are three types of aggression
- Repeated and stereotypic offending seen.

Chapter

31

Intermittent Explosive Disorder

Intermittent explosive disorder is seen in persons who have discrete episodes of losing control of aggressive impulses, resulting in serious assault or the destruction of property. The aggressiveness expressed is grossly out of proportion to any stressors that may have triggered the episodes. The symptoms occur as spells or attacks, appear within minutes or hours and, regardless of the duration, remit spontaneously and quickly. Each spell is usually followed by regret or self-reproach. Impulsivity or aggressiveness is absent between episodes. Schizophrenia, antisocial or borderline personality disorder, attention-deficit/hyperactivity disorder, conduct disorder, or substance intoxication also show spells of intermittent explosive conduct.

Some associated features suggest the possibility of an epileptoid state: the patient may experience an aura; postictal like changes in the sensorium, including partial or spotty amnesia; or hypersensitivity to photic, aural, or auditory stimuli. Persons with the disorder have a high incidence of hyperactivity, soft neurological signs, nonspecific electroencephalogram (EEG) findings, and accident-proneness.

Intermittent explosive disorder is more common in first-degree biological relatives of persons with the disorder than in the general population.

Disordered brain physiology, particularly in the limbic system, is involved in most cases of episodic violence. Predisposing factors in childhood include perinatal trauma, infantile seizures, head trauma, encephalitis, minimal brain dysfunction, and hyperactivity. The patient's childhood environments are often filled with alcoholics, beatings, threats to life, and promiscuity.

Compelling evidence indicates that serotonergic neurons mediate behavioral inhibition. Decrease in serotonergic transmission—as can be induced by inhibiting serotonin synthesis or antagonizing its effects—result in a decrease in punishment's effect as a deterrent to behavior.

The history is typically of a childhood in the midst of alcohol dependents, violence, and emotional instability. The patients' work histories are poor. The patients report job losses, marital difficulties, and trouble with the law. Most have sought psychiatric help in the past but without success. A high level of anxiety, guilt, and depression is usually present after an episode. Neurological examination sometimes reveals soft neurological signs, such as left-right ambivalence and perceptual reversal. EEG findings are frequently normal or show nonspecific changes. Psychological tests for organicity frequently result in normal findings.

The diagnosis of intermittent explosive disorder can be made only after disorders associated with the occasional loss of control of aggressive impulses have been ruled out. Those other disorders include psychotic disorders, personality change due to a general medical condition, antisocial or borderline personality disorder, conduct disorder, and intoxication with a psychoactive substance.

TREATMENT

A combined pharmacological and psychotherapeutic approach is indicated.

Anticonvulsants have long been used in treating explosive patients, with mixed results. Phenothiazines and antidepressants have been effective in some cases. Benzodiazepines have been reported to produce a paradoxical reaction of dyscontrol in some cases. Lithium carbonate has been reported to be useful in generally lessening aggressive behavior, and carbamazepine (tegretol) and phenytoin (dilantin) have also been reported to be helpful.

KLEPTOMANIA

The essential feature of kleptomania is a recurrent failure to resist impulses to steal objects not needed for personal use or their monetary value. The objects taken are often given away, returned surreptitiously, or kept and hidden.

The stealing is not planned and does not involve others. Although the thefts do not occur when immediate arrest is probable kleptomaniac persons do not always consider the chances of their apprehension, even though repeated arrests lead to pain and humiliation. In kleptomania the act of stealing is itself the goal.

Kleptomania appears to be more common among females than among males.

Etiology

Psychodynamic Factors

Those who focus on symbolism see meaning in the act itself, the object stolen, and the victim of the theft. Kleptomania is often associated with other disturbances such as mood disorders, obsessive-compulsive disorder, and eating disorders. The symptoms of kleptomania tend to appear in times of significant stress—for example losses, separations, and the ending of important relationships.

One theoretician described seven categories of stealing in chronically acting-out children: (1) as a means of restoring the lost mother-child relationship, (2) as an aggressive act, (3) as a defense against fears of being damaged (perhaps a search by females for a penis or a protection against castration anxiety in males), (4) as a means of seeking punishment, (5) as a means of restoring or adding to self-esteem, (6) in connection with and as a reaction to a family secret, and (7) as excitement and a substitute for a sexual act. One or more of those categories can also apply to adult kleptomania.

Biological Factors

Brain diseases and mental retardation have been associated with kleptomania, as they have with other disorders of impulse control.

Essential feature of kleptomania consists of recurrent, intrusive, and irresistible urges or impulses to steal unneeded objects. Kleptomaniac patients may also be distressed about the possibility or the actuality of their being apprehended and so manifest signs of depression and anxiety. Patients feel guilty, ashamed, and embarrassed about their behavior. They often have serious problems with interpersonal relation.

Most kleptomaniac patients steal from retail stores, but they may steal from family members in their own households or from their friends in a hostel.

Most kleptomaniac patients are referred for examination in connection with legal proceedings after apprehension, the clinical picture may be clouded by subsequent symptoms of depression and anxiety. Schizophrenic patients may steal in response to hallucinations and delusions, and patients with cognitive disorders may be accused of stealing because of their forgetting to pay for objects they have purchased.

Course and Prognosis

Kleptomania may begin in childhood, although most children and adolescents who steal do not become kleptomaniac adults. The course of the disorder waxes and wanes, but the disorder tends to be chronic. Many individuals seem never to have consciously considered the possibility of having to face the consequences of their acts, a feature in line with some descriptions of kleptomaniac patients as people who feel wronged and, therefore, entitled to steal.

Behavior therapy—including systematic desensitization, aversive conditioning, and a combination of aversive conditioning and altered social contingencies—has been reported to be successful, even when motivation was lacking.

PYROMANIA

Features of pyromania are deliberate and purposeful fire setting on more than one occasion; tension or affective arousal before setting the fires; fascination with, interest in, curiosity about, or attraction to fire and the activities and equipment associated with fire fighting; and pleasure, gratification, or relief when setting fires or when witnessing or participating in their aftermath. The patient may make considerable advance preparations before starting the fire.

Epidemiology

The disorder is found far more often in males than in females, and people who set fires are more likely to be mildly retarded than are the general population. Fire setters also tend to have a history of antisocial traits, such as truancy, running away from home, and delinquency. Enuresis has been considered a common finding in the history of fire setters, although controlled studies have failed to confirm the findings. However, studies have found an association between cruelty to animals and fire setting.

Etiology

Sigmund Freud saw fire as a symbol of sexuality. The warmth that is radiated by fire evokes the same sensation that accompanies a state of sexual excitation, and a flame's shape and movements suggest a phallus in activity. Other therapists have associated pyromania with an abnormal craving for power and social prestige. The incendiary act is a way to vent accumulated rage over the frustration caused by a sense of social, physical, or sexual inferiority. A number of studies have noted that the fathers of pyromanic patients were absent from their homes.

Promiscuity without pleasure and petty stealing, often approaching kleptomania, have been frequently noted to be delinquent trends in female fire setters.

Persons with pyromania are often regular watchers at fires in their neighbourhood, frequently set off false alarms, and show interest in fire-fighting paraphernalia.

Pyromania must also be separated from incendiary acts of sabotage carried out by dissident political extremists or paid torches, who are called arsonists in the legal system.

When fire setting occurs in conduct disorder and antisocial personality disorder, it is a deliberate act, rather than the failure to resist an impulse.

A diagnosis of pyromania should not be made when fires are set to make money from insurance agencies, to express a socio-political ideology, to conceal criminal activity, to express anger or vengeance, to improve one's living circumstances, or to respond to a delusion or a hallucination.

Pyromania usually begins in childhood. When the onset is in adolescence or adulthood, the fire setting tends to be deliberately destructive. The prognosis for treated children is good, and complete remission is a realistic goal. The prognosis for adults is guarded, because of their frequent use of denial, their refusal to take responsibility, and their concurrent alcohol dependence and lack of insight.

The treatment of fire setters has been difficult because of their lack of motivation. Incarceration may be the only method available to prevent a recurrence. Behavior therapy can be administered in the institution.

Carbamazepine has been reported to be successful in some cases.

PATHOLOGICAL GAMBLING

The essential feature of pathological gambling is persistent and recurrent maladaptive gambling behavior. Features include a preoccupation with gambling; the need to gamble with increasing amounts of money to achieve the desired excitement; repeated unsuccessful efforts to control, cut back, or stop gambling; gambling as a way of escaping from problems; gambling to recoup losses; lying to conceal the extent of the involvement with gambling; the commission of illegal acts to finance gambling; the jeopardizing or loss of personal and vocational relationships because of gambling; and a reliance on others for money to pay off debts.

Pathological gamblers are 1 to 3 percent of the adult United States population. The disorder is more common in men than in women. Alcohol dependence is more common among the parents of pathological gamblers than among the general population.

Etiology

The following may be predisposing factors for the development of the disorder; loss of a parent by death, separation, divorce, or desertion before the child is 15 years of age; inappropriate parental discipline (absence, inconsistency, or harshness); exposure to and availability of gambling activities for the adolescent; a family emphasis on material and financial symbols; and a lack of family emphasis on saving, planning and budgeting.

Diagnosis and Clinical Features

Pathological gamblers appear overconfident, somewhat abrasive, energetic, and free-spending, even when they have obvious signs of personal stress, anxiety, and depression. They commonly have the attitude that money is both the cause of and the solution to all their problems. As their gambling increases, they are usually forced to lie to obtain money and to continue gambling while holding the extent of their gambling behavior a secret. They make no serious attempt to budget or save money. When their borrowing resources are strained, they are likely to engage in antisocial behavior to obtain money for gambling. Their criminal behavior is typically nonviolent, such as forgery, embezzlement, or fraud. The conscious intent is to return or repay the money. Complications include alienation from family members and acquaintances, the loss of one's life accomplishments, suicide attempts, and association with fringe and illegal groups. Arrest for nonviolent crimes may lead to imprisonment.

Three phases are seen in pathological gambling: (1) The winning phase, ending with a big win, equal to about a year's salary, which hooks the patient; (2) The progressive-loss phase, in which patients structure their lives around gambling and move from being excellent gamblers to stupid ones (taking considerable risks, cashing in securities, borrowing money, missing work, and losing jobs); and (3) The desperate phase, with the patients gambling in a frenzy with large amounts of money, not paying debts, becoming involved with loan sharks, writing bad checks, and possibly embezzling. The disorder may take up to 15 years to reach the third phase, but then, within a year or two, the patients are totally deteriorated.

Treatment

Gamblers anonymous (GA) was founded in Los Angeles in 1957 and modelled on alcoholics anonymous (AA); it is accessible—at least in large cities—and is probably the most effective treatment for gambling. It is a method of inspirational group therapy, which involves public confession, peer pressure, and the presence of reformed gamblers available (as are sponsors in AA) to help members resist the impulse to gamble. Insight-oriented psychotherapy is the other option of treatment.

TRICHOTILLOMANIA

The essential feature of trichotillomania is the recurrent pulling out of one's hair, resulting in noticeable hair loss. Other clinical symptoms include an increasing sense of tension before pulling the hair and a sense of pleasure, gratification, or relief when pulling out the hair.

Etiology

Although trichotillomania is regarded as multi-determined, its onset has been linked to stressful situations in more than a quarter of all cases. Disturbances in mother-child relationships, fear of being left alone, and recent object loss are often cited as critical factors.

It has also been associated with obsessive compulsive disorder in some cases.

Trichophagy, mouthing of the hair, may follow the hair plucking. Complications of trichophagy include trichobezoars, malnutrition, and intestinal obstruction.

Characteristic histopathological changes in the hair follicle, known as trichomalacia, are demonstrated by biopsy and help distinguish trichotillomania from other causes of alopecia. Patients usually deny the behavior and often try to hide the resultant alopecia. Head banging, nail biting, scratching, gnawing, excoriation and other acts or self-mutilation may be present.

Treatment

Treatment usually involves psychiatrists and dermatologists in a joint endeavour. Psychopharmacological methods that have been used to treat psychodermatological disorders include topical steroids, hydroxyzine hydrochloride, an anxiolytic with antihistamine properties, anxiolytics-Specific Serotonin Reuptake Inhibitors (SSRIs) and antipsychotics.

Chapter

32

Oppositional Defiant Disorder

Oppositional defiant disorder is an enduring pattern of negativistic, hostile, and defiant behaviors in the absence of serious violations of social norms or the rights of others. The most common symptoms of oppositional defiant disorder include the following: often loses temper, often argues with adults, often actively defies or refuses to comply with adults' requests or rules, often deliberately does things that annoy other people, 'and often blames' others for his or her mistakes or misbehavior.

EPIDEMIOLOGY

Almost all parents of oppositional defiant disorder children are over-concerned with issues of power, control, and autonomy. Some families contain several obstinate children, controlling their depressed mothers, and passive-aggressive fathers. The patients may be unwanted children.

In late childhood, environmental trauma, illnesses, or chronic incapacity, such as mental retardation, may trigger oppositionalism as a defense against helplessness, anxiety, and loss of self-esteem. Another normative oppositional stage occurs in adolescence as an expression of the need to separate from the parents and to establish an autonomous identity.

Chronic oppositional defiant disorder almost always interferes with interpersonal relationships and school performance. The children are often friendless and perceive human relationships as unsatisfactory. Despite adequate intelligence, they do poorly or fail in school, as they withhold participation, resist external demands, and insist on solving problems without others' help.

Adolescents may abuse alcohol and illegal substances. Often, the disturbance evolves into a conduct disorder (30%), or into a mood disorder.

CONDUCT DISORDER: DIAGNOSIS (DSM-IV)

a. A repetitive and persistent pattern of behavior in which either the basic rights of others or major age-appropriate societal norms of rules are violated, as manifested by the presence of three (or more) of the following criteria in the past 12 months, with at least one criterion present in the past 6 months:

Aggression to people and animals:

1. Often bullies, threatens, or intimidates others
2. Often initiates physical fights
3. Has used a weapon that can cause serious physical harm to others (e.g. a bat, brick, broken bottle, knife, gun)
4. Has been physically cruel to people
5. Has been physically cruel to animals

6. Has stolen while confronting a victim (e.g. mugging, purse snatching, extortion, armed robbery)
7. Has forced someone into sexual activity

Destruction of property:

8. Has deliberately engaged in fire setting with the intention of causing serious damage.
9. Has deliberately destroyed others' property (other than by fire setting)

Deceitfulness or theft:

10. Has broken into someone else's house, building or car.
11. Often lies to obtain goods or favours or to avoid obligations (i.e. "cons" others)
12. Has stolen items of nontrivial value without confronting a victim. (e.g. shoplifting, but without breaking and entering; forgery)

Serious violations of rules:

13. Often stays out at night despite parental prohibitions, beginning before 13 years.
14. Has run away from home overnight at least twice while living in parental or parental surrogate home (or once without returning for a lengthy period).
15. Often truant from school beginning before age 13 years.

b. The disturbance in behavior causes clinically significant impairment in social, academic, or occupational functioning.

If the individual is age 18 years or older, criteria are not met for antisocial personality disorder.

Chapter

33

Mental Disability

Evidence for the recognition and treatment of intellectual disability dates to the earliest of medical writings. Hippocrates described microcephaly and craniostenosis, and Galen actively explored causes of cognitive disability. In the Middle Ages, Avicenna proposed treatments for meningitis and hydrocephalus and even defined levels of intellectual function.

The modern history for the field of **intellectual disability** begins in the late eighteenth and early nineteenth centuries. At that time, Jean-Marc Itard attempted a natural experiment to educate Victor, a "wild child" discovered in the forests of Aveyron, France. Although Itard judged his work with Victor a failure, this famous experiment marked the first time that anyone had considered the possibility that persons with such disabilities could be educated. Itard's efforts generated interest in educational and other interventions for persons with similar disabilities.

However, even more so than mental illness—which might be viewed as transient—having mental retardation is often regarded as a devastating and very stigmatizing disability.

DEFINITION OF INTELLECTUAL DISABILITY

Esquirol is credited as the first medical writer to have penned a definition, in 1843, and his seminal characterization of intellectual disability as a disorder of development instead of a disease is maintained in all modern definitions (which require an onset during childhood or adolescence).

In the latter half of the 20th century, deficits in adaptive behavior have been formally included in all definitions of intellectual disability. Although meanings vary, adaptive behavior is typically viewed as the performance of behaviors required for social and personal sufficiency.

Both the DSM-IV and the tenth revision of the World Health Organization's International Statistical Classification of Diseases and Related Health Problems (ICD-10) specify an IQ of 70 or less in the diagnostic criteria for intellectual disability. IQ scores are presumably derived from standardized intelligence tests that meet appropriate psychometric criteria for reliability and validity.

ICD-10	**Codes for mental retardation**	**(Axis 3)**
F70	Mild mental retardation	IQ 50–69
F71	Moderate mental retardation	IQ 35–49
F72	Severe mental retardation	IQ 20–34
F73	Profound mental retardation	IQ < 20

Prevalence of intellectual disability in the general population: 1–3%

Classification of causes of intellectual disability by etiology and frequency		
Etiology	*Examples*	*Estimated frequency (%)*
A. Prenatal causes		
1. **Genetic disorders**		4–28
Chromosomal aberrations	Down syndrome	
Monogenic mutations	Tuberous sclerosis, phenylketonuria and other metabolic disorders, fragile X syndrome	
Multifactorial	"Familial" mental retardation	
Malformation syndromes	Prader-Willi, Williams', Angelman's syndromes	
2. **Congenital malformations**		7–17
Malformations of the central nervous system	Neural tube defects	
Multiple malformation syndromes	Cornelia de Lange syndrome	
3. **Exposure**		5–13
Maternal infections	Congenital rubella, HIV	
Teratogens	Fetal alcohol syndrome	
Toxemia/placental insufficiency	Prematurity	
Other	Radiation, trauma	
B. Perinatal causes		2–1
1. Infections	Meningitis	
2. Delivery problems	Asphyxia	
3. Other	Hyperbilirubinemia	
C. Postnatal causes		3–12
1. Infections	Encephalitis	
2. Toxins	Lead poisoning	
3. Other postnatal causes	Traumas, brain tumors	
4. Psychosocial problems	Poverty, psychotic illness	
D. Unknown cause		30–50

ETIOPATHOLOGY OF MENTAL RETARDATION

Congenital Causes

Among chromosomal disorders Down's syndrome, Fragile-X syndrome and Prader-Willi syndrome are common.

Abnormalities in autosomal chromosome are associated with mental retardation, although aberration in sex chromosome are not always associated with mental retardation (such as Turner's syndrome with XO and Klinefelter's syndrome with XXY, XXXY and XXYY variation.)

Fragile X Syndrome

Fragile X syndrome, the most common inherited cause of intellectual disability, results in a wide range of learning and behavioral problems, with males being more often and more severely affected than females. As many as 1 in 4,000 males and 1 in 8,000 females are fully affected with the syndrome.

Clinical features: Long face, large ears, mid-face hypoplasia, high, arched palate, short stature, macro-orchidism, mitral valve prolapse, joint laxity, strabismus, hyperactivity, inattention, anxiety, stereotypies, speech and language delays, IQ decline, gaze aversion, social avoidance, shyness, irritability, learning disorder in some females, mild mental retardation in affected females, moderate to severe in males, verbal IQ > performance IQ.

Down's Syndrome

Down's syndrome has remained the most investigated and the most discussed syndrome in mental retardation. Children with the syndrome were originally called mongoloid because of their physical characteristics of slanted eyes, epicanthal folds, and flat nose.

Prevalence: 1 in 1,000 live births; 1 in 2,500 in women < 30 years old; 1 in 80 in women > 40 years old, 1 in 32 in women 45 years old.

Pathology: Three types of chromosomal aberration occur in this syndrome:

1. Trisomy 21 (three of chromosome 21, instead of the usual two.)
2. Non-disjunction of chromosome 21 is the most common cause, occurring after fertilization in any cell division results in mosaicism, a condition in which both normal and trisomic cells are found in various tissues.
3. In translocation there is a fusion of two chromosomes.

Clinical features of Down's syndrome: More than 80 clinical features characterize the phenotype of DS, including cognitive impairments, hypotonia, facial dysmorphisms, congenital heart disease, and other anomalies. The stereotype of a "Down personality" as being happy, good tempered, affectionate, placid, and stubborn has been difficult to verify. Intellectual disability is usually mild and these patients are often described as being socially adept and somewhat less prone to psychiatric disturbance than controls.

Co-morbidity with Intellectual Disability

Developmental disability is a significant risk factor for psychopathology in general. Individuals with IQ less than 70 have a two- to five-fold higher rate of psychiatric disorders overall compared with typically developing persons. Persons with intellectual disability are typically referred for evaluation because of self-injurious, aggressive, impulsive, or hyperactive behavior. If the behavior is of recent onset, it is more likely to consider an acute medical or psychiatric etiology. If the behavior is highly situational, occurring primarily in the context of the stress of task demands, the likelihood of a psychosis or mood disorder is probably reduced.

- ADHD is found in 9–18 percent of those with intellectual disability.
- Autism is reported in about 5 percent of patients with fragile X syndrome
- *Impulse control disorders:* Self-injury and aggression are the common reasons for referral for psychiatric consultations (up to 36 percent was reported in one study).
- Anxiety disorders including OCD and avoidant behavior are often seen but many of the intellectually disabled persons may be unable to articulate their subjective states or feelings. Reports on prevalence have been variable ranging from 1 to 25 percent.
- *Eating disorders:* Pica is perhaps the most common eating disorder reported.
- *Psychosis:* Patients with intellectual disability are at an increased risk for schizophrenia (approximately 1 per cent); bipolar disorders are not uncommon.

Prader-Willi Syndrome

Pathology: Prader-Willi syndrome is postulated to be the result of small deletion involving chromosome 15, usually occurring sporadically.

Signs: Compulsive eating behavior and often obesity, mental retardation, hypogonadism, small stature, hypotonic, small hands and feet. Children with the syndrome often have oppositional and defiant behavior.

Traumatic: Head Injury

The best known causes of head injury in children which produce developmental handicaps including seizures, are motor vehicle accidents, but more head injuries are caused by house hold accidents, such as falls from tables, from open windows and on stair ways.

Infective

Rubella

The children of affected mothers may show several abnormalities including congenital heart diseases, mental retardation, cataracts, deafness, microcephaly.

Timing is crucial as extent of frequency of the complications is inversely related to the duration of pregnancy at the time of maternal infections. When mothers are infected in the first trimester of pregnancy 10–15 percent, children are affected but the incidence rises to almost 50 percent, when the infections occur in the first month of pregnancy.

Cytomegalic Inclusion Disease

In many cases, cytomegalic inclusion disease remains dormant in the mother. Some children are stillborn, and others have jaundice, microcephaly, hepatosplenomegaly, and radiographic findings of intracerebral calcification. Children with mental retardation from the disease frequently have cerebral calcification, microcephaly or hydrocephalus. The diagnosis is confirmed by positive finding of virus in throat and urine cultures and by the recovery of inclusion-bearing cells in the urine.

Syphilis

Syphilis in pregnant women was once the main cause of various neuropathological changes in their offspring, including mental retardation.

Toxoplasmosis

Toxoplasmosis can be transmitted from the mother to the fetus. It causes mild or severe mental retardation and in severe cases, hydrocephalus, seizures, microcephaly and chorioretinitis.

Metabolic

Phenylketonuria

It is an inborn error of metabolism. Phenylketonuria (PKU) is transmitted as a simple recessive autosomal mendelian trait.

Pathalogy: The basic metabolic defect in phenylketonuria is an inability to convert phenylalanine, an essential amino acid, to paratyrosine because of the absence or inactivity of the liver enzyme phenylalanine hydroxylase, which catalyses the reaction.

Signs: Most patient with phenylketonuria are severely retarded but some are reported to have borderline or normal intelligence. Eczema, vomiting, convulsion are often present. Children suffering are typically hyperactive, exhibit erratic unpredictable behavior and are difficult to manage. Verbal and non-verbal communication is usually severely impaired or non-existent children's co-ordination is poor.

Lesch-Nyhan Syndrome

Lesch-Nyhan syndrome is a rare disorder caused by a deficiency of an enzyme involved in purine metabolism.

The disorder is X-linked; patients have mental retardation, microcephaly, seizures, choreoathetosis and spasticity. The syndrome also associated with severe compulsive self-mutilation by biting of the mouth and the fingers.

Lesch-Nyhan syndrome is an example of genetically determined syndrome in which a specific behavioral pattern is predictable.

Cretinism

Goitrous cretinism is a common cause of mental retardation in India. It is endemic in iodine-deficient areas like the goitrous Himalayan belt.

Early recognition and treatment is essential as it is a preventable cause of mental retardation.

Clinical features include goitre, dwarfism, coarse skin, ossification delays, apathy, hoarseness of voice, large tongue, subnormal temperature, potbelly, anaemia, hypotonia of muscles, hypertelorism and mental retardation.

Neurological

Cerebral Palsy

This is a syndrome consisting of a conglomeration of perinatal disorders of various etiologies, presenting with a common feature of paralysis of limbs.

The paralysis may be monoplegia, hemiplegia, triplegia, or quadriplegia. It is usually of upper motor neurone type, presenting with spasticity.

The extrapyramidal symptoms may be present and seizures occur often. Mental retardation is present in about 70 percent, of all cases and ranges from mild to severe.

Intoxication

Alcohol, Opium, Cocaine, Bromide, Lead

There is no doubt that severe lead intoxication can cause an encephalopathy with consequent intellectual impairment. It is less certain whether small amount of lead taken over longer periods (especially as a result of air pollution from lead additives in petrol) can cause intellectual impairment. It is known that children absorb lead more readily than adults and are therefore, at greater risk from environmental pollution. However, most of the studies have been of children from poor homes, and it is impossible to be certain how far findings of low intelligence (compared with children in other areas) are due to slightly raised levels in their blood, and how far to social influences.

Lewis (1929) distinguished two type of mental retardation

1. *Sub-cultural:* The lower end of the normal distribution curve often of intelligence in the population
2. *Pathological:* Due to specific disease process

In a study of 1280 mentally retarded people living in Colchester asylum, Penrose (1938) found that most cases were due not to a single cause, but due to interaction of inherited and environmental factors. Subsequent evidence has confirmed that mental retardation has multiple causes (Mackay 1982). This finding applies particularly to mild mental retardation in which it is unusual to find a single specific cause. Among the severely retarded, however, postmortem examination shows pathological causes in the majority (Crome and Stern 1972). Although not all these can be identified in life.

The relative frequencies of various causes show	
Environmental causes in	20%
Chromosomal	15%
Single gene disorder	10%
No cause found	60%

CLINICAL FEATURES OF MENTAL RETARDATION

1. *Mild mental retardation (IQ-50–70):* This group accounts for about four-fifth of the mentally retarded. Appearance is unremarkable and any sensory or motor deficits are slight. Mental retardation may not be identified until the start of schooling. They may need help under unusual stress.
2. *Moderate mental retardation (IQ-35–49):* This group accounts for about 12% of the mentally retarded. Most of them can talk or at least learn to communicate and most

can learn to care for themselves. They can undertake simple routine work.

3. *Severe mental retardation (IQ-20–34):* This group accounts for about 7% of mentally retarded. In pre-school year their development is usually greatly slowed. Many of them can be trained to look after themselves under close supervision and to communicate in a simple way. Adults can undertake simple tasks and engage in limited social activities.
4. *Profound mental retardation (IQ-<20):* This group accounts for less than 1% of mentally retarded. Few of them—learn to care for themselves completely, some eventually achieve simple behavior and social behavior.

ETIOPATHOLOGY OF MENTAL ILLNESS

A. Psychogenic

a. **Environmental:** First few years of life is accepted as formative part of life as most of the time of child is spent with parents. So a faulty guardianship with defective attitude/imbalanced behavior, lack of love and affection may affect mental make up.

b. **Mental:** Unsuccessful attempt to express mental conflicts between the instinctive desires and his wishes, ideas and ethical codes. When efforts to reconcile with these fails, anxiety and tension ensue leading to mental symptoms.

c. **Personality maladjustment:** Failure of a person to adjust with changing life situations may result in nervous breakdown.

B. Organic

a. Degenerative diseases—Senile degeneration, arteriosclerosis, case of head injury, cerebral haemorrhage

b. Metabolic disorders—Myxoedema, thyrotoxicosis, diabetes.

c. Miscellaneous—Addiction to alcohol

C. Heredity

As in case of Hutington's chorea, epilepsy, amaurotic family disease, idiocy, etc.

D. Congenital Anomalies

Intrauterine maldevelopment of central nervous system as seen in idiots, imbecile and morons.

E. Immediate Precipitating Factors

Failure in various spheres of life like love, marriages, business or work, anxiety over health, over work, fatigue, death of beloved relatives, etc. may lead to mental disorders.

PROCEDURE OF EXAMINATION

1. Preliminaries

Name
Age/Sex
Address
Place
Date of examination

2. Family History

To enquire whether any of his blood relations have any history of suffering from mental diseases, epilepsy, etc. or any one has committed suicide or was attacked by cerebral affection or syphilis.

3. Personal History

To be taken from patient himself and also from his relatives if available about:

- Duration of present complaint.
- History of any previous mental illness.
- Its nature, duration and how it got cured.
- Upbringing of the patient from childhood onwards.

Prenatal care and protection from childhood. Conflicts or maladjustment during childhood. Emotional fixation to parents, frustration in love and sex, inferiority complex, family trouble, financial or business worries. History of dependence on alcohol, cannabis, barbiturates, LSD, opium. History of head injury during birth in childhood or in later life. Usual sexual indulgence, masturbation, any change in habits, moods or sleep.

4. Socioeconomic History

Financial, Service position.

5. Behavioral Assessment

Based on observations by the clinical team of patient ability to care for himself, his social abilities including his ability to communicate, his sensory motor skills and any unusual behavior.

6. Psychiatric Assessment

a. ***Appearance:*** Manner of dressing, cleanliness, look-vacant or fixed, facial expression masked/making faces.
b. ***Posture and gait*** Hurried/Stealthy or aimless.
c. ***Mood:*** Whether emotional, excitable, irritable, exalted euphoric or apathetic or depresses or touchy, moody.
d. ***Speech arid talk:*** Any evidence of aphonia, asphyxia, thrilling, stammering, lisping, slurring, neologism, echolalia, coherent, meaningful relevant, wandering.
e. ***Memory and intelligence:*** Good or bad, capacity for apperception, degree of concentration and apperception, capacity for grasping.
f. ***Attention:*** whether attentive or fluctuating, careful or careless.
g. ***Writing:*** whether agraphic, intelligent or illegible, complete or incomplete. If writes obscene or insulting language, relevant or irrelevant.
h. ***Orientation:*** Present, absent or impaired.
i. ***Sleep:*** whether suffers from insomnia, hypo or hypersomnia, somnambulism, somnolentia.
j. ***Thought content:*** Any thought disorder, delusion, illusion, hallucination or obsession or thought process retarded, pre-occupied, ambivalent or double oriented.

7. Developmental Assessment

Based on a combination of clinical experience and standardized methods of measuring intelligence, language, motor performances and social skills. Although the IQ is the best general index of intellectual development, it is not reliable in very young.

8. Attitude to Opposite Sex

To ensure about any abnormal sex behavior, to opposite sex or same sex, sex perversions propensities to unnatural sex offences, like or dislike of talk on sex, sex related matters.

Physical Examination:

a. *Head*—any congenital anomalies as to shape size or other abnormality, microcephaly or cleft palate.
b. *Eyes*—any proptosis, defect of vision, pupils, accommodation, nystagmus
c. *Nose*—bridge-flattened or normal.
d. *Ears*—hearing-normal or defective.
e. *Tongue*—clean, foul or furred
f. *Limbs*—longer or shorter than normal
g. *Skin*—dry, moist more hairy, etc.
h. *Genitals*—any abnormality—congenital or acquired
i. ***Pulse/Respiration/Temperature/Blood Pressure.***

It is important to be alert for the physical signs of the many specific syndromes. The neurological examination should include particular attention to vision and hearing.

DIAGNOSIS

The diagnosis can be made by the following steps:

1. History
2. General physical examination
3. Detailed neurological examination
4. Mental status examination for associated

psychiatric disorders and clinical assessment of level of intelligence

5. Investigations:
   i. Routine investigations
   ii. Urine test, e.g. for phenylketonuria, maple syrup urine
   iii. EEG especially in presence of Epilepsy
   iv. Blood levels for inborn errors of metabolism
   v. Chromosomal studies—Downs syndrome
   vi. CT scan brain—Tuberous sclerosis, focal seizures, unexplained neurological syndrome, anomalies of skull configuration
   vii. Thyroid function tests: Cretinism
   viii. Liver function tests
6. **Psychological tests:** For assessment of intelligence
   i. Seguin form board test Stanford-Binnet, Binnet-Simon or Binnet-Kamath test.
   ii. Wechsler's intelligence scale for children—for 6.5 to 16 years of age.
   iii. Wechsler's pre-school and primary scale of intelligence for 4 to 6.5 years of age.
   iv. Raven's progressive matrices Assessment of adaptive behavior include
      - Vineland social maturity scale (VSMS)
      - Denever development screening test
      - Gessell development scale test

Differential Diagnosis

The diagnosis of the mental retardation is usually simple. However, while making this diagnosis following conditions must be kept in mind, as they can be and are many times mistaken for mental retardation, with disastrous results.

- Deaf and dumb (to be ruled out by clinical examination or audiometry).
- Deprived children with inadequate social stimulation (although this can also cause mental retardation. Many children become normal intellectually on providing adequate stimulation).
- Isolated speech defect.
- Psychiatric disorders like infantile autism, childhood onset schizophrenia. Systemic disorders (without mental retardation but with physical debiliation). Epilepsy.

CLASSIFICATION OF MENTAL ILLNESS

No satisfactory classification of mental illness can be given covering all aspects of various mental disease. Etiological classification suits the medicolegal purpose better than the clinical classification or WHO classification.

A. Clinical Classification

1. Developmental : Mental Deficiency or Amentia

a. Idiot
b. Imbecile
c. Feeble minded (moron)

2. Organic Disorders

i. Degenerative brain disease or dementia:
   a. Presenile dementia
   b. Senile, dementia
   c. Organic dementia
   d. Dementia paralyt
   e. Primary dementia or schizophrenia
   f. Dementia following head injury.

ii. Psychosis associated with organic diseases of nervous system:
   a. Epilepsy

iii. Due to syphilitic infection of CNS:
   a. GPI (General paralysis insane)

iv. Psychosis associated with other cerebral disorders:
   a. Cerebral arterial disorders

b. Hypertension with atherosclerosis
c. Lethargic encephalitis
d. Sydenhams chorea
e. Disseminated chorea

v. Psychosis associated with confusional insanity due to intoxication by:
a. Alcohol—Delirium tremens, Korsakoff psychosis
b. Opium groups
c. Cocaine
d. Bromide
e. Cannabis
f. Other habit-forming drugs.

vi. Mental illness due to intracranial infections and other disorders:
a. Viral and other infectious disease
b. Toxemias of pregnancy
c. Haemorrhages from various causes

vii. Mental illness due to metabolic and endocrine disorders:
a. Diabetes
b. Pernicious anaemia
c. Pellagra
d. Thyrotoxicosis
e. Myxedema
f. Tetany
g. Pituitary
h. Sexual disorders

3. Functional Psychosis

a. Schizophrenia: Simple-Schizoaffective —Hebephrenic—Latent—Catatonic—Residual—Paranoid—Unspecified

4. Affective Disorders

a. Excitement—Mania, Hypomania
b. Depression—X-Involuntary Melancholia
c. Y—Manic depressive reaction.
d. Anxiety

5. Neurosis

a. Anxiety neurosis
b. Hysterical neurosis
c. Phobic neurosis
d. Obsessive compulsive neurosis
e. Depressive neurosis
f. Depersonalization syndrome.

6. Personality Disorders

a. Psychopathic
b. Delinquent
c. Sexual deviations
d. Drug dependence.

WHO Classification

International statistical classification	
S. No. I	*Psychosis*
300	Schizophrenic disorders
301	Manic depressive reactions
302	Involutional melancholia
303	Paranoia and paranoid state
304	Senile psychosis
305	Presenile psychosis
306	Psychosis with cerebral arteriosclerosis
307	Alcoholic psychosis
308	Psychosis of other demonstrable etiology
309	Other unspecified psychosis
S.No.II	*Psychoneurotic reaction*
310	Anxiety reaction without mention of somatic symptoms
311	Hysterical reaction without mention of somatic symptoms
312	Phobic reaction
313	Obsessive compulsive reaction
314	Neurotic depressive reaction
315	Psychoneurosis with mention of somatic symptoms (affecting circulatory system)
316	Psychoneurosis with mention of somatic symptoms (affecting digestive system)
317	Psychoneurosis with somatic symptoms (affecting other systems)
318	Psychoneurotic disorders—others mixed and unspecified types

Contd.

Contd.

S. No.III.	*Disorders of character, behavior and intelligence*
319	Pathological personality
320	Immature personality
321	Alcoholism
322	Drug addiction
324	Primary childhood behavior
324	Mental deficiency
325	Other unspecified character, behavior, and intelligent disorders

INTELLIGENCE TEST

A patient (suspect) may be more intelligent than is suggested by the score, he obtains on an intelligence test. Anxiety, ill health, psychosis, unwillingness to co-operate, stimulation of mental disorder, lack of schooling, cultural isolation or a cultural background different from the group for whom the test was designed are factors, which may impair a person's function on an intelligence test. A skillful psychologist may be able to estimate the probable effects of such factors and thereby arrive at an approximate estimate of the suspect's potential intelligence.

The test behavior of the mental defective follows a definite predictable pattern, which is different from that of the malingerer. In general according to Hunt, the malinger will not fail the same items that the mental deficient does, and when he does fail the same items, he fails in a different fashion.

In reporting on the result of an intelligence test the psychologist should not confine himself to giving a bare statement of the IQ. He should indicate whether or not any factors were present, which might have interfered with the suspects test performance. The IQ figure should be further explained by stating whether the suspect is mentally defective or dull normal, average, bright normal, superior intelligence, borderline, mild, moderate or severe mentally retarded.

The diagnostic and statistical manual, mental disorders published by the American Pediatric Association states that a diagnosis of mild mental deficiency refers to functional [vocational] impairment, as would be expected with IQ of approximately 70–85. To refer a person with an IQ in this range as being mentally defective appears uncharitable.

The Wechsler Adult Intelligence Scale [WAIS] is more satisfactory for with criminal suspects than the Stanford-Binet Test [1937].

PERSONALITY TEST: THEMATIC APPERCEPTION TEST (TAT)

Thematic apperception test consists of 30 pictures of ambiguous social situations. The pictures are presented in a special sequence [specified order] to the subject [some of the pictures differs from men, women, boys and girls]. The subject is requested to tell a story about the picture indicating what he thinks is happening in the picture and what he thinks will be the outcome of the situation he has depicted.

The test differs from the Rorschach Test in so far as the stimulus material has a more obvious social meaning and concerns the interpersonal dynamics of the individual.

Nevertheless, the TAT in the hands of a skilled clinical psychologist can provide important evidence in the total clinical picture.

INTELLIGENCE QUOTIENT

Intelligence input all round efficiency of any subject's cognitive faculties. It is the combination of cognition (knowledge), affection (feeling), imagination, reasoning and judgment.

Intelligence quotient is shortly known as IQ. This is a process by which the intellectual capacity of a person is established. The mental age of a person is calculated, through performance of tests (Binnet-Simon test). When the mental age is divided by his actual age and multiplied by 100, it will denote IQ, i.e.

$$\frac{\text{Mental age}}{\text{Actual age}} \times 100 = \text{IQ}.$$

An IQ of 50 means that the individual's mental abilities are 50% of his age. Though with the increasing age the mental abilities will increase but generally the IQ will remain the same, i.e. at the age of 16 his abilities will be of 8 years.

Most of the intelligence test assumes a fixed age of 16 years for calculation of IQ.

Evaluation

Evaluation is based upon the classification of mental development: I.Q. Level:

1. 130 and above — veiy superior
2. 120–129 — superior
3. 110–119 — bright normal
4. 90–109 — average
5. 80–89 — dull normal
6. 70–79 — borderline
7. 50–69 — mild mental retardation
8. 35–49 — moderate mental retardation
9. 20–34 — severe mental retardation
10. < 20 — profound mental retardation

The evaluation is based on:

1. Thematic apperception test.
2. Rorschach-Binet test
3. Stanford Binet test
4. Wechsler adult intelligence scale (WAIS)
5. Binet-Kamath test of intelligence
6. Raven's progressive matrices
7. Bhatia's battery of intelligence
8. Welhsler child intelligence test
9. Questionnaire to the patient or guardian.

PROFORMA FOR THE DETAILED ASSESSMENT OF MENTALLY RETARDED PERSONS

Instructions: This is largely structured Proforma; hence all items should be filled, answered, even it is "not known" or "not applicable". If any elaboration of a particular item is needed the empty space in the end of each major section should be utilised.

I. Socio-demographic Data

Name: Income:
Sex: Mother Tongue:
Age: Address:
Date of assessment:

II. Complaints

a. Source of referral
b. Informant
c. Reliability: Reliable/unreliable Adequate/inadequate
d. Chronological list of complaints, with duration.

III. Family History

a. Genetic diagram

(Preferably three generations, with use of internationally accepted symbols and indicating abortions, perinatal deaths, twins, affected members, etc.)

b. Family history of illness
c. Consanguinity among parents: Father married to:

Sister's daughter, mother's brother's daughter, father's sister's daughter, mother's sister's daughter, father's brother's daughter (encircle the appropriate)

d. Parental background (Give age, education, occupation, any other relevant detail)

Father:

Mother:

e. Current living arrangement (Describe family setup)

IV. Prenatal Factors (State of Mother During Pregnancy)

Tick and describe the appropriate:

a. Nutritional status

b. Exposure to medication including drug abuse and irradiation

c. Infections (mention trimester):

1. Measles, mumps, chickenpox
2. Fever with or without other symptoms
3. Syphilis
4. Any other disease in mother:
   i. Diabetes ii. Pre-eclampsia
   iii. Toxemia iv. Anemia
   v. Psychiatric vi. Hypothyroidism
   vii. Any other.

V. Perinatal Factors (Including Neonatal)

a. *Labour*: Normal/abnormal (if abnormal, tick the appropriate and describe as follows)

i. Premature
ii. Postmature
iii. Prolonged labor
iv. Foetal distress
v. Assisted labor
vi. Abnormal
vii. Placenta previa, cord round the neck, etc.
viii. Induced labor
ix. others

b. *Child at birth*:

i. Birth weight
ii. Cry normal/delayed/no cry
iii. Cyanosis (APGAR score)
iv. Jaundice in available
v. Congenital anomalies

c. *First two weeks*:

i. Respiratory distress
ii. Cyanotic attacks
iii. Jaundice
iv. High fever
v. Fits
vi. Feeding problem
vii. Hypoglycemia,
viii. Other—Hypocalcemia

VI. Past Medical History (From 2 week to till date)

(Tick the relevant items and describe)

a. Feeding problems
b. Failure to thrive
c. Immunization history
d. Recurrent respiratory infections
e. Convulsion, epilepsy
f. Fever with loose motions and/or altere sensorium
g. Trauma or poisoning
h. Behavior disorders
i. Childhood neurotic traits
j. Autistic features
k. Self injurious behavior
l. Others (skin problems, abnormal smell of sweats, eczema, etc.)

VII. Developmental History

a. Delay first noticed at

b. Motor milestones:

i. Head control
ii. Sit with support
iii. Stand with support
iv. Walk with support
v. Walk without support
vi. Limb upstairs

c. Speech and language:

i. Babbling
ii. Two words
iii. Sentences
iv. Names, colors

d. Adaptive:

i. Grasp with whole hand

ii. Grasp between thumb and fingers
iii. Play with ball
iv. Avoid common dangers
v. Imaginative play
vi. Can write a few alphabets

e. Personal/Social:
i. Smiles at mother
ii. Can recognize father
iii. Responds to name
iv. Dress self
v. Toilet trained

f. Schooling:
i. Started at
ii. General performance
iii. Highest class achieved
iv. Specific reading, writing, arithmetic problems

g. Brief description of current level of development, including mother's estimation of the mental age.

VIII. Physical Examination

Under each item, some common anomalies are listed: The examiner should screen the child for these, or any other abnormalities and mention them below each item.

a. General

Facies: Mongoloid, gargoylism, round, elongated

Head circumference: cms: length/height and breadth of head.

Shape of the head Micro, macro, dolicho, oxycephaly

Physical growth : Height ________
Weight ________

Built: Short stature, dwarfism, gigantism, obese, emaciated

Skin: Abnormal color and thickness, pigmentation, naevi, cafe-are-lait spots, tuber, eczema, ichthyosis

Hair: Light or grey colored, sparse, excessive body hair, brittle

Vision: Diminished , absent, night blindness, refractive error

Eyes: Look for anomalies such as bushy eye brows, eyebrows meeting in center, slanting of palpebral fissure, epicanthic folds, hypertelorism, microcorneal clouding. Corneal opacities, cataract, nystagmus, squint, blue sclera, any other

Hearing: Partial or total deafness

Ears: Low set, posterior, simplified, malformed, lop-ears, long ears

Nose: Short, depressed bridge, flaring, beak shaped

Oral cavity: Look for cleft lip and palate, high arched palate, malformed dentition, fissured tongue, etc.

Other facial features: Long philtrum, submental region, forehead, etc.

Limbs: Short, long, asymmetric, increased carrying angle

Hand and feet: Simian crease, sidny line, poly or syndatly flat feet, weebing, little finger, anomalies-describe

Chest: Including heart and respiratory systems (pigeon chest, murmurs, pectus excavatum, pectus carinatum, gynecomastia, displaced nipple, etc.)

Abdomen: Distended, biumbilical, or inguinal hernia, hepatospleenomagaly

Neck and spine: Weabing, short neck, kyphoscoliosis, post anal dimple, spina bifida, gibbus

External genitalia: Hypospadias, undescended testis, large testis. Secondary sexual characters: Skeletal anomalies:

Neurologic: Specially look for hypotonia, cerebral palsy, movement disorders, posture, involuntary movements, extraocular movements, fundal examination, tone, bulk, reflexes, co-ordination gait, power, pupils

b. Behavioral

Attention: Dull, retarded, apathetic, distractible

Activity: Retarded, hyperkinetic, quiet

Sociability: Autistic features-describe

Mood: Irritable, smiling, temper-tantrums, tearful

Motor: Stereotypes, tics, self-injurious behavior

Any other: Has he/she any of the following behavioral problems? (Enquire each item)

1. Present 2. Absent
   a. Violent behavior
   b. Overactive, cannot sit at one place
   c. Sleep disturbances
   d. Muttering and laughing at self

IX. Development History

Current development of subject (enquire each item)

1. Yes 2. No

Motor Development

a. Holds head
b. Rolls over
c. Sits up
d. Crawls
e. Stands
f. Climbs stairs
g. Runs
h. Rides tricycles
i. Rides bicycles

Language

a. Cannot make comprehensible
b. Can talk in full sentences
c. Can hold a conversation
d. Any speech abnormality

Specially speech abnormalities like slurring stammering and echolalic.

Social Development

a. Toilet trained
b. Feeds self
c. Dresses self
d. Avoids common danger

General Abilities

a. Can identify common persons
b. Can identify common objects
c. Can follow simple instructions
d. Can identify colours
e. Can follow complex instructions
f. Can do simple calculations
g. Can do simple shopping

Other Abilities (Specify)

Clinical impression of mental retardation

1. Mild 2. Moderate
3. Severe 4. Profound

Psychological assessment:

1. Done 2. Not done

If assessment done:

A. Vineland social maturity scale:
   a. Social age (in months)
   b. Social quotient

B. Siguin form board test:
   a. Administered
   b. Could not be administered

If administered:
   a. Mental age (in months)
   b. IQ scores

Binnet—Kamath Intelligence Test:
   i. Administered
   ii. Could not administered

Specify reasons

If administered
   a. Mental age (in months)
   b. IQ scores

X. Comprehensive Diagnosis

1. Degree of retardation
2. Possible aetiology and/or syndromal diagnosis

3. Associated medical problems
4. Associated psychiatric problems
5. Impressions regarding parental knowledge and expectations

XI. Management Plan

a. Investigations:
   i. Further exploration of history
   ii. More detailed examination
      - Visual assessment
      - Hearing assessment
      - Pediatric assessment
      - Neurologic assessment
   iii. Biochemical (name)
   iv. Cytogenic study
   v. Radiological
   vi. Clinical photograph
   vii. Psychometric
   viii. Others (Skin biopsy, endocrinologic)

b. Intervention:
   i. Parental counselling (Individual)
   ii. Parental counselling (Group)
   iii. Speech therapy
   iv. Physiotherapy
   v. Nutritional counselling
   vi. Genetic counselling
   vii. Behavioral therapy
   viii. Referral to special school
   ix. Referral to occupational therapy and rehabilitation
   x. Admission to family ward
   xi. Self help group
   xii. Medication

XII. Name and Signature of the Person who Worked up the Case

XIII. Consultant Remarks

IDEAS

(INDIAN DISABILITY EVALUATION AND ASSESSMENT SCALE)

A scale for measuring and quantifying disability in mental disorders developed by the rehabilitation committee of the Indian Psychiatric Society 2002

I. Description of "IDEAS"

General Guidelines

- IDEAS is suited best for the purpose of measuring and certifying disability.
- It is, therefore, a brief and simple instrument, which can be used, even in busy clinical settings.
- Some training is required in the use of IDEAS.
- This is to be used only on out-patients and those living in the community, not appropriate for in-patients.
- Rating should be done only based on interviews of the primary care givers. Case records and patient's interviews can be used to supplement information.
- Only in rare instances when no primary care giver is available should the rating be based only on patient interview. This should then be documented.
- The gender specification "he" has been used for convenience and refers to both genders.
- Probe question help to guide one through the interview and to help identify dysfunction in one or more activities.

Diagnostic Categories

Patients with only the following diagnoses as per ICD or DSM criteria are eligible for disability benefits. Schizophrenia bipolar disorder dementia.

Obsessive Compulsive Disorder

Duration of Illness

The total duration of illness should be at least two years. For scoring, the number of months the patient was symptomatic in the (MI2Y-months of illness in the last two years) should be determined.

Who does the assessment?

Only the psychiatrist can do diagnosis and certification. Trained social workers, psychologist, or occupational therapist can do administration of IDEAS.

Frequency of Re-certification: Psychiatric disability will be re-assessed every two years and re-certified. The feasibility of doing this in the rural areas will however has to be examined. Items:

i. *Self care:* includes taking care of the body hygiene, grooming, health including bathing. Toileting, dressing, eating, and taking care of one's health.

ii. *Interpersonal Activities (Social Relationship):* Includes initiating and Maintaining interaction with others in a contextual and socially appropriate manner.

iii. *Communication and understanding:* Includes communication and conversation with others by producing and comprehending spoken/written/nonverbal messages.

iv. *Work*: These areas are Employment/Housework/Education measures and one aspect.

1. *Performing in work/job:* Performing in work/employment (paid)/self-employment/family concern and otherwise. Measure ability to perform tasks at employment completely and efficiently and in proper time, includes seeking employment.
2. *Performing in housework:* Maintaining in household including cooking, caring for other people at home, taking care of belongings, etc. Measure ability to take responsibility for and perform household tasks completely and efficiently and in proper time.
3. *Performing in school/college:* Measures Performance in education related tasks.

Scores of each item:

0 — no disability (none, absent, negligible)
1 — mild disability (slight, low)
2 — moderate disability (medium, fair)
3 — severe disability (high, extreme)
4 — profound disability (total, cannot do)
Total Score (range: 0–20)

Add scores of 4 items and obtain a total score MI2Y —months of illness in the last 2 years.

Interview with informant and case notes if available should be used to determine for how many months in the last two years the patient exhibited symptoms (Range: 1–4).

MI2Y—6 months: Score to be added is 1
7–12 months: Add 2
13–18 months: Add 3
18 months: Add 4

Global Disability

Total Disability score + MI2Y score = Global score (range: 1–20)

Percentage

For the purpose of welfare benefits, 40% will be cut off point. The score above 40% have been categorized as moderate, severe, profound based on the global disability score. The grading will be used to measure change over time. 1–7 Mild disability ≤ 40% and 8 above ≥ 40%

(8–13 moderate disability; 14–19 = severe disability; 20 = profound disability)

Manual for "IDEAS"

In order to score the instrument, information from all possible sources should be obtained. This will include interview of the patient, the care given and notes when available.

I. Self Care

This should be regarded as activity guided by social norms and conventions. The broad areas covered are:

a. Maintenance of personal hygiene and physical health.
b. Eating habits
c. Maintenance of personal belongings and living space.

Guiding Questions

a. Does he look after himself, wash his clothes regularly, take a bath and brush his teeth?
b. Does he have regular meals?
c. Does he take food of right quality and quantity?
d. Does he dress appropriately (weather condition, over dressing)
e. Does he take care of his personal belongings with reasonable standard of cleanliness and orderliness?

Scoring

0 = No disability

Patients level and pattern of self care are normal, within the sociocultural and economic context.

1 = Mild

Mild deterioration in self-care and appearance (not bathing, shaving, changing, clothes for the occasion as expected). Does not have adverse consequences such as hazards to his health. No embarrassment to family.

2 = Moderate

Lack of concern for self-care should be clearly established such as deterioration of physical health, obesity, tooth decay and body odours.

3 = Severe

Decline in self care should be marked in all areas. Patients wearing torn clothes, would only wash if made to and would only eat if told. Evidence of serious hazards to physical health (malnutrition, infection, patient unacceptable in public)

4 = Profound

Total or near total lack of self care (Example: risk to physical survival needs feeding, washing, putting on clothes, etc. constant supervision necessary.)

II. Inter-personal Activities

Includes patient's ability to form and maintain social relationships. This will be applicable to family, friends, colleagues and society at large. Ability for emotional response such as showing tolerance, responding to criticism or praise, and love and affection. Activities of engaging in physical intimacy. Ability to interact in a socially appropriate manner.

Guiding Questions

a. What is his behavior with others?
b. Do you think his behavior in social situations is appropriate?
c. What is the nature of his relationship with other family member?
d. Is he able to initiate social interaction on his own?
e. How does he behave with others?
f. Is he able to maintain friendship?
g. Does he show physical expression of affection and desire?

Scoring

0 = No

Patient gets along reasonably well with people. No friction in interpersonal relationships.

1 = Mild

Some difficulty in initiating and maintaining social interaction. Friction on isolated occasions. However his social behavior is generally acceptable to others.

2 = Moderate

Define difficulty in social interaction and interaction considered unhealthy. May be seen on more than one occasion. Could isolate himself from others and avoid company.

3 = Severe

Serious difficulty in initiating and maintaining social interaction. Behavior in social situations undesirable and generalized. Causes serious problems in daily living/or work. Patient is socially isolated.

4 = Profound

No attempts at engaging in any kind of social interaction. Family afraid of potential consequences.

III. Communication and Understanding

Understanding spoken messages as well as written and non-verbal messages. Ability to produce meaningful messages in order to communicate with others. Ability to converse in groups (such as chatting and discussing)

Use of communication devices such as telephone, e-mail, Internet, etc. Any reduction/excess of these behaviors should be considered. All modes of communication should be considered.

Guiding Questions

a. Does he avoid talking to people/talk excessively at times?
b. Is he able to start, maintain and end a conversion?
c. Does he indulge in reading, writing and other communication devices such as telephone, etc?
d. Are others able to comprehend his communication?
e. Do you need to encourage him to be more communicative?

Scoring

0 = No disability

Patient communicates with people as much as can be expected in his socio-cultural context. No difficulty in comprehension.

1 = Mild

Patient described as uncommunicative. Communication inappropriate (as in excitement). No active avoidance, but speaks only when spoken to.

2 = Moderate

A narrow range of communication. Communication can be too brief/in excess, incomplete or incomprehensible.

3 = Severe

Evidence of more generalized, active avoidance of any kind of communication, serious difficulty in comprehension.

4 = Profound

All communication is nil or a bare minimum. Communication totally incomprehensible.

IV. Work

This includes employment, house work and educational performance. (Score only one category in case of an overlap.)

Guiding Questions

a. Is he/she employed/unemployed/housewife/student?
b. If employed, does he goes to work regularly?
c. Does he like his job and is he coping well with it?
d. How is his competence at work?

Scoring

0 = No disability

Patient goes to work regularly and his output and quality of work performance are within acceptable levels for the job.

1 = Mild

Noticeable decline in patient's ability to work, cope with it and meet the demands of work, may threaten to quit.

2 = Moderate

Declining work performance, frequent absences, lack of concern about all this. Financial difficulties foreseen.

3 = Severe

Marked decline in work performance, disruptive at work, unwilling to adhere to disciplines of work. Threat of losing his job.

4 = Profound

Has been largely absent from his work, termination imminent. Unemployed, and making no efforts to find jobs.

Housewives

In similar ways, housewives should be rated on the amount, regularity and efficiency in which tasks in the following areas are completed. Consider the amount of help required completing these.

Acquiring daily necessities, making, storing and serving of food, cleaning the house, working with those helping with domestic duties such as maids, cooks, etc. looking after possessions and valuables in the house.

Students

Assess the score on performance in school/college, regularity, discipline, interest in future studies. Those who had to discontinue education on account of mental disability and unable to continue further should be given a score of 4.

The Indian Psychiatric Society through its taskforce has prepared simple assessment scale of mental disability for India. They have also enlisted the same by field study. It has been found by them that the face value, content value and criteria value have been quite acceptable, after the analysis of the field data and critical appraisal. Whether this is likely to be accepted into to by Government of India and other State and Union Territories in this country will become clear in due course. However, till then this document can have a place in the assessment for all people involved in the certification of psychiatric disability for the purpose of giving a percentage scoring. However the earlier system of certification may require to be continued till the administrative/legal obligation.

IDEAS

(INDIAN DISABILITY EVALUATION AND ASSESSMENT SCALE)
Scoring Sheet

Items
0
1
2
3
4

I. Self care
II. Interpersonal activities
III. Communication and understanding
IV. Work

A. Total score (I+II+III+IV) (Range 0–16)
B. MI2Y score (Range 1–4)
Global Score (A+B) (Range 1–20)
Percentage of disability (<40%/>40%)

Results of field studies

This was drawn from 8 centers all over the country. They were a good mixture of patients attending mental hospital, out-patient clinics of psychiatry in general hospital and rehabilitation centers. The four diagnostic groups were also included.

Total number of cases included in the field study = 1078
Centerwise distribution:

Bangalore (RFS) = 103

Kolkata (Antara) = 110

Chennai:

Imh = 160

Scarf = 260

Lucknow (KGM) = 100

Thrissur (GH) = 135

Trivandrum (GGH) = 100

Vellore (CMC) = 110

Gender and age distribution:

Males = 665 (61.6%)

Females = 413

Mean age of the patients + 37.4 ± 11.53
Mean duration of illness = 8.61 ± 6.55 years
This was the total duration of illness and not MI2Y.

Diagonostic Break-up
Schizophrenia = 560
Schizoaffective 13
Mood disorders:

- Depression =97
- Mania =116
- Bipolar disorder =198
- Dementia = 21
- OCD = 59
- Others = 14

Mean scores of items
N = 1078

Items	*Mean scores*	*Range*
Self care	0.97 ± 1.13	0–4
Interpersonal activities	1.54 ± 1.15	0–4
Communication and understanding	1.46 ± 1.18	0–4
Work	2.11 ± 1.42	0–4

a. Total score (Range 0–16) Mean = 6.05 ± 4.13
b. Total duration (Range 1–4) Mean = 2.88 ± 1.07
c. Global score (A + B) Mean = 8.93 ± 4.39
(Range 1–20)

- Please note that experience during field trails showed that it was rather difficult to compute total duration of illness in certain episodic illness. It was also felt that equating the duration of episodic disorders and chronic disorders would not be the right thing to do. Hence this has now been changed to months of illness during the last two years (MI2Y).

Reliability

Due to logistic reasons, it was not possible to conduct intercentre reliability exercises. Intercentre reliability was done in a few centers between two raters. The kappa value was 0.76 revealing the need for some training for the use of IDEAS.

Internal consistency was calculated. The alpha value was 0.8682 indicating good internal consistency between the items.

Validity

Face validity: The draft instrument was circulated among a team of mental health and disability professionals. Their opinions were sought as to whether at face value; the instrument appeared to be measuring the desired qualities. There was a general consensus on the 4 items of the instrument.

Content validity: During the work of some Indian centers on the ICIDH, several focus group discussions were held in SCARF for the purpose of this study. The group members consisting of, patients, families and professionals also felt that the items of the schedule were critical in the measurement of this disability.

Criterion validity was established by comparing IDEAS with SAPD (scheduled for the assessment of psychiatric disability), which has been standardized in India. Both these instruments were administered on 223 care givers at SCARF and also scored independently by two raters. Correlation for all the 4 items was good.

CONCLUSIONS

We now have a simple, but comprehensive instrument developed and standardized in India. It is primarily meant for measuring disability for the purpose of certification and, therefore, produces values, which can be converted into percentages similar to what is practiced for other disability. It can be used on the field in addition to busy clinical settings. It is largely dependent on the information provided by the primary care giver. Since it is on a 5-point scale, any changes occurring during re-assessments can be picked up.

Chapter

34

Marriage and Divorce

THE HINDU MARRIAGE ACT, 1955

Section 5. Conditions for a Hindu Marriage

5. A marriage may be solemnized between any two Hindus, if the following conditions are fulfilled, namely:

(i) **neither party** has a spouse living at the time of the marriage

1[(ii) at the time of the marriage, neither party

(a) is incapable of giving a valid consent to it in consequence of unsoundness of mind; or

(b) though capable of giving a valid consent, has been suffering from mental disorder of such a kind or to such an extent as to be unfit for marriage and the procreation of children; or

(c) has been subject to recurrent attacks of insanity or epilepsy.]

Section 13. Divorce

13. Divorce. (1) Any marriage solemnized, whether before or after the commencement of this Act, may, on a petition presented by either the husband or the wife, be dissolved by a decree of divorce on the ground that the other party;

1[(iii) has been incurably of unsound mind, or has been suffering continuously or intermittently from mental disorder of such a kind and to such an extent that the petitioner cannot reasonably be expected to live with the respondent.

Explanation: In this clause,

(a) the expression "mental disorder" means mental illness, arrested or incomplete development of mind, psychopathic disorder or any other disorder or disability of mind and includes schizophrenia;

(b) the expression "psychopathic disorder" means a persistent disorder or disability of mind (whether or not including subnormality of intelligence) which results in abnormally aggressive or seriously irresponsible conduct on the part of the other party, and whether or not it requires or is susceptible to medical treatment.]

MUSLIM MARRIAGE ACT, 1955

Divorce: The commonest mode of divorce by the husband is called Talaq.

Talaq confers on Muslim husband the privilege of being able to discard his wife whenever he chooses to do so for reasons good, bad or indifferent indeed for no reason at all.

The Dissolution of Muslim Marriage Act, 1939 enables a Muslim wife to seek divorce through court among other grounds, for impotency or insanity of the husband, and cruelty of the husband.

INDIAN CHRISTIAN DIVORCE ACT

The Indian Divorce Act deals with divorce among Christians. The reasons are almost similar to the ones under the Hindu Marriage Act. Roman Catholics do not come under the purview of any divorce proceedings since the Roman Catholic Church has not recognised divorce. The Divorce Act also does not contain any provision for divorce by mutual consent. Maintenance: During the period when the divorce case is in the court, the husband has to give one fifth of his salary for the maintenance of his wife. Later, maintenance can be given either yearly or once for all as total settlement. Custody: Custody of the child is decided by the court after going into the details of each individual case.

PART IV—NULLITY OF CHRISTIAN MARRIAGE

Section 18. *Petition for decree of nullity*: Any husband or wife may present a petition to the District Court or to the High Court, praying that his or her marriage may be declared null and void.

Section 19. *Grounds of decree*: Such decree may be made on any of the following grounds:

(1) that the respondent was impotent at the time of the marriage and at the time of the institution of the suit;

(3) that either party was a lunatic or idiot at the time of the marriage;

Nothing in this section shall effect the jurisdiction of the High Court to make decrees of nullity of marriage on the ground that the consent of either party was obtained by force or fraud.

CASE LAW

A S Mehta *vs* Bai Vasumati, AIR 1969 Guj.48: 10 Guj. LR 253

Insanity: Decree of nullity on the ground of unsoundness of mind of wife—It was found that wife was deaf and dumb by birth but was capable of managing herself and capable of discharging her marital obligations—In the circumstances, she cannot be held to be insane and marriage cannot be annulled.

Sudha Mehta vs Ravinder Mehta, 1990 Marriage L J 453 (P & H)

Insanity: Annulment of marriage on the ground that the wife suffered from recurrent attacks of epilepsy at the time of marriage—The doctors who examined her and diagnosed illness stated that she was suffering from epileptic attacks—Regarding condition of the wife it was stated by the doctor that fluid was coming out of the nose and froth from the mouth and the doctor advised the husband not to have intercourse with her and that it was attack of epilepsy—The medical evidence produced by the wife, did not rule out the fact that she was suffering from epilepsy—In the circumstances of the case the marriage was liable to be annulled.

Sunil Kumar *vs* Smt Jyoti alias Meena, 1988 Marriage L J 568 ((P & H)

Insanity—Annulment of marriage on the ground that the wife suffering from mental disorder since before the date of marriage and the same was concealed—The parties spent few days together for honeymoon immediately after marriage and the respondent though conceived but got aborted at the instance of the husband—Plea of insanity, therefore, rejected—Testimony of the doctor who examined the respondent also fell short of standard of proof to record a conclusion that the respondent was suffering from schizophrenia—The wife also offered to undergo any medical test—The plea of insanity therefore, rejected.

Bimla *vs* Baldev Raj, 1988 Marriage L J 1 (P & H)

Insanity: Husband pleading that the wife was suffering from mental disorder of such a kind that the petitioner could not be expected to live with her — It also came on the record that she was taken to mental hospital three or four times and was given electric shock and finally she was got admitted in mental hospital Amritsar as indoor patient and returned after 10 days being fully cured—There was no mention of electric shock being given in the record—therefore, nothing brought on the record that she was suffering from mental disorder at the time of marriage—Decree of divorce granted set aside.

V.Balakrishna *vs* V. Lalitha, AIR 1984 AP 225: 1984(1) APL J 32

Insanity: Annulment of marriage on the ground of epilepsy: The ground will be available only when the spouse had recurring attacks of epilepsy at the time of marriage—However, it is not true that recurrence as envisaged amounts to insanity only and not to epilepsy.

AIR 1982 Cal. 138: 1983 (1) DMC 457 (Del)

Insanity as a ground of annulment of marriage: Two elements are necessary: Firstly, the party concerned must be of unsound mind or intermittently suffering from mental disorder—Medical evidence showing that the wife was suffering from schizophrenia—Secondly, the parties were living together since 1975 and two children born out of wedlock—No such disease however, was found prior to July 1979—In these circumstances, the plea of insanity for annulling the marriage not accepted.

1980 Marriage L J 104 (P & H)

Insanity: Lunatic and idiot—Indicates total loss of reason of the last degree of mental disorder which incapacitates a person from marriage. Where the wife identified her husband in the court, her father and ten paise coin but could not total three ten paise coins, it can be said that she was not suffering from mental disorder and marriage could not be annulled being void—At the most it can be voidable.

AIR 1977 Punjab. 28. Insanity—Allegation of unsoundness of mind—No list of relatives filed by the husband as required under Order 32 Rule 3 CPC as applicable in Punjab and Haryana and the husband remained content by giving the description in the heading of the petition — Held, the decree of nullity will not be sustainable.

Insanity: Plea for annulment of marriage— Medical evidence showing that the mental ailment developed few days after the marriage and was not present at the time of marriage or even before the marriage—The statement of the wife before the doctor—She was having mental trouble from her childhood, will not be admissible—However, non-production of wife in the witness box on the advice of the doctor will not be fatal—In the circumstances, annulment of the marriage not granted.

Munishwar Datt vs Smt. Indra Kumari, AIR 1963 pb 449: ILR 1963 (2) pb. 263

Insanity as ground for dissolution of marriage, plea of insanity: Section. 12 (1) (b) of Hindu Marriage Act, 1955 lays down annulment of marriage in case one of the spouse was insane at the time of marriage—The onus is on the spouse taking plea of insanity—Where the permanent insanity is shown the burden is shifted on the respondent to show that the marriage was performed during lucid interval—The standard of proof in such cases must be beyond the reasonable doubt.

Munshwar Dutt vs Smt Indra Kumari AIR 1963 pb 449

Plea of insanity: Nature of unsoundness of mind: Attack of insanity when it amounts to mania or schizophrenia if it comes after marriage will not furnish a ground for annulling the marriage under section 12. Therefore, what is important is mental condition at the time of marriage, which is crucial time for determining the question of insanity as a ground for annulment.

Munishwar Dutt *vs* Smt. Indira Kumari, AIR 1963 SC pb. 449

Insanity: Standard of proof of insanity—In case it is shown that the respondent was suffering from permanent insanity, burden of proof to prove that marriage was solemnized during the period when the respondent was not under the attack of insanity will lie on the respondent.

The Times, 31 July 1963, MSL, January 1964, 55–56

Desertion—Insanity: In P *vs* P, the wife suffered from delusion that her husband intended to murder her, that he had broken her shoulder and that he had carried on various adulterous associations. After a short spell in hospital, she returned to her husband but then left him for good. Mr. Justice Llyod-Jones dismissed the husband's petition for divorce on the ground of desertion. He held that, although the wife knew she was leaving home she did not have an intention of deserting since she was acting under the force of her delusion that her husband intended to harm her.

(1962) 3 Wlr 422

Psychotic delusions: In Elphinstone v Elphinstone, a husband petitioned for divorce, on the grounds of cruelty. His wife had made various unfounded accusations against him and at a later stage of the marriage, physically attacked him. She was suffering from paranoid psychosis, which caused her to have delusions, that the husband was a hostile figure conspiring with others against her. In these accusations, she was wholly deluded, quite unable to appreciate that she was wrong; but save for the field covered by her delusions, she was a rational being, knew what she was doing and was able to distinguish right from wrong.

Ram Narain Gupta *vs* Rameshwari Gupta, (1998) 4 S.C.C.

For mental disorder to be a ground for divorce, the onus is to establish that its nature and degree is such that married life cannot be carried on.

The appellant approached the Court seeking the dissolution of his marriage on the ground of mental unsoundness, contained in Sec. 13 (1) (iii) of the Hindu Marriage Act, 1955. He alleged that the respondent suffered from a mental disorder of such a kind that it rendered the respondent unfit for married life and he could not be reasonably expected to live with her as had been decreed by the Court at the first instance but was dismissed by the High Court in Appeal.

Section 13 (1) (iii) of the Hindu Marriage Act, 1955 does not make the mere existence of a mental disorder of any degree sufficient in law to justify the dissolution of a marriage. The context in which the phrases 'unsoundness of mind' and 'mental disorder' occur in the section as grounds for dissolution of a marriage, require the assessment of the degree of the 'mental disorder'. Its degree must be such that the spouse seeking relief cannot reasonably be expected to live with the other. All mental abnormalities are not recognized as grounds for grant of decree. The personality disintegration that characterizes schizophrenia may be of varying degrees. The mere branding of a person as schizophrenic will not suffice. For purposes of Sec. 13 (1) (iii), 'Schizophrenia' is what schizophrenia does. Also the burden of proof of the existence of the requisite degree of mental disorder is on the spouse basing the claim on that state of facts.

Smt Asha Srivastava vs R.K. Srivastava, 1981 Marriage law JR 455 (Del)

Insanity: Annulment of marriage on the ground of mental health of the respondent:

- Medical evidence proving that the respondent was suffering from schizophrenia
- Though a marriage cannot be annulled on the basis of every misrepresentation or concealment, however, if there is a misrepresentation or concealment regarding a mental set concerning the respondent then the marriage can be annulled—Concealment about the ailment of schizophrenia which is a mental illness and is incurable according to the doctor, it would amount to obtaining the consent by fraud.

Gurnam Singh *vs* Chand Kaur @ Jaswinder Kaur, 1980 Marriage L J 104 (P & H)

Insanity: Allegation that the respondent was lunatic at the time of marriage and incapable of giving consent to the marriage and was unfit for marriage: However, no evidence produced to show that she was suffering from the said disease at the time of marriage—Mere mental disorder, is not sufficient for annulment of marriage—The doctor, a psychiatrist diagnosed that she was suffering from schizophrenia and prescribed drugs and she was given electroconvulsive therapy—According to the doctor, she was suffering from schizophrenia before she was married and even after marriage—According to Sec. 5 (of The Hindu Marriage Act, 1955) marriage cannot be solemnized if one of the party is suffering from mental disorder.

Schizophrenia as defined in Livingston's dictionary as a group of mental illnesses characterised by disorganization of the patient's personality resulting in chronic lifelong ill-health and hospitalization—Dementia praecox is a schizophrenic reaction which usually sets in between the ages of fifteen and thirty five years—However, inordinate delay of more than 9 years in filing the petition not explained and therefore, the annulment of the marriage refused.

Pranab Kumar Ghosh vs Krishna Ghosh, AIR 1975 Cal 109

Insanity: Wife suffering from schizophrenia at the time of marriage: Husband can seek annulment of marriage and curability of the disease would be immaterial—Held, further that all schizophrenia cases are lunatic though all lunatic persons may not suffer from schizophrenia.

Chapter

35

Intoxication

Relevancy of drunkenness where intention is a material factor in determining guilt of accused.

1. Where the intention with which an act is done is a material factor in determining the criminality of the act, it is obvious that the questions whether the accused was intoxicated at the time of the alleged offence and what was the degree and nature of the intoxication are relevant issues for determination. AIR 1938 Rang 219 (220): 39 Cri LJ 689 ** AIR 1928 Mad 196 (197): 29
2. The presumption under Sec. 86 that the voluntary drunkard who commits an offence has the same knowledge as he would have had if he had not been intoxicated given rise to a further presumption that he intended the ordinary and natural consequences of his act. (1912) 13 Cri LJ 864 (868) (FB) (Upp Bur) ** 1978 Cut LR (Cri) 219 (226,227) " 1978 Cri LJ NOC 260 (DB) **
3. Evidence of drunkenness short of incapacity to form a particular intent necessary to constitute the offence or to have the particular knowledge necessary to constitute the offence is not enough to rebut the presumption that every man must be presumed to intend the natural consequences of his act. AIR 1956 SC 488 (489, 490): 57 Cri LJ 919 ** 1979 Bom CR 507 (516) (DB) **

Voluntary intoxication incapacitating accused from forming particular intention which is necessary to constitute offence

Where a particular intention is essential to constitute an offence and the accused, by reason of intoxication, was incapable of forming the particular intention necessary to constitute the offence, he will not be guilty of the offence, in spite of the fact that the intoxication was voluntary. AIR 1956 SC 488 (489, 490): 1956 Cri LJ 919 (2) ** (1912) 13 Cri LJ 864 (868) (Low Bur) (FB) 1959 Ker LT 634 (636) **

1. The true test as to the state of intoxication contemplated by Sec. 86 is whether by reason of drunkenness the accused was incapable of forming the specific intention required to constitute the offence, and that it is not necessary to prove that the intoxication had made him absolutely incapable of understanding what he was doing or that he was doing what was either wrong or contrary to law. 1920 App Cas 479 ** 1931 Mad WN 113 (115) (DB).

Voluntary intoxication making accused excitable and violent.

1. The presumption that in spite of intoxication the accused intended natural

consequences of his act, cannot be rebutted by merely showing that the intoxication had made him excitable and predisposed to violence AIR 1957 All 667 (670): 1957 Cri LJ 1056 (DB) **

BURDEN OF PROOF

1. The burden of proof of involuntary intoxication which made the accused incapable of knowing what he was doing or that he was doing what was wrong or contrary to law, is on the accused. 1978 Cut LR (Cri) 202 (205): 1978 Cri LJ NOC 239 (DB) **
2. The onus of proof that by reason of intoxication the accused had become incapable of having the particular knowledge or forming the particular intention necessary to constitute the offence is on the accused 1978 Cut LR (Cri) 219 (226, 227): 1978 Cri LJ NOC 260 (DB) **

SENTENCE

1. Although voluntary intoxication is no defence to a criminal charge, such intoxication may be taken into consideration along with other facts and circumstances of the case in determining the appropriate sentence to be passed. ILR (1956) Trav –Co 658 ** AIR 1953 Raj 40 (42): 1953 Cri LJ 434 ** AIR 1941 Lah 454 (457): 43 Cri LJ 332 (DB) ** 1866 Pun Re (Cri) No. 41, P. 47 (47) (DB).

CANNABIS (GANJA) AND OTHER NARCOTICS—EFFECT

1. Hemp acts on the brain, causing usually excitement followed by confusion. If the drug is taken in small doses the effect produced is slight, consisting merely of some pleasurable stimulation of the higher centres. This in no way affects the individual's appreciation of the consequences of his acts. In large doses, hemp, like datura, causes a temporary insanity associated with hallucinations under the influence of which a person may be violent even to the extent of committing homicide AIR 1939 Cal 244 (248) (DB).
2. Where the prosecution was not able to prove motive for the accused to commit the murder of the deceased and there was no reliable evidence to show that accused were in possession of aluminium phosphide, or had the opportunity to mix up the same in the tea before the same was served to the deceased, in the circumstances the accused would be entitled to acquittal. (1989) 1 Rec Cri R 432 (435): (1989) 1 All Cri LR 620 (DB) (P & H) (1999) 1 Raj Cri C 530 (534)
3. In a case of death of wife by consuming poison, when there is no evidence to prove that accused husband aided or abetted offence of suicide, and when the testimony of interested witness is not reliable, the accused is entitled to acquittal especially when co-accused, his mother was acquitted and no appeal was also preferred by State Government. 1993 Cri LJ 2724 (2730) (P & H)

   [See also (1999) 1 East Cri C 1147 (1154) (Pat) (Where death of the deceased was alleged to be caused by administering the poison by accused persons and there was nothing specific against the accused that he alone had administered poison and there was no eye witness of the occurrence and further the poison has also not been detected during chemical examination, conviction of the accused for offence would not be proper particularly when the other co-accused were acquitted in the case)].

HOMICIDE DONE UNDER INFLUENCE OF HYPNOTIC DRUGS

A person under the influence of hypnotic drug may lose his cognitive faculties, fail to understand the nature and consequences of his act and also cannot distinguish right from wrong. His criminal responsibility will thus be regulated as per provisions of Sec. 84 IPC. Same thing holds good in respect of "Running amok" in case of Chronic Cannabis Psychosis.

Explanation

In Rex *vs* Salkeld, Salkeld shot a woman in a dancing hall, after he consumed a number of hypnotic tablets following sleeplessness and a fit of depression. The learned judge while convicting the accused to five years' imprisonment, lessening the charge of murder to manslaughter, opined that owing to the defendant's habit and taking the drug at the material moment, he was in a muddled state of mind, so that he was not in a position to make intention to kill vide Birmingham post, July 18, 1946.

CASE LAW

Insanity Caused by Excessive Drinking, Smoking Ganja, etc.

1. Where insanity is caused by excessive drinking (although voluntary) or by excessive smoking of ganja, etc., such insanity will also amount to " unsoundness of mind" under this section, and where it makes a person incapable of understanding what he is doing or that he is doing something which is either wrong or contrary to law, it would be a good defence under this section to a criminal charge, provided that such state of mind at that time existed when the accused did the act which is charged as an offence AIR 1956 SC 488 (491): 1956 Cri LJ 919(2).
2. The mere loss of self-control due to drinking, smoking ganja, etc. will not be "insanity" in the sense of this section. AIR 1955 Punj 13 (15): 1955 Cri LJ (DB) **
3. Where the intoxication is not voluntary, and has deprived the accused of his capacity to distinguish between right and wrong, Sec. 85 will afford him protection from criminal liability for his acts while he was in that state, although his condition may not have amounted to actual insanity. (1912) 13 Cri LJ 167 (167,168) (Nag) (DB). [Bue see 1920 APP Cas 479 (500): 89 LJKB 437.]

Mavari Surya Satyanarayana *vs* State of A.P. 1995 Cri L J 689 (AP)

Insanity as plea of defence: Mental faculties of the accused cannot be said to be completely dominated by intoxication. Therefore, where the accused after consuming liquor, scolded his wife and then poured kerosene on her body and set her on fire, he would be liable to be convicted under Sec. 302 IPC.

Ennique F. Rio *vs* State, 1975 Cri L J 1337

Offence committed under the influence of intoxication: Where the offence was committed when the accused was highly intoxicated and requisite intention to commit the offence not proved it was necessary to examine whether the accused was beside his mind altogether as a result of heavy drinking. The learned trial court observed that under the influence of intoxication the accused magnified the small provocation and this fact brings out the state of mind of the accused. Showing that he was incapable of forming requisite intention so as to bring the offence under Sec. 300 and therefore, the case will come under IPC Sec. 304, part II since the accused at least caused the death of the deceased with the knowledge that his act was likely to cause death but without having any intention to cause death.

J.C. Nager P.S. Bangalore *vs* Santanam, 1998 Cr. L.J. 3045 at page No. 3049

Legal Aspects in view of Alcohol

While accidents govern and add to the criminal responsibility of the driver in case he is found drunk, but if the victim is also found drunk or found intoxicated, instantly the responsibility is mitigated to that extent in respect of accident.

Kunjami Ayatu *vs* State of M.P., 1987 (2) Crimes 232

Where both parties consumed liquor: The accused under the influence of liquor beat the victim to death. However, there was no evidence that on account of the liquor he had lost equilibrium of mind. However the accused continued beating even after he fell down. The blows given only to vital parts of the body. It showed that he was not incapacitated to know the nature of the acts done by him. Therefore, the accused was convicted under Sec. 302, IPC.

State (Delhi Administration) *vs* Sube singh, 1985 Cri L J 1190

Clinical examination: Reliance on the evidence of clinical examination where the doctor examined and issued a certificate that he smelt alcohol will not mean that the opinion was not correct. Where the blood of the accused is sent for chemical examination and the result of chemical analysis was suppressed from the court, the court will be justified in ignoring the evidence of chemical examination.

Ennique F. Rio *vs* State, 1975 Cri LJ 1337

In another very important case—Bachubhai *vs* State, 1971 (3) SCC 930—The Hon'ble Court has observed that blood and urine test are very important. Drunkenness cannot be based merely on the breath of the appellant, unsteadiness of gait and dilation of pupils and with the conclusion that the conviction of the accused person on such grounds is in no way justice.

Evidence of intoxication—The question will be whether the evidence established that mind of the accused was so affected by intoxicant that he more easily gave way to violent passion. However, there is difference between insanity and influence of intoxication. There is distinction between the defence of insanity in the true sense caused by excessive drunkenness and defence of drunkenness which produces a condition such that the mind of the drunken man becomes incapable of forming an intention. If the actual insanity supervenes the result of alcoholic excess, it will furnish a defence on the ground of insanity but if it fell short of insanity, evidence of drunkenness rendering the accused incapable of forming specific intent to constitute the crime, it must be proved whether or not he has such intention.

Maniram Ganju *vs* State of Assam, AIR 1970 Assam 49

The test for determining the influence of intoxication—The accused was examined by medical officer who found smell of alcohol was present and eyes were congested and gait was unsteady and speech was incoherent. In the opinion of the doctor the accused had taken alcohol which was sufficient to make him intoxicated. Mere smell of alcohol however, is not sufficient because the smell of alcohol may be due to the fact that the accused had contravened the part of Sec. 13(b) of prohibition Act or that he had taken alcohol which fell under the unenforceable and inoperative part of the section.

AIR 1969 Cal 304: 1978 HLR 206 (Del)

Karan Singh Balubha vs State of Gujarat, AIR 1967 Guj. 219

Test to find out as to whether a person was under intoxication: In order to ascertain whether a particular individual is drunk or not, quantity taken is not determining factor. If the prosecution relies solely on the report of the chemical analyser to prove the fact of concentration of blood which had been collected and sent for chemical analysis, the certificate of chemical analyser could be the evidence if the certificate is obtained in the prescribed form.

State *vs* Ramsingh Dessasingh, AIR 1963 Bom. 68

The question whether a person was under the influence of intoxication and to what extent: Where the Medical Officer issued a certificate stating that the accused smelt of liquor and his pupils were dilated the eyes were congested, and blood from his body was sent to chemical analyser. According to the chemical analyser report, blood contained 0.292 percent W/V of ethyl alcohol. Such certificate can be accepted in evidence if the same is not challenged but the court cannot refuse to consider the evidence furnished by the certificate, merely because it did not mention the date on the basis of which the chemical analyzer arrived at the percentage of alcohol mentioned in his certificate. However, without examining the chemical analyser, it cannot be held that charge against the accused was not proved.

Ukha Kolhe *vs* State of Maharashtra, AIR 1963 SC 1531: 1963 (2) Cri LJ 418

Determination of fact of intoxication: Report of chemical examiner in respect of blood collected in the course of investigation of an offence under Bombay Prohibition Act, otherwise when in the manner shut out under the said Act cannot be used as evidence—To that extent Sec. 510 of CrPC is superseded by Sec. 129 B of the Bombay Act. But the report of the Chemical analyser relating to examination of blood of an accused person collected at a time when no investigation was pending or at the instance of police officer or prohibition officer, would be admissible under Sec. 510 CrPC.

Prabhu Nath *vs* State of UP AIR 1957 All 66: 1957 Cri LJ 1056

Offence committed under the influence of intoxication: Effect of influence of intoxication. If the intoxication is taken voluntarily, it cannot be taken as a defence.

Palani Goudan In Re AIR 1957 Mad. 546: 1957 Cri LJ 976

Test for determination of intoxication: The doctor observed smelling of alcohol redness of eyes, dilatation of pupils, tongue was clean and dry, speech was incoherent and gait was staggering. On these symptoms the doctor formed the opinion that the accused consumed liquor and was under the influence of intoxication. The doctor examined the accused, found that he was suffering from Asthma and chronic bronchitis, prescribed some tonic which contained slight alcohol. The tonic contained 12 percent of alcohol. According to the doctor if the mixture and tonic is taken together the smell of alcohol will continue for one hour. Thus smelling of alcohol will not suffice to prove intoxication.

Dass Kandha *vs* The State, 1976 Cri L J 2010

State of intoxication: It must be such as would render the accused incapable of forming specific intent essential to constitute the crimes and therefore, mere proof of drinking of some liquor would not be proof of intoxication. The onus will be squarely on the accused to lead evidence independently or to bring by cross-examination that he was in such a state of intoxication.

Thimmiah *vs* State of Mysore, AIR 1957 Mysore 83

Effect of intoxication: The petitioner intended that he had taken the cough syrup B.G. Phos and symptoms found on him were due to the fact that he consumed that medicine. The evidence of the doctor however negatives the pleas of the accused having consumed B.G. Phos. According to the doctor, the breath smelt of alcohol, pupils dilated and eyes were congested. The pulse was 92 per minute and the speech was incoherent and the gait was staggering. In the opinion of the doctor, the petitioner had taken alcohol and he was also intoxicated. According to the doctor, the petitioner was incapable of taking care of himself. According to the doctor even if a person taken whole bottle of B.G. Phos, he will not smell of alcohol and he will not be intoxicated. Therefore the plea of the accused not accepted.

In Rex *vs* Meade (1909) I.K.B. 895, the accused in a state of drunkenness did beat a woman so violently that she died as a result of rupture of intestines. In Lower Court, the defence of drunkenness was set aside. In Court of Criminal Appeal, it could be successfully pleaded that the accused was so intensely drunk that he was not capable of understanding, that what he was doing was dangerous to life and was likely to cause death, and a verdict of manslaughter was substituted.

In the case of King Emperor *vs* Bishan Singh, the principle of Rex *vs* Beard was followed, where the accused was convicted for having murdered 3 persons by using a fire-arm in an intoxicated state, causing such injuries which in ordinary course of nature were likely to cause death-*Vide* Lahore High Court, Criminal Appeal No. 201 of 1928.

In Rex *vs* Donoghue Simpson K. (1954) Police, J, 27, 110, the accused, killed his best friend Meaney by stabbing him with a bayonet on his head and neck under the impression that Meaney was a dummy, placed fully clothed in his bed as a practical joke. The story was that both the friends spent the preceding evening by drinking in a pub and both retired to the room of Donoghue to sleep it off. On waking up in the early hours of morning, still intoxicated, Donoghue found himself sitting in a chair with clothes on. On going to bed he found the "dummy" in his bed, dragged it off to the floor, where if fell like a "sack of coal"; then by taking up the bayonet used for cutting bread, he inflicted stab injuries on the "dummy"; then he dragged the dummy on the landing, where the body was found on the next morning. When Donoghue finally woke up, he found blood on the floor and then realised, what had really happened.

Donoghues's story was largely believed, as during autopsy, the blood alcohol of Meaney was found to be 347 mgm percent, urine alcohol was 450 percent. This value was considered to be a greater saturation than is compatible with life in many people. When both the friends were last seen, it was reported that Meaney was more sober than Donoghue and thus it could be very well presumed that Donoghue could not have less blood alcohol saturation.

In the trial, it could be successfully proved that the accused was too much drunk to make any malicious intent to kill, as under such blood alcohol saturation, he could not have been capable of clear thinking and to make an intention to kill. The accused was a quiet inoffensive respectable little man, was very friendly with his friend, whom he killed and he made no attempt to evade his responsibility. The prison medical officer deposed that under such degree of drunkenness, one could mistakenly believe that he was stabbing a dummy and not a human being.

Donoghue was convicted with a sentence of 3 years' imprisonment.

Basdev *vs* State of Pepsu, 1956 SCR 363: 1956 Cri L J 919: 1956 SCA 695: AIR 1956 SC 488

Extent of intoxication: Offence of murder under the influence of drink. There was no evidence to show that the accused was incapacitated to form requisite intention as required for committing murder under Sec. 302. In the absence of such evidence the accused will be liable under Sec. 302 and not under Sec. 304, part-II.

State *vs* Mehbob Maulabux, AIR 1956 Bom 270

Test for determination of extent of intoxication: where the doctor examined the petitioner and found there was smell of liquor in the mouth and pupil dilated and eyes were red and pulse was excited and the doctor was of the opinion that the accused was under intoxication.

In Re. Suruthayyam, 1954 Cri L J 672

Extent of intoxication: The state of intoxication as envisaged in Sec. 86 is in anyway different from that contemplated in Sec. 85. Both Secs. 85 and 86 lay down the law relating to drunkenness as bearing of their, the wrongful acts committed by persons. The absence of qualifying words in Sec. 86 cannot be lead to infer that even if the insobriety is not such as to impair the reasons of the offender the requisite intent cannot be presumed.

Satyarao *vs* State, AIR 1954 And 4: 1954 Cri L J 1929

Determination of intoxication fact: The expression intoxication is synonymous with the drunkenness—According to the dictionary meaning poisoning or action of poisoning whether of drug, bacterial or other toxic substance, and a condition resulting from such poisoning is termed as intoxication. It is thus clear that intoxication implied to excessive amount of drunkenness.

Balaswami *vs* State, 1952 (1) Mad. L J 772

Intoxication a defence: Section 85, IPC provides intoxication as defence. If a person is rendered incapable of knowing the nature of the act, done by him, when a person voluntarily drinks and is in a state of intoxication, he shall be dealt with as if he had the same knowledge as he would have had if he had not been intoxicated. If a person in the state of complete intoxication is found in the house of another during night time, it cannot be presumed that he had the intention of committing theft or the offence of which he is charged. Sec. 86 no doubt imputes to him the knowledge to enter another man's house, but that is not enough for criminal trespass and there must be further proof that he had the intention to commit particular offence.

Public Prosecutor *vs* Channippa Pujari, AIR 1951 Mad 703

Determination of influence of intoxication: Sub-inspector of the police found that the accused was smelling of the liquor and sent him for medical examination which found the accused having consumed alcohol. Lower court held that mere smelling of alcohol was not sufficient because it could be for the reasons other than the liquor such as by the taking medication like asava or aristha. Redness of the eyes was also explained saying that it may be due to weeping, etc. The order of acquittal approved.

In D.P.P. *vs* Beard (1920) A.C. p 479, the accused was convicted on charge of murder of a girl of 13 years who died from suffocation while being raped, as the accused put his hand over her face to prevent her from shouting. The defence of drunkenness was put to the jury to lessen the charge of murder to manslaughter. House of Lords held that drunkenness could not be a defence here, unless it could be established that the accused at the time of committing the crime was too drunk to form an intention to commit it. Death resulted from suffocation by the way of putting hand on the face to prevent her from crying. This felonious act was in continuity and furtherance of the other felonious act of rape. A person cannot be convicted of crime unless the mens mens rea (mind is guilty, criminal intent, guilty knowledge and wilfulness). In this case, drunkenness fell short of proved incapacity to form intent to commit the crime. Drunkenness cannot be accepted as a defence, unless it rendered the accused incapable of forming the intention to rape. Hence, the plea of drunkenness was rejected and conviction of murder was restored.

Khandu *vs* Emperor, 1934 Cri L J 1096

Determination of intoxication and its effect: Where the accused petitioner was arrested and was sent to medical officer, being suspected of intoxication with liquor, according to the medical certificate, his pupils were dilated, gait was unsteady, speech was incoherent and he smelt alcohol. However, mere smell of alcohol could not show that he was under the influence of intoxication. Intercourse with animal is also unnatural offence—Where carnal intercourse committed with a bullock through nose, it amounts to bestiality and punishable under Sec. 377 IPC—In this case, the accused was seen having carnal intercourse by placing his penis inside the nostril of bullock which was tied to a tree—Held, he was punishable under Sec. 377.

The following two points are very important to be noted.

- When the person has himself consumed alcohol and on account of the effect of alcohol commits any crime, the truth is, he would be responsible for his criminal act...
- When the person has been given alcohol to make him drunk or intoxicated up to the extent that he does not know the difference between right and wrong, the criminal responsibility of such person is instantly over.

Symptoms to assess whether the person is drunk.

While the person is drunk his condition becomes such that:

1. His breath smells of liquor
2. Has excited pulse
3. Red eyes
4. Dilated pupils
5. Excitement with happy signs or a feeling of wild excitement
6. Equilibrium of mind is lost
7. Has incoherent speech and staggering gait.

Chapter

36

Draft Mental Health Care Act 2010 (06 Dec 2010)

MINISTRY OF HEALTH AND FAMILY WELFARE GOVERNMENT OF INDIA, NEW DELHI

Mental Health Care Act (MHCA), 2010 under preparation due to periodic amendments to the Mental Health Act 1987.

DESCRIPTION

An Act to provide access to mental health care for persons with mental illness and to protect and promote the rights of persons with mental illness during the delivery of mental health care.

STATEMENT OF OBJECTS AND REASONS

Recognizing that:

- Persons with mental illness constitute a vulnerable section of society and are subject to discrimination in our society.
- Families bear disproportionate financial, emotional and social burden of providing treatment and care for their relatives with mental illness.
- Persons with mental illness should be treated like other persons with health problems and the environment around them should be made as conducive to facilitate recovery, rehabilitation and full participation in society.
- The Mental Health Act, 1987 has failed to protect the rights of persons with mental illness and promote access to mental health care in the country.

And in order to:

- Protect and promote the rights of persons with mental illness during the delivery of health care in institutions and in the community.
- Ensure health care treatment and rehabilitation to persons with mental illness is provided in the least restrictive environment possible, and in a manner that does not intrudes on their rights and dignity. Community-based solutions, preferably in the vicinity of the person's usual place of residence, are preferred to institutional solutions.
- Provide treatment, care and rehabilitation to improve the capacity of the person to develop his or her full potential and to facilitate his or her integration into community life.
- Fulfill the obligations under the Constitution of India and the obligations under various International Conventions ratified by India.
- Regulate the public and private mental health sectors within a rights framework to achieve the greatest public health good.
- Improve accessibility to mental health care by mandating sufficient provision of quality public mental health services and non-discrimination in health insurance.
- Establish a mental health system integrated into all levels of general health care.

- Promote principles of equity, efficiency and active participation of all stakeholders in decision making.

CHAPTERS IN MHCA 2010

1. Preliminary
2. Rights of Persons with Mental Illness
3. Duties of Government
4. Mental Health Review Commission
5. State Mental Health Authority
6. Mental Health Facilities
7. Admission, Treatment and Discharge
8. Responsibilities of Other Agencies
9. Penalties and Miscellaneous provisions

Chapter I: Preliminary

Section 1: Short title, extent and commencement

Section 2: Definitions

a. Care-giver
b. Family
c. Informed Consent
d. Least Restrictive Alternative or Less Restrictive Option
e. Magistrate
f. Medical Officer in Charge
g. Medical Practitioner
h. Mental Health Facility
i. Mental Health Professional
j. Minor
k. Notification
l. Prescribed
m. Prisoner with Mental Illness"
n. Psychiatrist
o. Relative
p. Mental Health Review Commission and District Panel of the Mental Health Review Commission
q. State Mental Health Authority

Section 3: Mental Illness

Section 4: Competence

Section 5: Advance Directive

Section 6: Nominated Representative

Chapter II: Rights of Persons with Mental Illness

Section 7: Right to Access Mental Health Care

Section 8: Right to Community Living

Section 9: Right to Protection from Cruel, Inhuman and Degrading Treatments

Section 10: Right to Equality and Nondiscrimination

Section 11: Right to Information

Section 12: Right to Confidentiality

Section 13: Access to Medical Records

Section 14: Right to Personal Contacts and Communication

Section 15: Right to Legal Aid

Section 16: Right to make Complaints about Deficiencies in Provision of Services

Chapter III: Duties of Government

Section 17: Promotion of Mental Health and Preventive Programmes

Section 18: Creating Awareness about Mental Health and Illness and Reducing Stigma associated with Mental Illness

Section 19: Human Resources and Training

Section 20: Co-ordination within the Government

Chapter IV: Mental Health Review Commission

Section 21: Constitution of a Mental Health Review Commission

Section 22: Constitution of District Panels of the Mental Health Review Commission

Section 23: Disqualification and Removal

Section 24: Terms and Conditions of Service

Section 25: Decisions of the Commission and the District Panels

Section 26: Applications to District Panel

Section 27: Proceedings before the District Panel

Section 28: Functions of the Mental Health Review Commission and District Panel of the Mental Health Review Commission

Section 29: Appeals

Section 30: Budgetary Provisions for the Commission and District Panels

Section 31: Power to make regulations

Chapter V: State Mental Health Authority

Section 32: State Mental Health Authority

Section 33: Composition of the State Mental Health Authority

Section 34: Chairperson and Executive Officer of the State Mental Health Authority

Section 35: Functions of the State Mental Health Authority
Section 36: Proceedings of the State Mental Health Authority
Section 37: Budgetary Provisions
Section 38: Power to Make Regulations

Chapter VI: Mental Health Facilities

Section 39: Registration and Standards for Mental Health Facilities
Section 40: Procedure for Registration and Inspection of Mental Health Facilities
Section 41: Certificates, Fees and Register of Mental Health Facilities

Chapter VII: Admission, Treatment and Discharge

Section 42: Independent (without Support) Admission and Treatment

Section 43: Admission of a Minor

Section 44: Discharge of Independent Patients

Section 45: Admission and Treatment of Persons with Mental Illness, with High support Needs, in a Mental Health Facility, up to 30 days (Supported Admission)

Section 46: Admission and Treatment of Persons with Millness Illness, with High Support needs, in a Mental Health Facility, beyond 30 days (Supported Admission beyond 30 days)

Section 47: Leave of Absence

Section 48: Absence without Leave or Discharge

Section 49: Transfer of Persons with Mental Illness from one Mental Health Facility to Another Mental Health Facility

Section 50: Emergency Treatment

Section 51: Prohibited Treatments

Section 52: Restriction on Psychosurgery for Persons with Mental Illness

Section 53: Restraints and Seclusion
Section 54: Discharge Planning
Section 55: Research

Chapter VIII: Responsibilities of Other Agencies

Section 56: Duties of Police Officers in Respect of Persons with Mental Illness
Section 57: Order in case of Person with Mental Illness who is Ill Treated or Neglected
Section 58: Conveying or Admitting a Person with Mental Illness to a Mental Health Facility by a Magistrate
Section 59: Prisoners with Mental Illness
Section 60: Question of Mental Illness in Judicial Process

Chapter IX: Penalties and Miscellaneous Provisions

Section 61: Penalties for Establishing or Maintaining a Mental Health Facility in Contravention of Chapter VI

Section 62: General Provision for Punishment of offences

Section 63: Special Relaxation in requirements for States of the North East Council

Section 64: Protection of Action Taken in Good faith

Section 65: Effect of Act on other Laws

Section 66: Power to Remove Difficulty

Section 67: Repeal and Saving

- A copy of the proposed amendments is available on the Ministry's website for wider consultations and for eliciting views of all stakeholders.
- Responses/views/comments may be mailed to amendmentstomha1987@gmail.com

Chapter

37

Mental Health and Postpartum Psychosis

MENTAL HEALTH

That while imprisonment restricts the right to liberty, it does not restrict the human rights of convicts. "It is time to ensure that a convict who leaves the correction home/prison is restored to the society as a law-abiding citizen" (Delhi High Court).

The World Psychiatric Association in the General Assembly of its 23rd World Congress in Vienna (30 September 2023) approved a Position Statement recommending that the death penalty should not be imposed on any person with mental illness or intellectual and developmental disabilities. In the coeval times, the term "health" is not only limited to the physical aspect of the body but also includes mental and spiritual well-being. The concept in itself has attracted colossal credibility and has encouraged the government to look after the existing facilities and make way for up-to-the-minute developments taking place in terms of mental health care.

Psychopathy is considered to be an aggravating rather than a mitigating factor in determining criminal responsibility (Delhi High Court).

A Delhi High Court bench comprising of Justice Pradeep Nandrajog and Justice Mukta Gupta, while affirming the death sentence awarded to three men accused of raping and brutally murdering a 17-year-old girl, prodded on the question of psychopathic crimes and effect of such tendencies while awarding a punishment. The Court asserted: "It is the dominant view among psychiatrists and the law."

In The Supreme Court of India Criminal Appellate Jurisdiction BR Gavai; J., M.M. Sundresh; J. Criminal Appeal No. 2010 of 2010. 12 January, 2023 In Prakash Nayi @ Sen versus State of Goa Indian Penal Code, 1860; Section 84: Indian Evidence Act, 1872; Section 105, 8: The burden of proof does lie on the accused to prove to the satisfaction of the Court that one is insane while doing the act prohibited by law. Such a burden gets discharged based on a prima facie case and reasonable materials produced on his behalf. The extent of probability is one of preponderances. This is for the reason that a person of unsound mind is not expected to prove his insanity beyond a reasonable doubt. Secondly, it is the collective responsibility of the person concerned, the Court and the prosecution to decipher the proof of insanity by not treating it as adversarial. Though a person is presumed to be sane, once there are adequate materials available before the Court, the presumption gets discharged: The behaviour and conduct before, during and after the occurrence has to be looked into. (Para 8–9) Indian Penal Code, 1860; Section 84: The existence of an unsound mind is a sine qua non to the applicability of the provision. A mere unsound mind *per se* would not suffice, and it should be to the extent of not knowing the nature of the act: A mere medical insanity cannot be said to mean unsoundness of mind. There may be a case where a person suffering from medical insanity would have committed an act, however, the test is one of legal insanities to attract the mandate of Section 84 of the IPC. There must be an inability of a person in knowing the nature of the act or to understand it to be either wrong or contrary to the law. Code of Criminal Procedure, 1973: In finding out whether an accused would be sound enough to stand a trial, it is the mandatory duty of the Court. The whole idea under the provisions discussed is to facilitate a person of unsound mind to stand trial, not only because of his reasoning capacity, but also to treat him as the one who is having a disability. The role of the Court is to find the remedial measures and do complete justice. "If Hamlet from himself be taken away, and when he is not himself does wrong Laertes, then Hamlet does it not; Hamlet denies it. Who does it, then? His madness. If it be so, Hamlet is of the faction that is wrong'd; His madness is poor Hamlet's enemy." -William Shakespeare (*Source:* Hamlet, W.S. (Play) Act-5 Scene-2 Line-245) 2 1. While acknowledging the hurt that he has caused to Laertes for causing the death of his father, whom he murdered by way of a mistaken identity, Hamlet pleads temporary madness. While pleading so, he disassociates himself from the act as if it was done by a third person and he was made to suffer the consequence. He thus pleads to treat him as a victim rather than an offender. Though the act of Hamlet does constitute a culpable homicide coming within the definition of Section 300 of the Indian Penal Code, 1860 an act of unsound mind would not attract the same. Through these lines, Shakespeare brings out the agony of a man having to justify his act of madness. 2. Raising the plea of insanity on the mandate of Section 84 of the Indian Penal Code, 1860 (hereinafter 'the IPC'), the appellant seeks reversal of the order of conviction passed by the Division Bench of the High Court of Bombay at Goa, confirming the order of the Additional Sessions Judge, S.G. Margao-II. As we are dealing with the seminal issue of applicability of Section 84 of the IPC and in the light of the focus made by the counsel for the appellant, we do not propose to go into the merits. Section 84 of The Indian Penal Code, 1860 "84. Act of a person of unsound mind. "Nothing is an offence which is done by a person who, at the time of doing it, by reason of unsoundness of mind, is incapable of knowing the nature of the act, or that he is doing what is either wrong or contrary to law." Section 84 of the IPC recognizes only an act which could not be termed as an offence. It starts with the words "nothing is an offence". The said words are a clear indication of the intendment behind this laudable provision. Such an act shall emanate from an unsound mind. Therefore, the existence of an unsound mind is a sine qua non to the applicability of the provision. A mere unsound mind *per se* would not suffice, and it should be to the extent of not knowing the nature of the act. Such a person is incapable of knowing the nature of the said act. Similarly, he does not stand to reason as to whether an act committed is either wrong or contrary to law. Needless to say, the element of incapacity emerging from an unsound mind shall be present at the time of commission. The provision speaks about the act of a person of unsound mind. It is a very broad provision relatable to the incapacity. The test is from the point of view of a prudent man. Therefore, a mere medical insanity cannot be said to mean unsoundness of mind. There may be a case where a person suffering from medical insanity would have committed an act, however, the test is one of legal insanities to attract the mandate of Section 84 of the IPC. There must be an inability of a person in knowing the nature of the act or to understand it to be either wrong or contrary to the law. The aforesaid provision is founded on the maxim, actus non reum facit nisi mens sit rea, i.e., an act does not constitute guilt unless done with a guilty intention. It is a fundamental principle of criminal law that there has to be an element of *mens rea* in forming guilt with intention. A person of an unsound mind, who is incapable of knowing the consequence of an act, does not know that such an act is right or wrong. He may not even know that he has committed that act. When such is the position, he cannot be made to suffer punishment. This act cannot be termed as a mental rebellion constituting a deviant behaviour leading to a crime against society. He stands as a victim in need of help, and therefore, cannot be charged and tried for an offence. His position is that of a child not knowing either his action or the consequence of it. An accused who seeks exoneration from liability of an act under Section 84 of the Penal Code is to prove legal insanity and not medical insanity. Expression "unsoundness of mind" has not been defined in the Penal Code and it has mainly been treated as equivalent to insanity. But the term "insanity" carries different meaning in different contexts and describes varying degrees of mental disorder. "Every person who is suffering from mental disease is not ipso facto exempted from criminal liability. The mere fact that the accused is conceited, odd, irascible and his brain is not quite all right, or that the physical and mental ailments from which he suffered had rendered his intellect weak and affected his emotions or indulges in certain unusual acts, or had fits of insanity at short intervals or that he was subject to epileptic fits and there was abnormal behaviour or the behaviour is queer are not sufficient to attract the application of Section 84 of the Penal Code." Section 84 lays down the legal test of responsibility in cases of alleged unsoundness of mind. There is no definition of "unsoundness of mind" in the IPC. The courts have, however, mainly treated this expression as equivalent to insanity. But the term 'insanity' itself has no precise definition. It is a term used to describe varying degrees of mental disorder. So, every person, who is mentally diseased, is not *ipso facto* exempted from criminal responsibility. A distinction is to be made between legal insanity and medical insanity. A court is concerned with legal insanity, and not with medical insanity..." Section 84 embodies the fundamental maxim of criminal law, i.e. actus non reum facit nisi mens sit rea (an act does not constitute guilt unless done with a guilty intention). In order to constitute an offence, the intent and act must concur; but in the case of insane persons, no culpability is fastened on them as they have no free will (furios is nulla voluntas est). The section itself provides that the benefit is available only after it is proved that at the time of committing the act, the accused was labouring under such a defect of reason, from disease of the mind, as not to know the nature and quality of the act he was doing, or that even if he did not know it, it was either wrong or contrary to law then this section must be applied. The crucial point of time for deciding whether the benefit of this section should be given or not, is the material time when the offence takes place. In coming to that conclusion, the relevant circumstances are to be taken into consideration, it would be dangerous to admit the defence of insanity upon arguments derived merely from the character of the crime. It is only unsoundness of mind which naturally impairs the cognitive faculties of the mind that can form a ground of exemption from criminal responsibility. If a person cut off the head of a sleeping man because it would be great fun to see him looking for it when he woke up, would obviously be a case where the perpetrator of the act would be incapable of knowing the physical effects of his act. The law recognizes nothing but incapacity to realise the nature of the act and presumes that where a man's mind or his faculties of ratiocination are sufficiently dim to apprehend what he is doing, he must always be presumed to intend the consequence of the action he takes. When a person is accused of any offence, the burden of proving the existence of circumstances bringing the case within any of the General Exceptions in the Indian Penal Code (45 of 1860), or within any special exception or proviso contained in any other part of the same Code, or in any law defining the offence, is upon him, and the Court shall presume the absence of such circumstances. The burden of proof does lie on the accused to prove to the satisfaction of the Court that one is insane while doing the act prohibited by law. Such a burden gets discharged based on a prima facie case and reasonable materials produced on his behalf. The extent of probability is one of preponderances. This is for the reason that a person of unsound mind is not expected to prove his insanity beyond a reasonable doubt. Secondly, it is the collective responsibility of the person concerned, the Court and the prosecution to decipher the proof qua insanity by not treating it as adversarial. Though a person is presumed to be sane, once there are adequate materials available before the Court, the presumption gets discharged. Section 105 of the Indian Evidence Act, which places the burden of proving, has its exceptions. Though, as a general principle, the onus is upon the person accused to bring his case under the exception, dealing with the case under Section 84 of the IPC, one has to apply the concept of preponderance of probabilities. The aforesaid provision has to be read along with Section 8 of the Indian Evidence Act. The better way to reconcile the aforesaid provision would be to have a look into the behaviour and conduct before, during and after the occurrence. As Section 84 of the IPC has its laudable objective behind it, the prosecution and the Court have their distinct roles to play. The agency has to take up the investigation from the materials produced on behalf of the person claiming unsoundness. It has to satisfy itself that the case would not come within the purview of Section 84 of the IPC. The Court on its part has to satisfy itself as to whether the act was done by a person with an unsound mind within the rigour of Section 84 of the IPC. It is better to place reliance on the classical decision in Dahyabhai Chhaganbhai Thakkar v. State of Gujarat (AIR 1964 SC 1563), wherein the Court held that: "The doctrine of burden of proof in the context of the plea of insanity may be stated in the following propositions: The prosecution must prove beyond reasonable doubt that the accused had committed the offence with the requisite mens rea; and the burden of proving that always rests on the prosecution from the beginning to the end of the trial. There is a rebuttable presumption that the accused was not insane, when he committed the crime, in the sense laid down by Section 84 of the Indian Penal Code: The accused may rebut it by placing before the court all the relevant evidence oral, documentary or circumstantial, but the burden of proof upon him is no higher than that rests upon a party to civil proceedings. Even if the accused was not able to establish conclusively that he was insane at the time he committed the offence, the evidence placed before the court by the accused or by the prosecution may raise a reasonable doubt in the mind of the court as regards one or more of the ingredients of the offence, including mens rea of the accused and in that case the court would be entitled to acquit the accused on the ground that the general burden of proof resting on the prosecution was not discharged. The onus of proving unsoundness of mind is on the accused. But where during the investigation previous history of insanity is revealed, it is the duty of an honest investigator to subject the accused to a medical examination and place that evidence before the court and if this is not done, it creates a serious infirmity in the prosecution case and the benefit of doubt has to be given to the accused. The onus, however, has to be discharged by producing evidence as to the conduct of the accused shortly prior to the offence and his conduct at the time or immediately afterwards, also by evidence of his mental condition and other relevant factors. Mere abnormality of mind or partial delusion, irresistible impulse or compulsive behaviour of a psychopath affords no protection under Section 84. Behaviour, antecedent, attendant and subsequent to the event, may be relevant in finding the mental condition of the accused at the time of the event, but not that remote in time. It is difficult to prove the precise state of the offender's mind at the time of the commission of the offence, but some indication thereof is often furnished by the conduct of the offender while committing it or immediately after the commission of the offence. A lucid interval of an insane person is not merely a cessation of the violent symptoms of the disorder, but a restoration of the faculties of the mind sufficiently to enable the person soundly to judge the act. But the expression does not necessarily mean complete or perfect restoration of the mental faculties to their original condition. If there is such a restoration, the person concerned can do the act with such reason, memory and judgment as to make it a legal act; but merely a cessation of the violent symptoms of the disorder is not sufficient." "Section 84 IPC carves out an exception, that an act will not be an offence, if done by a person, who at the time of doing the same, by reason of unsoundness of mind, is incapable of knowing the nature of the act, or what he is doing is either wrong or contrary to law. But this onus on the accused, under Section 105 of the Evidence Act is not as stringent as on the prosecution to be established beyond all reasonable doubts. The accused has only to establish his defence on a preponderance of probability, as observed in Surendra Mishra v. State of Jharkhand (2011) 11 SCC 495: (2011) 3 SCC (Cri) 232, after which the onus shall shift on the prosecution to establish the inapplicability of the exception. But, it is not every and any plea of unsoundness of mind that will suffice. The standard of test to be applied shall be of legal insanity and not medical insanity, as observed in State of Rajasthan v. Shera Ram (2012) 1 SCC 602: (2012) 1 SCC (Cri) 406, as follows: (Shera Ram, SCC p. 614, para 19) "19...Once, a person is found to be suffering from mental disorder or mental deficiency, which takes within its ambit hallucinations, dementia, loss of memory and self-control, at all relevant times by way of appropriate documentary and oral evidence, the person concerned would be entitled to seek resort to the general exceptions from criminal liability." 12. The crucial point of time for considering the defence plea of unsoundness of mind has to be with regard to the mental state of the accused at the time the offence was committed collated from evidence of conduct which preceded, attended and followed the crime. It is now well settled that the crucial point of time at which unsoundness of mind should be established is the time when the crime is actually committed and the burden of proving this lies on the accused. In Dahyabhai Chhaganbhai Thakkar v. State of Gujarat (1964) 7 SCR 361: AIR 1964 SC 1563, it was laid down that 'there is a rebuttable presumption that the accused was not insane. When he committed the crime, in the sense laid down by Section 84 of the Penal Code, the accused may rebut it by placing before the court all the relevant evidence—oral, documentary or circumstantial, but the burden of proof upon him is no higher than that which rests upon a party to civil proceedings'. If from the materials placed on record, a reasonable doubt is created in the mind of the Court with regard to the mental condition of the accused at the time of occurrence, he shall be entitled to the benefit of the reasonable doubt and consequent acquittal. There is not even a need for an application under Section 329 of Cr.P.C. in finding out as to whether an accused would be sound enough to stand a trial, rather it is the mandatory duty of the Court. Under Section 330, the Court can even go to the extent of discharging such a person if his inability to stand trial continues with a rigid chance of improvement. As per Section 334 of Cr.P.C., the judgment of the Court shall include a specific finding that the act was committed due to unsoundness of mind, though it was actually done. The reason is simple as there cannot be an acquittal on the ground of unsoundness of mind unless the act is actually done. The whole idea under the provisions discussed is to facilitate a person of unsound mind to stand trial, not only because of his reasoning capacity, but also to treat him as the one who is having a disability. The role of the Court is to find the remedial measures and do complete justice. If a friendly approach is required to be followed during the trial, when adequate powers have been conferred upon the Court to even discharge an accused on the ground of an unsound mind, the same reasoning will have to be applied with much force when it comes to Section 84 of the IPC. We find adequate materials on the assessment and evaluation of legal and medical insanity, which are totally different from each other. Forensic psychiatry attempts to help Courts determine the mental condition of the accused to determine whether the person could have intended to commit the crime and whether he is in a fit state to stand the trial. Medical insanity and legal insanity are not necessarily congruent. A mental illness that requires institutional care or administration of therapeutic care for medical insanity may not still be sufficient insulate the person from consequences of a criminal act and punishment if she/he is not legally insane. The assessment shall be to elicit such information as the law qualifies the general exception for proof of culpability under Section 84 of IPC. Is the accused mentally unsound? Is the mental unsoundness such that s/he is not capable of knowing (i) the nature of act; or (ii) the act is wrong, or (iii) contrary to law? These questions are directly related to testing the requirement of law. Is she/he capable of understanding the nature of proceedings in Court and stand trial? This shall be necessary to ensure that he has sufficient ability to consult with is counsel instruct him for a fair trial and defence. Every accused is bound to know the nature of proceedings against him/her. What was the mental condition of the accused, when the crime took place? Is it likely that the accused is malingering mental illness? The answers will point out to fixing the criminal responsibility to the acts attributed to him/her. Post-trial care may issue questions like: What is prognosis for cure for the mental illness? Will she/he be dangerous not to be let at large? In many a foreign jurisdiction, the questions may vary depending on the nature of proof of insanity and its intensity that is relevant under law to appraise criminal responsibility for the act: Could there have been an irresistible impulse to commit the act charged with? Was the mental condition so severe that s/he had no capacity to control his/her behaviour? 7 Was s/he under any form of delusion to inflict the criminal assault to fend off falsely perceived personal harm or injury? The evaluation process: The evaluation process generally includes, broadly, three major components or sources of data: (a) An interview with the accused (b) forensic assessment instruments, and (c) third party information including (but by no means limited to) collateral reports, witness statements, victim statements, police reports, and records of various sorts (i.e. mental health, treatment, school, medical, crime scene, etc.). Along with these sources, the role of delusions in evaluations of criminal responsibility (as the nature and quality of the accused 'delusionality') is often central in determining the extent of impairment in mental state at the time of the offence, especially in contested cases that may have a bearing on limiting responsibility if not completely exonerating him from the offence charged with. The role of the expert is not to present legal conclusions or formal psychopathological diagnoses. Rather, the role of examiner, as expert, is to import state of-the-art/science knowledge about the existence of various psychopathological conditions and their relationship to various behavioural, perceptual, cognitive and judgmental capacities into the legal/moral decisional process.

Schizophrenia

The term 'schizophrenia' means disintegration of mind. The term dementia praecox was changed because it implied that the disease always ended in dementia, which it did not. The term praecox meant that the disease developed at the time of puberty or adolescence, but in many cases developed outside that period. Since it was thought that the disease always ended in dementia, it meant a hopeless prognosis, which created a spirit of defeatism in the minds of people. "Schizophrenia n. a severe *mental illness characterised by a disintegration of the process of thinking, of contact with reality, and of emotional responsiveness. Positive symptoms, such as delusions and hallucinations (especially of voices), are common, and any Schneiderian first rank symptoms are particularly indicative of the illness. Negative symptoms include social withdrawal, impairment of ego boundaries, and loss of energy and initiative. Schizophrenia is diagnosed only if symptoms persist for at least one month. The illness can spontaneously remit, run a course with infrequent or frequent relapses, or become chronic. The prognosis has improved with *anti-psychotic drugs and with vigorous psychological and social management and rehabilitation. The many causes include genetic factors, environmental stress, and possibly illicit drug use. "Schizophrenia spectrum and other psychotic disorders include schizophrenia, other psychotic disorders, and schizotypal (personality) disorder. They are defined by abnormalities in one or more of the following five domains: Delusions, hallucinations, disorganized thinking (speech), grossly disorganized or abnormal motor behavior (including catatonia), and negative symptoms. Schizophrenia is certainly an over-powering mental illness.

Facts and Analysis

The case of the prosecution is that the appellant attacked the deceased at a store in which he was working, which belonged to the brother of his grandfather, who did not have any issue. There was no motive and the overt act attributed is that he assaulted the deceased with an iron locking plate without any provocation and premeditation. The occurrence took place on 14.05.2004 at 6:00 a.m. It was seen by PW2. He took the material object and came out of the shop and went to the bus stand. Thereafter, he came back to the shop and left it there. He once again walked to the bus stand and was sitting on a chair. He neither moved away from the said place nor made any attempt to leave. A treatment was indeed given to him at the GMC Hospital, Bhiwani in the State of Haryana prior to the occurrence. He was taken as an in-patient for a period from 17.11.2003 till 26.11.2003. He was suffering from anxiety neurosis with reactive depression and had symptoms of acid peptic disease and mild hypertension. The treatment given to him was akin to one meant for schizophrenia. Accordingly, he was prescribed the medicine 'Thioril'. Before the Court of Sessions, an application under

Section 329 of Cr.P.C. was filed on behalf of the appellant. Even while considering the application for bail, the Court noticed the inability of the appellant to understand the ongoing proceedings. Two doctors were examined as AWs 1 and 2, for the fact that he was indeed suffering from schizophrenia. AW2 was examined to show that he was taking the treatment earlier at GMC Hospital at Bhiwani. AW1 is the doctor who examined him after the occurrence on the orders of the trial court. She had deposed that he was indeed suffering from chronic schizophrenia. She was further examined as DW1. She once again made a clear deposition in tune with the certificate issued by her earlier that he was suffering from schizophrenia, and it must have been from the age of 14 or 15 years. The fact that he was unable to understand the act committed, and his subsequent incarceration was taken note of. While issuing the first certificate, this Government doctor in clear terms had stated that the appellant was not fit enough to stand the trial. However, she gave another certificate after treating him as an in-patient to the effect that he could stand trial thereafter. The Court of Sessions and the High Court rendered the conviction on merits. The plea of insanity was also taken. It was accordingly rejected on the ground that, the brother of the grandfather of the appellant, did not find any abnormality and that his mother has not been examined. The doctor who physically examined the accused after the incident, stated that the accused was mentally well. However, the evidence of the Government doctor who deposed, who was the uncle of the accused, and clearly spoke about the earlier treatment received by the accused. The evidence was not even taken note of. The conduct, though subsequent, of the appellant, was ignored. Before this Court, a report was called for from the District and Sessions Judge, Bhiwani as the medicine prescription and other documents could not be deciphered, and there was no discussion on the prior treatment given. We are of the view, that the aforesaid exercise would not have been warranted, had the evidence, which could be deciphered from the records furnished before us, been brought to the notice of the Court. In the report, it was stated that it could not be confirmed that the appellant was suffering from schizophrenia. We may note that the statements of the doctors were recorded after 16 years of the occurrence. In fact, they had also found it difficult to remember the nature of the treatment given to the appellant. In any case, that is a material which actually will go in favour of the appellant as the factum of treatment is not in dispute, particularly when it is corroborated by the evidence on more than one occasion. We may also add that this report merely records the statements of the doctors who have not been examined before the Court. Suffice it to say, that the evidence of the Government doctor as who withstood cross examination ought to have been accepted. The mere fact that the appellant subsequently became fit to face the trial is sufficient enough to render an order of acquittal as it is indicative of his prior insanity. We do feel that both the Trial Court and the High Court were influenced by the nature of the act while ignoring the condition of the appellant and the fact that the burden on the accused is one of preponderance of probability. We have also been informed that the appellant has recovered fully and mixed well with the society. For the aforesaid reasons, we are unable to give our imprimatur to the conviction rendered against the appellant as he is certainly entitled to the benefit conferred under Section 84 of the IPC. The order dated 25.07.2006 of the trial court of conviction and sentence of the appellant punishable under Section 302 of the IPC and the judgment and order dated 02.06.2008 of the High Court affirming the same are set aside. The appellant is acquitted of all the charges charged with. The bail bonds of the accused shall stand discharged. Pending application(s), if any, shall stand disposed of.

(The Supreme Court of India Criminal Original Jurisdiction Suo Motu Writ Petition (CRL.) No.1 of 2022 In Re: Framing Guidelines Regarding Potential Mitigating Circumstances to be Considered While Imposing Death Sentences Judgments. Ravindra Bhat, J.) This order is necessitated due to a difference of opinion and approach amongst various judgments, on the question of whether, after recording conviction for a capital offence, under law, the court is obligated to conduct a separate hearing on the issue of sentence. 2. Section 235 of the Code of Criminal Procedure, 1973 (hereinafter, "CrPC" or "Code") reads as follows: "235. Judgment of acquittal or conviction. (1) After hearing arguments and points of law (if any), the Judge shall give a judgment in the case. (2) If the accused is convicted, the Judge shall, unless he proceeds in accordance with the provisions of Section 360, hear the accused on the question of sentence, and then pass sentence on him according to law." Section 235, as it exists in the statute today, was Section 309 of the erstwhile Code (of 1898). It was introduced on account of the recommendations of the 48th Report of the Law Commission of India, on Some Questions Under the Code of Criminal Procedure Bill, 1970 (dated July 1972). Additionally, Section 309 of the CrPC is also relevant. It reads as follows: "309. Power to postpone or adjourn proceedings. (1) In every inquiry or trial, the proceedings shall be held as expeditiously as possible, and in particular, when the examination of witnesses has once begun, the same shall be continued from day to day until all the witnesses in attendance have been examined, unless the Court finds the adjournment of the same beyond the following day to be necessary for reasons to be recorded. (2) If the Court, after taking cognizance of an offence, or commencement of trial, finds it necessary or advisable to postpone the commencement of, or adjourn, any inquiry or trial, it may, from time to time, for reasons to be recorded, postpone or adjourn the same on such terms as it thinks fit, for such time as it considers reasonable, and may by a warrant remand the accused if in custody: Provided that no Magistrate shall remand an accused person to custody under this section for a term exceeding fifteen days at a time: Provided further that when witnesses are in attendance, no adjournment or postponement shall be granted, without examining them, except for special reasons to be recorded in writing: 1 Provided also that no adjournment shall be granted for the purpose only of enabling the accused person to show cause against the sentence proposed to be imposed on him. Explanation 1. If sufficient evidence has been obtained to raise a suspicion that the accused may have committed an offence, and it appears likely that further evidence may be obtained by a remand, this is a reasonable cause for a remand. Explanation 2. The terms on which an adjournment or postponement may be granted include, in appropriate cases, the payment of costs by the prosecution or the accused." 3. In Bachan Singh v. State of Punjab1 this court, in its majority judgment, upheld the constitutionality of the death sentence, on the condition that it could be imposed in the "rarest of rare" cases. The court was conscious of the safeguard of a separate hearing, on the question of sentence, and articulated such a safeguard as a valuable right, which insures to a convict, to urge why in the circumstances of his or her case, the extreme penalty of death ought not to be imposed. This court, in Bachan Singh, observed as follows: "151. Section 354 (3) of the CrPC, 1973, marks a significant shift in the legislative policy underlying the Code of 1898, as in force immediately before April 1, 1974, according to which both the alternative sentences of death or imprisonment for life provided for murder and for certain other capital offences under the Penal Code, were normal sentences. Now according to this changed legislative policy which is patent on the face of Section 354 (3), the normal punishment for murder and six other capital 1 1983 (1) SCR 145 3 offences under the Penal Code, is imprisonment for life (or imprisonment for a term of years) and death penalty is an exception. The Joint Committee of Parliament in its Report, stated the object and reason of making this change, as follows: 'A sentence of death is the extreme penalty of law and it is but fair that when a Court awards that sentence in a case where the alternative sentence of imprisonment for life is also available, it should give special reasons in support of the sentence. Accordingly, Sub-section (3) of Section 354 of the current Code provides: "When the conviction is for an offence punishable with death or, in the alternative with imprisonment for life or imprisonment for a term of years, the judgment shall state the reasons for the sentence awarded, and, in the case of sentence of death, the special reasons for such sentence." In the context, we may also notice Section 235 (2) of the Code of 1973, because it makes not only explicit, what according to the decision in Jagmohan's case was implicit in the scheme of the Code, but also bifurcates the trial by providing for two hearings, one at the pre-conviction stage and another at the pre-sentence stage. It requires that: "If the accused is convicted, the Judge shall, unless he proceeds in accordance with the provision of Section 360, hear the accused on the question of sentence, and then pass sentence on him according to law." The Law Commission in its 48th Report had pointed out this deficiency in the sentencing procedure: "It is now being increasingly recognised that a rational and consistent sentencing policy requires the removal of several deficiencies in the present system. One such deficiency is the lack of comprehensive information as to characteristics and background at the offender. The aims of sentencing:- Themselves obscure become all the more so in the absence of information on which the correctional process is to operate. The public as well as the courts themselves are in the dark about judicial approach in this regard. We are of the view that the taking of evidence as to the circumstances relevant to sentencing should be encouraged and both the prosecution and the accused should be allowed to co-operate in the process." By enacting Section 235 (2) of the new Code, Parliament has accepted that recommendation of the Law Commission. Although Sub-section (2) of Section 235 does not contain a specific provision as to evidence and provides only for hearing of the accused as to sentence, yet it is implicit in this provision that if a request is made in that behalf by either the prosecution or the accused, or by both, the Judge should give the party or parties concerned an opportunity of producing evidence or material relating to the various factors bearing on the question of sentence. "Of course,", as was pointed out by this Court in Santa Singh v State of Punjab AIR 1976 SC 2386 "care would have to be taken by the Court to see that this hearing on the question of sentence is not turned into an instrument for unduly protracting the proceedings. The claim of due and 4 proper hearing would have to be harmonised with the requirement of expeditious disposal of proceedings." 153. We may also notice Sections 432, 433 and 433A, as they throw light as to whether life imprisonment as currently administered in India, can be considered an adequate alternative to the capital sentence even in extremely heinous cases of murder. 154. Sections 432 and 433 of the Code of 1973 continue Sections 401 and 402 of the Code of 1898, with necessary modifications which bring them in tune with Articles 72 and 161 of the Constitution. Section 432 invests the "appropriate Government" as (defined in Sub-section (7) of that section) with power to suspend or remit sentences. Section 433 confers on the appropriate Government power to commute sentence, without the consent of the person sentenced. Under Clause (a) of the section, the appropriate Government may commute a sentence of death, for any other punishment provided by the Indian Penal Code. 155. With effect from December 18, 1978, the Cr. PC (Amendment) Act, 1978, inserted new Section 433A which runs as under: "433A. Restriction on power of remission or commutation in certain cases.- Notwithstanding anything contained in Section 432, where a sentence of imprisonment for life is imposed on conviction of a person for an offence for which death is one of the punishments provided by law, or where a sentence of death imposed on a person has been commuted under Section 433 into one of imprisonment for life, such person shall not be released from prison unless he had served at least fourteen years of imprisonment." It may be recalled that in Jagmohan this Court had observed that, in practice, life imprisonment amounts to 12 years in prison. Now, Section 433A restricts the power of remission and commutation conferred on the appropriate Government under Sections 432 and 433, so that a person who is sentenced to imprisonment for life or whose death sentence is commuted to imprisonment for life must serve actual imprisonment for a minimum of 14 years. We may next notice other provisions of the extant Code (corresponding to Sections 374, 375, 376 and 377 of the repealed Code) bearing on capital punishment. Section 366 (i) of the Code requires the Court passing a sentence of death to submit the proceedings to the High Court, and further mandates that such a sentence shall not be executed unless it is confirmed by the High Court. On such a reference for confirmation of death sentence, the High Court is required to proceed in accordance with Sections 367 and 368. Section 367 gives power to the High Court to direct further inquiry to be made or additional evidence to be taken. Section 368 empowers the High Court to confirm the sentence of death or pass any other sentence warranted by law; or to annul or alter the conviction or order a new trial or acquit the accused. Section 369 enjoins that in every case so submitted, the confirmation of the sentence, or any new sentence or order passed by the High Court, shall, when such court consists of two or more Judges, be made, passed and signed by at least two of them. Section 370 provides that where any such case is heard before a Bench of Judges and such Judges are equally divided in opinion, the case shall be referred to a third Judge. In this fasciculus of sections relating to confirmation proceedings in the High Court, the Legislature has provided valuable safeguards of the life and liberty of the subject in cases of capital sentences. These provisions seek to ensure mat where in a capital case, the life of the convicted person if at stake, the entire evidential material bearing on the innocence as guilt of the accused and the question of sentence must be scrutinised with utmost caution and care by a superior Court. Section 235 provides for a bifurcated trial and specifically gives the accused person a right of pre-sentence hearing, at which stage, he can bring on record material or evidence, which may not be strictly relevant to or connected with the particular crime under inquiry. Section 354 facilitates on the choice of sentence. The present legislative policy discernible from Section 235 read with Section 354 is that in fixing the degree of punishment or making the choice of sentence for various offences, including one under Section 302, Penal Code, the Court considers the circumstances connected with particular crime. The normal rule is that the offence of murder shall be punished with the sentence of life imprisonment. The court can depart from that rule and impose the sentence of death only if there are special reasons for doing so. Such reasons must be recorded in writing before imposing the death sentence, While considering the question of sentence to be imposed for the offence of murder under Section 302 Penal Code; the court must have regard to every relevant circumstance relating to the crime as well as the criminal. If the court finds, but not otherwise, that the offence is of an exceptionally depraved and heinous character and constitutes, on account of its design and the manner of its execution, a source of grave danger to the society at large, the court may impose the death sentence. The first requirement that there should be a bifurcated proceeding at which the sentencing authority is apprised of the information relevant to the imposition of sentence is met by the enactment of Section 235, sub-section (2), but the second requirement that the sentencing authority should be provided with standards to guide its use of the information is not satisfied and the imposition of death penalty under Section 302 of the Penal Code, 1860 read with Section 354, sub-section (3) of the Code of Criminal Procedure, 1973 must therefore be held to be arbitrary and capricious and hence violative of Articles 14 and 21." Plainly, therefore, the majority in Bachan Singh took note that convicts would be afforded a separate hearing, to urge why capital sentence ought not to be resorted to. The majority concluded: "157-A. In this fasciculus of sections relating to confirmation proceedings in the High Court, the legislature has provided valuable safeguards of the life and liberty of the subject in cases of capital sentences. These provisions seek to ensure that where in a capital case, the life of the convicted person is at stake, the entire evidential material bearing on the innocence or guilt of the accused and the question of sentence must be scrutinised with utmost caution and care. Therefore, was an important consideration to uphold the validity of death sentence, in the rarest of rare cases. It is realised that sentencing is an important stage in the process of administration of criminal justice—as important as the adjudication of guilt—and it should not be consigned to a subsidiary position as if it were a matter of not much consequence. It should be a matter of some anxiety to the court to impose an appropriate punishment on the criminal and sentencing should, therefore, receive serious attention of the court... The reason is that a proper sentence is the amalgam of many factors, the circumstances—extenuating or aggravating—of the offence, the prior criminal record, if any, of the offender, the age of the offender, the record of the offender as to employment, the background of the offender with reference to education, home life, sobriety and social adjustment, the emotional and mental condition of the offender, the prospects for the rehabilitation of the offender, the possibility of return of the offender to a normal life in the community, the possibility of treatment or training of the offender, the possibility that the sentence may serve as a deterrent to crime by the offender or by others and the current community need, if any, for such a deterrent in respect to the particular type of offence. Hence the new provision in Section 235. We are, therefore, of the view that the hearing contemplated by Section 235 is not confined merely to hearing oral submissions, but it is also intended to give an opportunity to the prosecution and the accused to place before the court facts and material relating to various factors bearing on the question of sentence and if they are contested by either side, then to produce evidence for the purpose of establishing the same. Of course, care would have to be taken by the court to see that this hearing on the question of sentence is not abused and turned into an instrument for unduly protracting the proceedings. The claim of due and proper hearing Santa Singh v. State of Punjab, (1976) SCC 190. It would have to be harmonised with the requirement of expeditious disposal of proceedings." In Muniappan v. State of Tamil Nadu, a two-judge bench of this court held that Section 235 was not a formality which could be dispensed with, and required consideration after conviction was confirmed: "The obligation to hear the accused on the question of sentence which is imposed by Section 235 of the Criminal Procedure Code is not discharged by putting a formal question to the accused as to what he has to say on the question of sentence. All admissible evidence is before the judge but that evidence itself often furnishes a clue to the genesis of the crime and the motivation of the criminal. It is the bounden duty of the judge to cast aside the formalities of the court scene and approach the question of sentence from a broad, sociological point of view. The occasion to apply the provisions of Section 235 arises only after the conviction is recorded. Questions which the judge can put to the accused under Section 235 and the answers which the accused makes to those questions are beyond the narrow constraints of the Evidence Act. The Sessions Judge, in the instant case, complied with the form and letter of the obligation which Section 235 imposes, forgetting the spirit and substance of that obligation." The death sentence provided for by Section 302 is an alternative to the sentence of life imprisonment; secondly, that special reasons have to be stated if the normal rule is departed from and the death sentence has to be imposed; and, thirdly, because the accused is entitled, under Section 235 of the Code of Criminal Procedure, to be heard on the question of sentence. It is because the court has an option to impose either of the two alternative sentences, subject to the rule that the normal punishment for murder is life imprisonment, that it is important to hear the accused on the question of sentence. If the law provides a mandatory sentence of death as Section 303 of the Penal Code does, neither Section 235 nor Section 354 of the Code of Criminal Procedure can possibly come into play. If the court has no option save to impose the sentence of death, it is meaningless to hear the accused on the question of sentence and it becomes superfluous to state the reasons for imposing the sentence of death". The court thus reiterated that the accused is entitled to be heard on the question of sentence before its imposition. "The requirement of hearing the accused is intended to satisfy the rule of natural justice. It is a fundamental requirement of fair play that the accused who was hitherto concentrating on the prosecution evidence on the question of guilt should, on being found guilty, be asked if he has anything to say or any evidence to tender on the question of sentence. This is all the more necessary since the courts are generally required to make the choice from a wide range of discretion in the matter of sentencing. The said provision therefore satisfies a dual purpose; it satisfies the rule of natural justice by according to the accused an opportunity of being heard on the question of sentence and at the same time helps the court to choose the sentence to be awarded. Since the provision is intended to give the accused an opportunity to place before the court, all the relevant material having a bearing on the question of sentence there can be no doubt that the provision is salutary and must be strictly followed. It is clearly mandatory and should not be treated as a mere formality. In a case of life or death as stated earlier, the presiding officer must show a high decree of concern for the statutory right of the accused and should not treat it as a mere formality to be crossed before making the choice of sentence. If the choice is made, as in this case, without giving the accused an effective and real opportunity to place his antecedents, social and economic background, mitigating and extenuating circumstances, etc., before the court, the court's decision on the sentence would be vulnerable. We need hardly mention that in many cases a sentencing decision has far more serious consequences on the offender and his family members than in the case of a purely administrative decision;

a fortiori, therefore, the principle of fair play must apply with greater vigour in the case of the former than the latter. An administrative decision having civil consequences, if taken without giving a hearing is generally struck down as violative of the rule of natural justice. The sentencing court must approach the question seriously and must endeavour to see that all the relevant facts and circumstances bearing on the question of sentence are brought on record. Only after giving due weight to the mitigating as well as the aggravating circumstances placed before it, it must pronounce the sentence. As a general rule the trial courts should after recording the conviction adjourn the matter to a future date and call upon both the prosecution as well as the defence to place the relevant material bearing on the question of sentence before it and thereafter pronounce the sentence to be imposed on the offender." The court held that the hearing should be intended to afford an opportunity to place materials to show mitigating circumstances—and, for the prosecution, aggravating circumstances and that "sufficient time must be given to the accused... on the question of sentence". A bifurcated hearing for convicting and sentencing is necessary to provide an effective opportunity to the accused. Scarce information about the accused at the time of sentencing, severely disadvantages the process of considering mitigating circumstances. It is clarified that mere mention of these circumstances by counsel, serve no purpose—rather, they must be connected to the possibility of reformation and assist principled judicial reasoning (as required under S. 235(2) CrPC). Constrained by this lack of assistance, this court (as mentioned above) in Rajesh Kumar [Rajesh Kumar v. State (2011) 13 SCC 706] has even gone so far as to hold that the very fact that the state had not given any evidence to show that the convict was beyond reform and rehabilitation was a mitigating circumstance, in itself. It is unfortunate to note that both the trial Court, and High Court, failed to provide an effective sentencing hearing to the accused, at the relevant stage, which is a right under Section 235(2) CrPC recognised by this court in several cases. In fact, it was argued by the accused that the trial court in contravention of this court's judgments, had proceeded to hear on sentencing almost immediately, depriving the accused of the opportunity to put forth their case for a less stringent sentence. The trial court order on sentencing, records in passing—the plea of 'young age' and 'socio-economic factors' as mitigating circumstances, but reflects, at best, a mechanical consideration of the same. Swayed by the brutality of the crime and "shock of the collective and judicial conscience", the High Court affirmed imposition of the death penalty solely on the basis of the aggravating circumstances of the crime, with negligible consideration of mitigating circumstances of the criminal. The Court may, in appropriate cases, have to adjourn the matter in order to give to the accused sufficient time to produce the necessary data and to make his contentions on the question of sentence. That, perhaps, must inevitably happen where the conviction is recorded for the first time by a higher court." This was in turn, followed by another three-judge bench in Tarlok Singh v. State of Punjab. Another case, where a similar conclusion was arrived at, but on differing reasoning was Ramdeo Chauhan v. State of Assam , where in a review petition, a bench of three judges, upheld the death penalty by a 2:1 majority. In this case, the proviso to Section 309(2) of CrPC was considered, in relation to Section 235(2). The court observed that the previous rulings had not taken note of the second proviso 15 to Section 309 of the Code. The court held that the mandate of the proviso under Section 309 was not to adjourn the hearing for affording a separate proceeding on sentence, however in cases where death sentence was one of the choices of punishment, the court had discretion to adjourn the hearing for a separate proceeding on sentence: "In a case punishable with death or imprisonment for life, there is no difficulty for the court where the sentence proposed to be imposed is an alternative sentence of life imprisonment but if it proposes to award the death sentence, it has discretion to adjourn the case in the interests of justice as held in Sukhdev Singh case [(1992) 3 SCC 700 : 1992 SCC (Cri) 705] . I have no doubt in holding that despite the bar of third proviso to sub-section (2) of Section 309, the court, in appropriate cases, can grant adjournment for enabling the accused persons to show cause. It was held that while the accused facing the possibility of death sentence was not entitled to an adjournment, nothing barred the court from granting the same. Many cases have grappled with the question as to the choice between the two. The approach of this Court needs to be rationalised and understood in the light of cautionary approach discussed above. The common thread that runs through all these decisions is the express acknowledgment that meaningful, real and effective hearing must be afforded to the accused, with the opportunity to adduce material relevant for the question of sentencing. The question of what constitutes 'sufficient time' at the trial court stage, in this manner appears not to have been addressed in the light of the express holding in Bachan Singh. This, in the court's considered opinion, requires consideration and clarity.

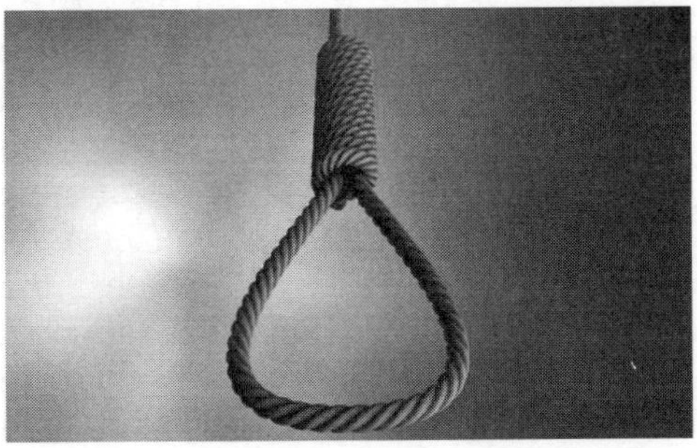

A former Army Officer has been sentenced to death by an Additional Sessions Court in Haryana's Palwal for murdering six people in 2018. The convict, Naresh Dhankar, was found guilty and convicted under Sections 302, 307, 332, 353, and 186 of the Indian Penal Code. Dhankar brutally killed six people in one night, using an iron pipe to repeatedly inflict blows that resulted in fatality.

The term "serial killing" is 'murder' simpliciter and no other offence is mentioned anywhere. It clearly indicates that the Legislation has intended to cover only the 'actual killer' under the definition of 'hardcore prisoner' and not the 'conspirator'. In order to cover a prisoner under the definition of 'hardcore prisoner', it is necessary that he must have participated in actual commission of the substantive offence of murder under Section 302 IPC and the aiding offence of criminal conspiracy under Section 120-B read with Section 302 IPC will not be covered under the category of 'hardcore prisoner'. The interpretation of hardcore prisoner has to be appreciated in view of subsequent convictions, therefore, status of Gurmit Ram Rahim at the threshold of definition in Section 2(aa)(i) of the Act does not depend upon the fact whether subsequent sentences have in fact started or not. The Statute identifies an offence of murder simpliciter and not a conspiracy to murder or abetment thereof.

POSTPARTUM DEPRESSION

The petitioner is a married woman of twenty-seven years. She and her husband have two children, the younger of which is about one-year-old. She filed the petition under Article 32 for directions to the respondents to permit a medical termination of her ongoing pregnancy. The petitioner states that she did not discover that she was pregnant until after twenty weeks of the pregnancy had elapsed because she had lactational amenorrhea. As a result of lactational amenorrhea, women who are breastfeeding do not menstruate. She therefore did not realize that the absence of menstruation was indicative of pregnancy. The petitioner states that she visited the gynaecologist for the first time after the delivery of her second child because she was feeling weak, nauseous, dizzy and experiencing abdominal discomfort. She underwent an ultrasound scan, upon which she realized that she was pregnant. The pregnancy was estimated to be around twenty-four weeks at that time. The petitioner avers that she and her husband attempted to medically terminate the pregnancy at various hospitals but that they were unable to because of the Medical Termination of Pregnancy Act 1971 read with the Medical Termination of Pregnancy Rules 20032 (as amended in 2021). She therefore 1 "MTP Act" 2 "MTP Rules" 4 approached this Court by invoking its writ jurisdiction. She sought permission for the medical termination of her pregnancy on the following grounds: a. **She suffers from post-partum depression and her mental condition does not permit her to raise another child**; and b. Her husband is the only earning member of their family and they already have two children to care for. Additionally, they have other family members who depend on them. As per the current status, the baby is viable and has a reasonable chance of survival. The chances of postpartum psychosis of which the couple is worried of, are present even at this gestation following delivery. The mother is a previous 2 LSCS and the chances of complications due to hysterotomy are there at this gestation. In such a scenario, the termination of pregnancy may be reconsidered. The option of antenatal care and delivery at AIIMS, New Delhi, has been discussed with the couple. 6. Physical fitness of the woman for the termination of pregnancy: (a) Yes ( ) (b) No ( ) " By its order dated 9 October 2023, this Court allowed the petition and permitted the medical termination of the pregnancy on the ground that continuing with the pregnancy could seriously imperil the mental health of the petitioner. The order was pronounced in Court and the reasons were to follow later. 5. On 10 October 2023, a doctor from AIIMS (who was a member of the Medical Board which examined the petitioner) emailed Ms. Aishwarya Bhati, learned ASG, stating that the foetus has a strong chance of survival and seeking directions from this Court as to whether the foetal heartbeat ought to be stopped. The email also stated that if the foetal heartbeat was not stopped, the baby would be placed in an intensive care unit and that there was a high possibility of immediate and long-term physical and mental disability. AIIMS sought a direction from the Court as to whether a foeticide should be carried out. The email is extracted below: This is regarding the Supreme Court order dated 9.10.2023, regarding termination of pregnancy of Ms ... This is not a termination, but a preterm delivery where the baby born will be provided treatment and care. A baby who is born preterm and also of such low birth weight will have a long stay in intensive care unit, with a high possibility of immediate and long term physical and mental disability which will seriously jeopardise the quality of life of the child. In such a scenario, a directive needs to be given as to what is to be done with the baby? If the parents agree to keep the child this will take a major physical, mental, emotional and financial toll on the couple. If it is to go for adoption, the process needs to be spelt out clearly as to needs to clear that baby who comes into the world will have a better chance at life if the delivery happens after at least 8 weeks. It is also to be kept in mind that the consequences of delivery which have happened in the previous two babies can happen at this time also, with a delivery now at this time. We would be obliged if a directive on these is given by the Hon Supreme Court to ease out the process. Ms. Bhati mentioned the case at 4 pm on 10 October 2023 before the Bench presided over by the Chief Justice. Ms Bhati informed this Court that in view of the email extracted above and the ensuing urgency, she mentioned the matter before Kohli, J (Nagarathna J was presiding over another Bench) and requested that it be listed. Kohli, J. orally informed Ms. Bhati that she was functus officio after passing the order dated 9 October 2023 and that the matter ought to be mentioned before the Chief Justice of India so that he may exercise his powers on the administrative side and constitute a bench to hear the matter. As stated above, Ms. Bhati mentioned the matter before the Bench presided over by the Chief Justice. The ASG stated that she would move a recall application, before the same bench which had heard the petition earlier the urgency arising as a result of the fact that the Court had directed an MTP to be carried out immediately upon the petitioner reporting to AIIMS. This was the appropriate course on the part of the ASG to follow since the Judges who had heard the petition (Justices Kohli and Nagarathna) were not sitting as a Bench thereafter and a special Bench had to be constituted. This lay within the powers of the Chief Justice on the administrative side. The Chief Justice constituted the same two-Judge Bench comprising of Kohli, J. and Nagarathna, J. to hear the application for recall of the order dated 9 October 2023 and the case was directed to be notified on the next day in the sitting list of 11 October 2023. The two-Judge Bench heard the counsel for the petitioners as well as the ASG. At this juncture, the petitioner filed an affidavit which stated, "I have made a wilful and conscious decision to medically terminate my pregnancy and don't want to keep the baby even if survives." The judges were unable to agree when the application moved by the ASG was heard and delivered a split verdict. In her judgment, Kohli, J. held that her judicial conscience prevented her from allowing the prayer in view of the email sent to Ms. Bhati. Nagarathna, J., on the other hand, held that the order dated 9 October 2023 ought not to be overturned for the following reasons: The interest of the mother, who already had two children and would deliver a third child within a year of delivering the second, must be given preference; The socio-economic conditions and the mental state of the petitioner must be considered by this Court; The decision of the petitioner ought to be respected and must not be substituted by the decision of this Court; and d. A foetus is dependent on the mother and cannot be recognized as a personality apart from that of the mother as its very existence is owed to the mother. Following the split verdict, the petition was directed to be listed before the present three judge Bench, in view of the difference of opinion between the two judges on the application for recall of the order dated 9 October 2023. On 13 October 2023, this Court passed an order calling for a further report from AIIMS on certain specific issues. They were formulated thus: "(i) Whether the fetus is suffering from any abnormality as provided by Subsection 2(b) of Section 3 of the Act. Though the earlier report mentions that the fetus is normal, nonetheless, in order to place the matter beyond doubt, we request a further report to be submitted on the above aspect; (ii) Whether the continuance of the pregnancy of the petitioner to full term would be jeopardised by the drugs which may be prescribed for the alleged condition from which the petitioner is stated to be suffering; and (iii) The medical professionals at AIIMS would be at liberty to carry out their own diagnosis in regard to the alleged medical condition and to indicate their own independent evaluation of the mental and physical condition of the petitioner. Upon doing so, we request **the doctors to apprise this Court if the petitioner is found to be suffering from postpartum psychosis** and whether any alternate administration of medication consistent with the pregnancy would be available so as to neither jeopardise the well-being of the petitioner or the foetus in that regard. This exercise shall be carried out during the course of the day. The Medical Board constituted by AIIMS comprised of nine doctors, including in the fields of obstetrics and gynaecology, paediatrics, and psychiatry. The conclusions in the report submitted by the Medical Board to this Court are extracted below: 1. As assessed by USG and Foetal Echo, the foetus **does not have any structural anomaly** at the present time. Here the board would also like to put on record that all abnormalities cannot be picked up on USG scans. 2. The continuation of pregnancy to full term while the woman is on the revised medications (as advised by the psychiatrist on the board) is not likely to significantly increase the risk of adverse outcomes for the mother and foetus as compared to other pregnant woman. 3. On a psychiatric assessment the board is of the opinion that she has a past history of postpartum psychosis, currently controlled on medications. Her medications have been reviewed and revised for an optimal management. It is felt that with proper care and treatment under appropriate medical supervision, the mother and baby can be managed well during pregnancy and postpartum as has been previously evidenced by her response to medications in case of worsening of symptoms, she may be admitted and treated." 11. Hence, the points put to the Medical Board for determination were answered in the following terms: a. No abnormality has been detected in the foetus; b. The continuation of the pregnancy would not be jeopardised by the medication which the petitioner is currently taking; and c. The petitioner has a history of postpartum psychosis which is currently being controlled on medication. A revised medication regime was prescribed for optimal management of the postpartum psychosis. The issues which arise for the consideration of this Court are: a. What is the nature of the jurisdiction under which this Court is adjudicating this case; and b. Can the relief sought in the writ petition be granted? B. Medical termination of pregnancies. The termination of pregnancies is governed by the MTP Act and the rules framed under it. The MTP Act is a progressive legislation which regulates the manner in which pregnancies may be terminated. Section 3 spells out certain conditions which must be satisfied before a pregnancy can be terminated. The "Section 3: When pregnancies may be terminated by registered medical practitioners (1) Notwithstanding anything contained in the Indian Penal Code (45 of 1860), a registered medical practitioner shall not be guilty of any offence under that code or under any other law for the time being in force, if any pregnancy is terminated by him in accordance with the provisions of this Act. [(2) Subject to the provisions of sub-section (4), a pregnancy may be terminated by a registered medical practitioner, (a) where the length of the pregnancy does not exceed twenty weeks, if such medical practitioner is, or (b) where the length of the pregnancy exceeds twenty weeks but does not exceed twenty-four weeks in case of such category of woman as may be prescribed by rules made under this Act, if not less than two registered medical practitioners are, of the opinion, formed in good faith, that (i) the continuance of the pregnancy would involve a risk to the life of the pregnant woman or of grave injury to her physical or mental health; or (ii) there is a substantial risk that if the child were born, it would suffer from any serious physical or mental abnormality. Explanation 1: For the purposes of clause (a), where any pregnancy occurs as a result of failure of any device or method used by any woman or her partner for the purpose of limiting the number of children or preventing pregnancy, the anguish caused by such pregnancy may be presumed to constitute a grave injury to the mental health of the pregnant woman.

Explanation 2: For the purposes of clauses (a) and (b), where any pregnancy is alleged by the pregnant woman to have been caused by rape, the anguish caused by the pregnancy shall be presumed to constitute a grave injury to the mental health of the pregnant woman. (2A) The norms for the registered medical practitioner whose opinion is required for termination of pregnancy at different gestational age shall be such as may be prescribed by rules made under this Act. (2B) The provisions of sub-section (2) relating to the length of the pregnancy shall not apply to the termination of pregnancy by the medical practitioner where such termination is necessitated by the diagnosis of any of the substantial foetal abnormalities diagnosed by a Medical Board. (2C) Every State Government or Union territory, as the case may be, shall, by notification in the Official Gazette, constitute a Board to be called a Medical Board for the purposes of this Act to exercise such powers and functions as may be prescribed by rules made under this Act. (2D) The Medical Board shall consist of the following, namely: (a) a Gynaecologist; (b) a Paediatrician; (c) a Radiologist or Sonologist; and (d) such other number of members as may be notified in the Official Gazette by the State Government or Union Territory, as the case may be. 11 conditions depend upon the length of the pregnancy. Where the length of the pregnancy does not exceed twenty weeks, one Registered Medical Practitioner must be of the opinion, formed in good faith, that: 6 a. The continuance of the pregnancy would involve a risk to the life of the pregnant woman or of grave injury to her physical or mental health. The anguish caused by a pregnancy which occurs due to the failure of a contraceptive method is presumed to constitute a grave injury to the mental health of the woman; 8 or b. There is a substantial risk that if the child were born, it would suffer from any serious physical or mental abnormality. Where any pregnancy is alleged by the pregnant woman to have been caused by rape, the anguish caused by the pregnancy is presumed to constitute a grave injury to the mental health of the woman. The presumption adverted to in (a) above makes it evident that the MTP Act recognizes the autonomy of the pregnant woman and respects her right to choose the course of her life. (3) In determining whether the continuance of a pregnancy would involve such risk of injury to the health as is mentioned in Sub-section (2), account may be taken of the pregnant woman's actual or reasonably foreseeable environment. (4) (a) No pregnancy of a woman, who has not attained the age of eighteen years, or, who having attained the age of eighteen years, is a mentally ill person, shall be terminated except with the consent in writing of her guardian. (b) Save as otherwise provided in clause (a), no pregnancy shall be terminated except with the consent of the pregnant woman." 5 "RMP" as defined under Section 2(d) of the MTP Act Section 3(2)(a), MTP Act 7 Section 3(2)(b)(i), MTP Act 8; Explanation 1 to Section 3(2), MTP Act 9 Section 3(2)(b)(ii), MTP Act 10; Explanation 2 to Section 3(2), MTP Act 12 14. Where the length of the pregnancy exceeds twenty weeks but does not exceed twenty-four weeks, two RMPs must be of the opinion discussed in the preceding paragraph. The categories of women where a pregnancy beyond 20 weeks and up to 24 weeks may be terminated are permitted to be prescribed by rules made by the delegate of the legislature. Rule 3B of the MTP Rules (as amended in 2021) provides grounds for the termination of a pregnancy up to twenty-four weeks. The termination may be allowed in the following cases or for the following persons: a. Survivors of sexual assault or rape or incest; b. Minors; c. Change of marital status during the ongoing pregnancy (widowhood and divorce); d. Women with physical disabilities with a major disability in terms of the criteria laid down under the

Rights of Persons with Disabilities Act 2016; e. Mentally ill women including mental retardation; f. Foetal malformation that has a substantial risk of being incompatible with life or where in the event of birth, the child may suffer from physical or mental abnormalities and be seriously handicapped; and 11 Section 3(2)(b), MTP Act 13 g. Women with pregnancy in humanitarian settings or disaster or emergency situations as may be declared by the Government.12 In X v. Principal Secretary, Department of Health and Family Welfare, GNCTD, 13 this Court held that the benefits of Rule 3B(c) extend equally to both single and married women and that the benefits of Rule 3B extend to all women who undergo a change in their material circumstances. 15. Significantly, if in the opinion of an RMP, the termination of a pregnancy is immediately necessary to save the life of a pregnant woman, the provisions of Section 3 which relate to the length of the pregnancy and the opinion of two RMPs shall not apply.14 Section 4 (which concerns the place at which a pregnancy may be terminated) shall not apply to such cases as well. The design of the statute makes it evident that saving the life of the pregnant woman is of paramount importance, notwithstanding the length of the pregnancy. 12 Rule 3B, MTP Rules: 3-B. Women eligible for termination of pregnancy up to twenty-four weeks. The following categories of women shall be considered eligible for termination of pregnancy under Clause (b) of Sub-section (2) Section 3 of the Act, for a period of up to twenty-four weeks, namely— **(a) survivors of sexual assault or rape or incest; (b) minors; (c) change of marital status during the ongoing pregnancy (widowhood and divorce); (d) women with physical disabilities [major disability as per criteria laid down under the Rights of Persons with Disabilities Act, 2016 (49 of 2016)]; (e) mentally ill women including mental retardation; (f) the foetal malformation that has substantial risk of being incompatible with life or if the child is born it may suffer from such physical or mental abnormalities to be seriously handicapped; and (g) women with pregnancy in humanitarian settings or disaster or emergency situations as may be declared by the Government**. 2022 SCC On Line SC 1321 14 Section 5, MTP Act: Sections 3 and 4 when not to apply.—(1) The provisions of Section 4, and so much of the provisions of sub-section (2) of Section 3 as relate to the length of the pregnancy and the opinion of not less than two registered medical practitioners, shall not apply to the termination of a pregnancy by a registered medical practitioner in a case where he is of opinion, formed in good faith, that the termination of such pregnancy is immediately necessary to save the life of the pregnant woman. .... The provisions of Section 3(2) relating to the length of the pregnancy shall not apply to the termination of a pregnancy by an RMP, where such termination is necessitated by the diagnosis of any of the substantial foetal abnormalities diagnosed by a Medical Board. The Medical Board has the power to allow or deny the termination of a pregnancy the length of which is beyond twenty-four weeks. It may do so only after ensuring that the procedure would be safe for the woman at that gestation age and after considering whether the foetal malformation leads to a substantial risk of the foetus being incompatible with life, or where the child (if it is born) may suffer from such physical or mental abnormalities as to be seriously handicapped. Therefore, the outer temporal limit within which a pregnancy may be terminated is lifted in some cases. The position of law can therefore be summarized as follows: Length of the pregnancy; Requirements for termination Up to twenty weeks: Opinion of one RMP in terms of Section 3(2): Between twenty and twenty-four weeks: Opinion of two RMPs in terms of Section 3(2) read with Rule 3B: Beyond twenty-four weeks If the termination is required to save the life of the pregnant woman, the opinion of one RMP in terms of Section 5. If there are substantial foetal abnormalities, with the approval of the 15 Section 3(2B), MTP Act 16 Rule 3A(a)(i), MTP Rules 17 Ibid 15 Medical Board in terms of Section 3(2B) read with Rule 3A(a)(i) C. Analysis i. The jurisdiction of this Court to hear this case 18. Having described the factual background, the procedural history, and the framework of law, we turn to the issues raised in this case. As noticed in the first segment of this judgment, the Union of India filed an application for the recall of the order dated 9 October 2023 passed by a two-Judge Bench of this Court on the ground that one of the doctors on the Medical Board emailed the learned ASG, seeking a clarification of that order. It is trite law that once a judgment or order attains finality, a party seeking to challenge the decision rendered may do so only by taking recourse to one of the following: a. Invoking the jurisdiction of the court to review the judgment or order; b. Preferring an appeal against the judgment or order (where an appeal lies); or c. In the case of the Supreme Court, filing a curative petition. The reason for the availability of a limited number of routes by which a judgment can be challenged is that there must be quietus to a dispute. Unlimited modes by which judgments or orders can be challenged would result in chaos, uncertainty, and unpredictability. This is also the reason why an application for recall of an order or judgment cannot be entertained by this Court, save and except in exceptional circumstances such as where a party which is directly affected was not served with notice of the proceedings. Otherwise, the hearing and disposal of an application for recall may even have the effect of creating an intra-court appeal, which is impermissible and wholly unknown to this Court. Indeed, this Court has repeatedly deprecated the practice of filing applications for recall and noted that they may sometimes be an abuse of the process of the law. In the present case, the Union of India filed an application for recall because certain aspects of the situation at hand were brought to its attention after the petition was disposed of by the order dated 9 October 2023. We have no doubt that there was no intention to abuse the process of the law. However, the appropriate procedure which it ought to have followed would be to file a Review Petition, accompanied by an application for urgent listing and an application for hearing in open court, given the urgency of the matter. The Bench consisting of Kohli and Nagarathna, JJ agreed to hear the matter. The immense urgency at that time did not permit this Court to address the reasons for doing so. The reasons are addressed presently. Under Article 142 of the Constitution, this Court has the power to pass such decree or make such order as is necessary for doing complete justice in any cause Delhi Admn. v. Gurdip Singh Uban, (2000) 7 SCC 296; Order dated 3 September 2020 in M.A. No.1434 of 2020 in Misc. Application Diary No.15272 of 2020 in Suo Moto Contempt Petition (Criminal) No. 2 of 2019 17 or matter pending before it. In State v. Kalyan Singh, this Court observed that Article 142 permitted it to relax the application of law depending upon the particular facts and circumstances of the case: This article gives a very wide power to do complete justice to the parties before the Court, a power which exists in the Supreme Court because the judgment delivered by it will finally end the litigation between the parties. It is important to notice that Article 142 follows upon Article 141 of the Constitution, in which it is stated that the law declared by the Supreme Court shall be binding on all courts within the territory of India. Thus, every judgment delivered by the Supreme Court has two components—the law declared which binds courts in future litigation between persons, and the doing of complete justice in any cause or matter which is pending before it. It is, in fact, an Article that turns one of the maxims of equity on its head, namely, that equity follows the law. By Article 142, as has been held in State of Punjab [State of Punjab v. Rafiq Masih, (2014) 8 SCC 883: (2014) 4 SCC (Civ) 657: (2014) 6 SCC (Cri) 154: (2014) 3 SCC (L&S) 134] judgment, equity has been given precedence over law. But it is not the kind of equity which can disregard mandatory substantive provisions of law when the court issues directions under Article 142. While moulding relief, the court can go to the extent of relaxing the application of law to the parties or exempting altogether the parties from the rigours of the law in view of the peculiar facts and circumstances of the case. This being so, it is clear that this Court has the power, nay, the duty to do complete justice in a case when found necessary. ... " (emphasis supplied). In the present case, this Court is justified in exercising its jurisdiction under Article 142 in view of the following circumstances: a. This is not an ordinary civil case. Rather, it is one which concerns the viability of a medical termination of a pregnancy and the course of action to be adopted by the doctors on the basis of the development of the foetus; b. Certain aspects of the case which ought to have been brought to the attention of this Court came to light after the order dated 9 October 2023 19 (2017) 7 SCC 444 18 had been passed. This was not within the control of any of the parties to the case but was the result of the actions of a third party altogether (the Medical Board). However, this information could have had a bearing on the directions issued by this Court; and c. There was immense urgency in this matter. ii. Decision on the prayer. We now turn to the issue of whether the relief sought in the writ petition can be granted. As noticed above, the length of the pregnancy has crossed twenty-four weeks. It is now approximately twenty-six weeks and five days. A medical termination of the pregnancy cannot be permitted for the following reasons: a. Having crossed the statutory limit of twenty-four weeks, the requirements in either of Section 3(2B) or Section 5 must be met; b. There are no "substantial foetal abnormalities" diagnosed by a Medical Board in this case, in terms of Section 3(2B). This Court called for a second medical report from AIIMS to ensure that the facts of the case were accurately placed before it and no foetal abnormality was detected; and c. Neither of the two reports submitted by the Medical Boards indicates that a termination is immediately necessary to save the life of the petitioner, in terms of Section 5. Under Article 142 of the Constitution, this Court has the power to do complete justice. However, this power may not be attracted in every case. If a medical termination were to be conducted at this stage, the doctors would be faced with a viable foetus. One of the options before this Court, which the email from AIIMS has flagged, is for it to direct the doctors to stop the heartbeat. This Court is averse to issuing a direction of this nature for the reasons recorded in the preceding paragraph. The petitioner, too, did not wish for this Court to issue such a direction. This was communicated by her to the court during the course of the hearing. In the absence of a direction to stop the heartbeat, the viable foetus would be faced with a significant risk of lifelong physical and mental disabilities. The reports submitted by the Medical Board speak for themselves. For these reasons, we do not accede to the prayer for the medical termination of the pregnancy. The delivery will be conducted by AIIMS at the appropriate time. The Union Government has undertaken to pay all the medical costs for the delivery and incidental to it. Should the petitioner be inclined to give the child up for adoption, the Union Government has stated through the submission of the ASG that they shall ensure that this process takes place at the earliest, and in a smooth fashion. The decision of whether to give the child up for adoption is entirely that of the parents.

Appendices

APPENDIX I

The Protection of Children from Sexual Offences Act 2012

No. 32 of 2012 (19th June, 2012)

An Act to protect children from offences of sexual assault, sexual harassment and pornography and provide for establishment of special courts for trial of such offences and for matters connected therewith or incidental there to.

WHEREAS clause (3) of Art. 15 of the Constitution, inter alia, empowers the State to make special provisions for children.

AND WHEREAS, the Government of India has acceded on the 11th December, 1992 to the Convention on the Rights of the Child, adopted by the General Assembly of the United Nations, which has prescribed a set of standards to be followed by all State parties in securing the best interests of the child.

AND WHEREAS it is necessary for the proper development of the child that his or her right to privacy and confidentiality be protected and respected by every person by all means and through all stages of a judicial process involving the child.

AND WHEREAS it is imperative that the law operates in a manner that the best interest and well being of the child are regarded as being of paramount importance at every stage, to ensure the healthy physical, emotional, intellectual and social development of the child.

AND WHEREAS the State parties to the Convention on the Rights of the Child are required to undertake all appropriate national, bilateral and multilateral measures to prevent:

a. the inducement or coercion of a child to engage in any unlawful sexual activity.
b. the exploitative use of children in prostitution or other unlawful sexual practices.
c. the exploitative use of children in pornographic performances and materials.

AND WHEREAS sexual exploitation and sexual abuse of children are heinous crimes and need to be effectively addressed.

BE it enacted by Parliament in the Sixty-third Year of the Republic of India as follows:

Chapter I

Preliminary

1. **Short title, extent and commencement:**
   a. This Act may be called the **Protection of Children from Sexual Offences Act 2012**.
   b. It extends to the **whole of India**, except the State of Jammu and Kashmir.
   c. It shall come into force on such date as the Central Government may, by notification in the Official Gazette, appoint.

2. **Definitions:**
   a. In this Act unless the context otherwise requires:
      i. "aggravated penetrative sexual assault" has the same meaning as assigned to it in Sec. 5.
      ii. "aggravated sexual assault" has the same meaning as assigned to it in Sec. 9.

iii. "armed forces or security forces" means armed forces of the Union or security forces or police forces, as specified in the Schedule.

iv. "child" means any person below the age of eighteen years.

v. "domestic relationship" shall have the same meaning as assigned to it in clause (f) of Sec. 2 of the Protection of Women from Domestic Violence Act 2005 (43 of 2005).

vi. "penetrative sexual assault" has the same meaning as assigned to it in Sec. 3.

vii. "prescribed means" prescribed by rules made under this Act.

viii. "religious institution" shall have the same meaning as assigned to it in the Religious Institutions (Prevention of Misuse) Act 1988 (41 of 1988).

ix. "sexual assault" has the same meaning as assigned to it in Sec. 7.

x. "sexual harassment" has the same meaning as assigned to it in Sec. 11.

xi. "shared household" means a household where the person charged with the offence lives or has lived at any time in a domestic relationship with the child.

xii. "special court" means a court designated as such under Sec. 28.

xiii. "special public prosecutor" means a public prosecutor appointed under Sec. 32.

b. The words and expressions used herein and not defined but defined in the Indian Penal Code (45 of 1860), the Code of Criminal Procedure, 1973 (2 of 1974), the Juvenile Justice (Care and Protection of Children) Act 2000 (56 of 2000) and the Information Technology Act 2000 (21 of 2000) shall have the meanings respectively assigned to them in the said Codes or the Acts.

Chapter II

Sexual Offences Against Children

A. Penetrative sexual assault and punishment therefor:

3. Penetrative sexual assault: A person is said to commit "penetrative sexual assault" if:

a. he penetrates his penis, to any extent, into the vagina, mouth, urethra or anus of a child or makes the child to do so with him or any other person; or

b. he inserts, to any extent, any object or a part of the body, not being the penis, into the vagina, the urethra or anus of the child or makes the child to do so with him or any other person; or

c. he manipulates any part of the body of the child so as to cause penetration into the vagina, urethra, anus or any part of body of the child or makes the child to do so with him or any other person; or

d. he applies his mouth to the penis, vagina, anus, urethra of the child or makes the child to do so to such person or any other person.

4. Punishment for penetrative sexual assault: Whoever commits penetrative sexual assault shall be punished with imprisonment of either description for a term which shall not be less than seven years but which may extend to imprisonment for life, and shall also be liable to fine.

B. Aggravated penetrative sexual assault and punishment therefor:

5. Aggravated penetrative sexual assault:

a. whoever, being a police officer, commits penetrative sexual assault on a child:

i. within the limits of the police station or premises at which he is appointed; or

ii. in the premises of any station house, whether or not situated in the police station, to which he is appointed; or

iii. in the course of his duties or otherwise; or

iv. where he is known as, or identified as, a police officer.

b. whoever being a member of the armed forces or security forces commits penetrative sexual assault on a child:

i. within the limits of the area to which the person is deployed; or
ii. in any areas under the command of the forces or armed forces; or
iii. in the course of his duties or otherwise; or
iv. where the said person is known or identified as a member of the security or armed forces.

c. whoever being a public servant commits penetrative sexual assault on a child; or
d. whoever being on the management or on the staff of a jail, remand home, protection home, observation home, or other place of custody or care and protection established by or under any law for the time being in force, commits penetrative sexual assault on a child, being inmate of such jail, remand home, protection home, observation home, or other place of custody or care and protection; or
e. whoever being on the management or staff of a hospital, whether Government or private, commits penetrative sexual assault on a child in that hospital; or
f. whoever being on the management or staff of an educational institution or religious institution, commits penetrative sexual assault on a child in that institution; or
g. whoever commits gang penetrative sexual assault on a child.

   Explanation: *When a child is subjected to sexual assault by one or more persons of a group in furtherance of their common intention, each of such persons shall be deemed to have committed gang penetrative sexual assault within the meaning of this clause and each of such person shall be liable for that act in the same manner as if it were done by him alone; or*

h. whoever commits penetrative sexual assault on a child usings deadly weapons, fire, heated substance or corrosive substance; or
i. whoever commits penetrative sexual assault causing grievous hurt or causing bodily harm and injury or injury to the sexual organs of the child; or
j. whoever commits penetrative sexual assault on a child, which:
   - physically incapacitates the child or causes the child to become mentally ill as defined under clause (b) of Sec. 2 of the Mental Health Act 1987 (14 of 1987) or causes impairment of any kind so as to render the child unable to perform regular tasks, temporarily or permanently; or
   - in the case of female child, makes the child pregnant as a consequence of sexual assault;
   - inflicts the child with human immunodeficiency virus or any other life-threatening disease or infection which may either temporarily or permanently impair the child by rendering him physically incapacitated, or mentally ill to perform regular tasks.
k. whoever, taking advantage of a child's mental or physical disability, commits penetrative sexual assault on the child; or
l. whoever commits penetrative sexual assault on the child more than once or repeatedly; or
m. whoever commits penetrative sexual assault on a child below twelve years; or
n. whoever being a relative of the child through blood or adoption or marriage or guardianship or in foster care or having a domestic relationship with a parent of the child or who is living in the same or shared household with the child, commits penetrative sexual assault on such child; or
o. whoever being, in the ownership, or management, or staff, of any institution providing services to the child, commits penetrative sexual assault on the child; or

p. whoever being in a position of trust or authority of a child commits penetrative sexual assault on the child in an institution or home of the child or anywhere else; or

q. whoever commits penetrative sexual assault on a child knowing the child is pregnant; or

r. whoever commits penetrative sexual assault on a child and attempts to murder the child; or

s. whoever commits penetrative sexual assault on a child in the course of communal or sectarian violence; or

t. whoever commits penetrative sexual assault on a child and who has been previously convicted of having committed any offence under this Act or any sexual offence punishable under any other law for the time being in force; or

u. whoever commits penetrative sexual assault on a child and makes the child to strip or parade naked in public, is said to commit aggravated penetrative sexual assault.

6. Punishment for aggravated penetrative sexual assault:

Whoever, commits aggravated penetrative sexual assault, shall be punished with rigorous imprisonment for a term which shall not be less than ten years but which may extend to imprisonment for life and shall also be liable to fine.

C. Sexual assault and punishment therefor:

7. Sexual assault:

Whoever, with sexual intent touches the vagina, penis, anus or breast of the child or makes the child touch the vagina, penis, anus or breast of such person or any other person, or does any other act with sexual intent which involves physical contact without penetration is said to commit sexual assault.

8. Punishment for sexual assault:

Whoever, commits sexual assault, shall be punished with imprisonment of either description for a term which shall not be less than three years but which may extend to five years, and shall also be liable to fine.

D. Aggravated sexual assault and punishment therefor:

9. Aggravated sexual assault:

a. Whoever, being a police officer, commits sexual assault on a child:
   i. within the limits of the police station or premises where he is appointed; or
   ii. in the premises of any station house whether or not situated in the police station to which he is appointed; or
   iii. in the course of his duties or otherwise; or
   iv. where he is known as, or identified as a police officer.

b. whoever, being a member of the armed forces or security forces, commits sexual assault on a child:
   i. within the limits of the area to which the person is deployed; or
   ii. in any areas under the command of the security or armed forces; or
   iii. in the course of his duties or otherwise; or
   iv. where he is known or identified as a member of the security or armed forces.

c. whoever being a public servant commits sexual assault on a child; or

d. whoever being on the management or on the staff of a jail, or remand home or protection home or observation home, or other place of custody or care and protection established by or under any law for the time being in force commits sexual assault on a child being inmate of such jail or remand home or protection home or observation home or other place of custody or care and protection; or

e. whoever being on the management or staff of a hospital, whether Government or private, commits sexual assault on a child in that hospital; or

f. whoever being on the management or staff of an educational institution or religious institution, commits sexual assault on a child in that institution; or

g. whoever commits gang sexual assault on a child.

Explanation: *When a child is subjected to sexual assault by one or more persons of a group in furtherance of their common intention, each of such persons shall be deemed to have committed gang sexual assault within the meaning of this clause and each of such person shall be liable for that act in the same manner as if it were done by him alone;* or

h. whoever commits sexual assault on a child using deadly weapons, fire, heated substance or corrosive substance; or

i. whoever commits sexual assault causing grievous hurt or causing bodily harm and injury or injury to the sexual organs of the child; or

j. whoever commits sexual assault on a child, which:
   - physically incapacitates the child or causes the child to become mentally ill as defined under clause l of Sec. 2 of the Mental Health Act 1987 (14 of 1987) or causes impairment of any kind so as to render the child unable to perform regular tasks, temporarily or permanently; or
   - inflicts the child with human immunodeficiency virus or any other life-threatening disease or infection which may either temporarily or permanently impair the child by rendering him physically incapacitated, or mentally ill to perform regular tasks.

k. whoever, taking advantage of a child's mental or physical disability, commits sexual assault on the child; or

l. whoever commits sexual assault on the child more than once or repeatedly; or

m. whoever commits sexual assault on a child below twelve years; or

n. whoever, being a relative of the child through blood or adoption or marriage or guardianship or in foster care, or having domestic relationship with a parent of the child, or who is living in the same or shared household with the child, commits sexual assault on such child; or

o. whoever, being in the ownership or management or staff, of any institution providing services to the child, commits sexual assault on the child in such institution; or

p. whoever, being in a position of trust or authority of a child, commits sexual assault on the child in an institution or home of the child or anywhere else; or

q. whoever commits sexual assault on a child knowing the child is pregnant; or

r. whoever commits sexual assault on a child and attempts to murder the child; or

s. whoever commits sexual assault on a child in the course of communal or sectarian violence; or

t. whoever commits sexual assault on a child and who has been previously convicted of having committed any offence under this Act or any sexual offence punishable under any other law for the time being in force; or

u. whoever commits sexual assault on a child and makes the child to strip or parade naked in public, is said to commit aggravated sexual assault.

10. Punishment for aggravated sexual assault: Whoever, commits aggravated sexual assault shall be punished with imprisonment of either description for a term which shall not be less than five years but which may extend to seven years, and shall also be liable to fine.

E. Sexual harassment and punishment therefor

11. Sexual harassment:

A person is said to commit sexual harassment upon a child when such person with sexual intent:

a. utters any word or makes any sound, or makes any gesture or exhibits any object or part of body with the intention that such word or sound shall be heard, or such gesture or object or part of body shall be seen by the child; or

b. makes a child exhibit his body or any part of his body so as it is seen by such person or any other person; or
c. shows any object to a child in any form or media for pornographic purposes; or
d. repeatedly or constantly follows or watches or contacts a child either directly or through electronic, digital or any other means; or
e. threatens to use, in any form of media, a real or fabricated depiction through electronic, film or digital or any other mode, of any part of the body of the child or the involvement of the child in a sexual act; or
f. entices a child for pornographic purposes or gives gratification therefor.

Explanation: *Any question which involves sexual intent shall be a question of fact.*

12. Punishment for sexual harassment: Whoever, commits sexual harassment upon a child shall be punished with imprisonment of either description for a term which may extend to three years and shall also be liable to fine.

Chapter III

Using Child for Pornographic Purposes and Punishment therefor

13. Use of child for pornographic purposes: Whoever, uses a child in any form of media (including programme or advertisement telecast by television channels or internet or any other electronic form or printed form, whether or not such programme or advertisement is intended for personal use or for distribution), for the purposes of sexual gratification, which includes:

a. representation of the sexual organs of a child;
b. usage of a child engaged in real or simulated sexual acts (with or without penetration);
c. the indecent or obscene representation of a child, shall be guilty of the offence of using a child for pornographic purposes.

Explanation: *For the purposes of this section, the expression "use a child" shall include involving a child through any medium like print, electronic, computer or any other technology for preparation, production, offering, transmitting, publishing, facilitation and distribution of the pornographic material.*

14. Punishment for using child for pornographic purposes:

a. Whoever, uses a child or children for pornographic purposes shall be punished with imprisonment of either description which may extend to five years and shall also be liable to fine and in the event of second or subsequent conviction with imprisonment of either description for a term which may extend to seven years and also be liable to fine.

b. If the person using the child for pornographic purposes commits an offence referred to in Sec. 3, by directly participating in pornographic acts, he shall be punished with imprisonment of either description for a term which shall not be less than ten years but which may extend to imprisonment for life, and shall also be liable to fine.

c. If the person using the child for pornographic purposes commits an offence referred to in Sec. 5, by directly participating in pornographic acts, he shall be punished with rigorous imprisonment for life and shall also be liable to fine.

d. If the person using the child for pornographic purposes commits an offence referred to in Sec. 7, by directly participating in pornographic acts, he shall be punished with imprisonment of either description for a term which shall not be less than six years but which may extend to eight years, and shall also be liable to fine.

e. If the person using the child for pornographic purposes commits an offence referred to in Sec. 9, by directly participating in pornographic acts, he shall be punished with imprisonment of either description for a term which shall not be less than eight years but which may extend to ten years, and shall also be liable to fine.

15. Punishment for storage of pornographic material involving child:

Any person, who stores, for commercial purposes any pornographic material in any form involving a child shall be punished with imprisonment of either description which may extend to three years or with fine or with both.

Chapter IV

Abetment of and Attempt to Commit an Offence

16. Abetment of an offence:

A person abets an offence, who

First.

Instigates any person to do that offence; or

Secondly.

Engages with one or more other person or persons in any conspiracy for the doing of that offence, if an act or illegal omission takes place in pursuance of that conspiracy, and in order to the doing of that offence; or

Thirdly.

Intentionally aids, by any act or illegal omission, the doing of that offence.

Explanation I: *A person who, by willful misrepresentation, or by willful concealment of a material fact, which he is bound to disclose, voluntarily causes or procures, or attempts to cause or procure a thing to be done, is said to instigate the doing of that offence.*

Explanation II: *Whoever, either prior to or at the time of commission of an act, does anything in order to facilitate the commission of that act, and thereby facilitates the commission thereof, is said to aid the doing of that act.*

Explanation III: *Whoever employ, harbours, receives or transports a child, by means of threat or use of force or other forms of coercion, abduction, fraud, deception, abuse of power or of a position, vulnerability or the giving or receiving of payments or benefits to achieve the consent of a person having control over another person, for the purpose of any offence under this Act is said to aid the doing of that act.*

17. Punishment for abetment:

Whoever abets any offence under this Act if the act abetted is committed in consequence of the abetment, shall be punished with punishment provided for that offence.

Explanation: *An act or offence is said to be committed in consequence of abetment, when it is committed in consequence of the instigation, or in pursuance of the conspiracy or with the aid, which constitutes the abetment.*

18. Punishment for attempt to commit an offence:

Whoever attempts to commit any offence punishable under this Act or to cause such an offence to be committed, and in such attempt, does any act towards the commission of the offence, shall be punished with imprisonment of any description provided for the offence, for a term which may extend to one-half of the imprisonment for life or, as the case may be, one-half of the longest term of imprisonment provided for that offence or with fine or with both.

Chapter V

Procedure for Reporting of Cases

19. Reporting of offences:

a. Notwithstanding anything contained in the Code of Criminal Procedure, 1973 (2 of 1974), any person (including the child), who has apprehension that an offence under this Act is likely to be committed or has knowledge that such an offence has been committed, he shall provide such information to:
   a. the Special Juvenile Police Unit; or
   b. the local police.
b. Every report given under sub-section (1) shall be:
   i. ascribed an entry number and recorded in writing;

ii. be read over to the informant;
iii. shall be entered in a book to be kept by the Police Unit.

c. Where the report under Sub-section (1) is given by a child, the same shall be recorded under Sub-section (2) in a simple language so that the child understands contents being recorded.
d. In case contents are being recorded in the language not understood by the child or wherever it is deemed necessary, a translator or an interpreter, having such qualifications, experience and on payment of such fees as may be prescribed, shall be provided to the child if he fails to understand the same.
e. Where the Special Juvenile Police Unit or local police is satisfied that the child against whom an offence has been committed is in need of care and protection, then, it shall, after recording the reasons in writing, make immediate arrangement to give him such care and protection (including admitting the child into shelter home or to the nearest hospital) within twenty-four hours of the report, as may be prescribed.
f. The Special Juvenile Police Unit or local police shall, without unnecessary delay but within a period of twenty-four hours, report the matter to the Child Welfare Committee and the Special Court or where no Special Court has been designated, to the Court of Session, including need of the child for care and protection and steps taken in this regard.
g. No person shall incur any liability, whether civil or criminal, for giving the information in good faith for the purpose of Sub-section (1).

20. Obligation of media, studio and photographic facilities to report cases:

Any personnel of the media or hotel or lodge or hospital or club or studio or photographic facilities, by whatever name called, irrespective of the number of persons employed therein, shall, on coming across any material or object which is sexually exploitative of the child (including pornographic, sexually-related or making obscene representation of a child or children) through the use of any medium, shall provide such information to the Special Juvenile Police Unit, or to the local police, as the case may be.

21. Punishment for failure to report or record a case:

a. Any person, who fails to report the commission of an offence under Sub-section (1) of Sec. 19 or Sec. 20 or who fails to record such offence under Sub-section 2 of Sec. 19 shall be punished with imprisonment of either description which may extend to six months or with fine or with both.
b. Any person, being in-charge of any company or an institution (by whatever name called) who fails to report the commission of an offence under Sub-section (1) of Sec. 19 in respect of a subordinate under his control, shall be punished with imprisonment for a term which may extend to one year and with fine.
c. The provisions of Sub-section (1) shall not apply to a child under this Act.

22. Punishment for false complaint or false information:

a. Any person, who makes false complaint or provides false information against any person, in respect of an offence committed under Secs. 3, 5, 7 and Sec. 9, solely with the intention to humiliate, extort or threaten or defame him, shall be punished with imprisonment for a term which may extend to six months or with fine or with both.
b. Where a false complaint has been made or false information has been provided by a child, no punishment shall be imposed on such child.
c. Whoever, not being a child, makes a false complaint or provides false information against a child, knowing it to be false, thereby victimising such

child in any of the offences under this Act shall be punished with imprisonment which may extend to one year or with fine or with both.

23. Procedure for media:

a. No person shall make any report or present comments on any child from any form of media or studio or photographic facilities without having complete and authentic information, which may have the effect of lowering his reputation or infringing upon his privacy.

b. No reports in any media shall disclose, the identity of a child including his name, address, photograph, family details, school, neighbourhood or any other particulars which may lead to disclosure of identity of the child: Provided that for reasons to be recorded in writing, the Special Court, competent to try the case under the Act may permit such disclosure, if in its opinion such disclosure is in the interest of the child.

c. The publisher or owner of the media or studio or photographic facilities shall be jointly and severally liable for the acts and omissions of his employee.

d. Any person who contravenes the provisions of Sub-section (1) or Sub-section (2) shall be liable to be punished with imprisonment of either description for a period which shall not be less than six months but which may extend to one year or with fine or with both.

Chapter VI

Procedures for Recording Statement of the Child

24. Recording of statement of a child:

a. The statement of the child shall be recorded at the residence of the child or at a place where he usually resides or at the place of his choice and as far as practicable by a woman police officer not below the rank of sub-inspector.

b. The police officer while recording the statement of the child shall not be in uniform.

c. The police officer making the investigation, shall, while examining the child, ensure that at no point of time the child come in the contact in any way with the accused.

d. No child shall be detained in the police station in the night for any reason.

e. The police officer shall ensure that the identity of the child is protected from the public media, unless otherwise directed by the Special Court in the interest of the child.

25. Recording of statement of a child by Magistrate:

a. If the statement of the child is being recorded under Sec. 164 of the Code of Criminal Procedure, 1973 (2 of 1974) (herein referred to as the Code), the Magistrate recording such statement shall, notwithstanding anything contained therein, record the statement as spoken by the child: Provided that the provisions contained in the first proviso to Sub-section (1) of Sec. 164 of the Code shall, so far it permits the presence of the advocate of the accused shall not apply in this case.

b. The Magistrate shall provide to the child and his parents or his representative, a copy of the document specified under Sec. 207 of the Code, upon the final report being filed by the police under Sec. 173 of that Code.

26. Additional provisions regarding statement to be recorded:

a. The Magistrate or the police officer, as the case may be, shall record the statement as spoken by the child in the presence of the parents of the child or any other person in whom the child has trust or confidence.

b. Wherever necessary, the Magistrate or the police officer, as the case may be, may take the assistance of a translator or an interpreter, having such qualifications, experience and on payment of such fees as may be prescribed, while recording the statement of the child.

c. The Magistrate or the police officer, as the case may be, may, in the case of a child having a mental or physical disability, seek the assistance of a special educator or any person familiar with the manner of communication of the child or an expert in that field, having such qualifications, experience and on payment of such fees as may be prescribed, to record the statement of the child.

d. Wherever possible, the Magistrate or the police officer, as the case may be, shall ensure that the statement of the child is also recorded by audio-video electronic means.

27. Medical examination of a child:

a. The medical examination of a child in respect of whom any offence has been committed under this Act shall, notwithstanding that a First Information Report or complaint has not been registered for the offences under this Act be conducted in accordance with Sec. 164A of the Code of Criminal Procedure, 1973 (2 of 1974).

b. In case the victim is a girl child, the medical examination shall be conducted by a woman doctor.

c. The medical examination shall be conducted in the presence of the parent of the child or any other person in whom the child reposes trust or confidence.

d. Where, in case the parent of the child or other person referred to in Sub-section (3) cannot be present, for any reason, during the medical examination of the child, the medical examination shall be conducted in the presence of a woman nominated by the head of the medical institution.

Chapter VII
Special Courts

28. Designation of special courts:

a. For the purposes of providing a speedy trial, the State Government shall in consultation with the Chief Justice of the High Court, by notification in the Official Gazette, designate for each district, a Court of Session to be a Special Court to try the offences under the Act: Provided that if a Court of Session is notified as a children's court under the Commissions for Protection of Child Rights Act 2005 (4 of 2006) or a Special Court designated for similar purposes under any other law for the time being in force, then, such court shall be deemed to be a Special Court under this section.

b. While trying an offence under this Act a Special Court shall also try an offence [other than the offence referred to in Sub-section (1)], with which the accused may, under the Code of Criminal Procedure, 1973 (2 of 1974), be charged at the same trial.

c. The Special Court constituted under this Act notwithstanding anything in the Information Technology Act 2000 (21 of 2000), shall have jurisdiction to try offences under Sec. 67B of that Act in so far as it relates to publication or transmission of sexually explicit material depicting children in any act, or conduct or manner or facilitates abuse of children online.

29. Presumption as to certain offences:
Where a person is prosecuted for committing or abetting or attempting to commit any offence under Secs. 3, 5, 7 and Sec. 9 of this Act the Special Court shall presume, that such person has committed or abetted or attempted to commit the offence, as the case may be unless the contrary is proved.

30. Presumption of culpable mental state:

a. In any prosecution for any offence under this Act which requires a culpable mental state on the part of the accused, the Special Court shall presume the existence of such mental state but it shall be a defence for the accused to prove the fact that he had no such mental state with respect to the act charged as an offence in that prosecution.

b. For the purposes of this section, a fact is said to be proved only when the Special Court believes it to exist beyond reasonable doubt and not merely when its existence is established by a preponderance of probability.

Explanation: *In this section, "culpable mental state" includes intention, motive, knowledge of a fact and the belief in, or reason to believe, a fact.*

31. Application of Code of Criminal Procedure, 1973 to proceedings before a Special Court:

Save as otherwise provided in this Act the prov or the purposes of the said provisions, the Special Court shall be deemed to be a Court of Sessions and the person conducting a prosecution before a Special Court, shall be deemed to be a Public Prosecutor.

32. Special Public Prosecutors:

a. The State Government shall, by notification in the Official Gazette, appoint a Special Public Prosecutor for every Special Court for conducting cases only under the provisions of this Act.

b. A person shall be eligible to be appointed as a Special Public Prosecutor under Sub-section (1) only if he had been in practice for not less than seven years as an advocate.

c. Every person appointed as a Special Public Prosecutor under this section shall be deemed to be a Public Prosecutor within the meaning of clause (u) of Sec. 2 of the Code of Criminal Procedure, 1973 (2 of 1974) and provision of that Code shall have effect accordingly.

Chapter VIII
Procedure and Powers of Special Courts and Recording of Evidence

33. Procedure and powers of Special Court:

a. A Special Court may take cognizance of any offence, without the accused being committed to it for trial, upon receiving a complaint of facts which constitute such offence, or upon a police report of such facts.

b. The Special Public Prosecutor, or as the case may be, the counsel appearing for the accused shall, while recording the examination-in-chief, cross-examination or re-examination of the child, communicate the questions to be put to the child to the Special Court which shall in turn put those questions to the child.

c. The Special Court may, if it considers necessary, permit frequent breaks for the child during the trial.

d. The Special Court shall create a child-friendly atmosphere by allowing a family member, a guardian, a friend or a relative, in whom the child has trust or confidence, to be present in the court.

e. The Special Court shall ensure that the child is not called repeatedly to testify in the court.

f. The Special Court shall not permit aggressive questioning or character assassination of the child and ensure that dignity of the child is maintained at all times during the trial.

g. The Special Court shall ensure that the identity of the child is not disclosed at any time during the course of investigation or trial: Provided that for reasons to be recorded in writing, the Special Court may permit such disclosure, if in its opinion such disclosure is in the interest of the child.

Explanation: *For the purposes of this Sub-section, the identity of the child shall include the identity of the child's family, school, relatives, neighbourhood or any other information by which the identity of the child may be revealed.*

h. In appropriate cases, the Special Court may, in addition to the punishment, direct payment of such compensation as may be prescribed to the child for any physical or mental trauma caused to him or for immediate rehabilitation of such child.

i. Subject to the provisions of this Act a Special Court shall, for the purpose of the trial of any offence under this Act have all the powers of a Court of Session and shall try such offence as if it were a Court of Session, and as far as may be, in accordance with the procedure specified in the Code of Criminal Procedure, 1973 (2 of 1974) for trial before a Court of Session.

34. Procedure in case of commission of offence by child and determination of age by Special Court:

a. Where any offence under this Act is committed by a child, such child shall be dealt with under the provisions of the Juvenile Justice (Care and Protection of Children) Act 2000 (56 of 2000).

b. If any question arises in any proceeding before the Special Court whether a person is a child or not, such question shall be determined by the Special Court after satisfying itself about the age of such person and it shall record in writing its reasons for such determination.

c. No order made by the Special Court shall be deemed to be invalid merely by any subsequent proof that the age of a person as determined by it under Sub-section (2) was not the correct age of that person.

35. Period for recording of evidence of child and disposal of case:

a. The evidence of the child shall be recorded within a period of thirty days of the Special Court taking cognizance of the offence and reasons for delay, if any, shall be recorded by the Special Court.

b. The Special Court shall complete the trial, as far as possible, within a period of one year from the date of taking cognizance of the offence.

36. Child not to see accused at the time of testifying:

a. The Special Court shall ensure that the child is not exposed in any way to the accused at the time of recording of the evidence, while at the same time ensuring that the accused is in a position to hear the statement of the child and communicate with his advocate.

b. For the purposes of Sub-section (1), the Special Court may record the statement of a child through video conferencing or by utilising single visibility mirrors or curtains or any other device.

37. Trials to be conducted in camera:

The Special Court shall try cases in camera and in the presence of the parents of the child or any other person in whom the child has trust or confidence: Provided that where the Special Court is of the opinion that the child needs to be examined at a place other than the court, it shall proceed to issue a commission in accordance with the provisions of Sec. 284 of the Code of Criminal Procedure, 1973 (2 of 1974).

38. Assistance of an interpreter or expert while recording evidence of child:

a. Wherever necessary, the Court may take the assistance of a translator or interpreter having such qualifications, experience and on payment of such fees as may be prescribed, while recording the evidence of the child.

b. If a child has a mental or physical disability, the Special Court may take the assistance of a special educator or any person familiar with the manner of communication of the child or an expert in that field, having such qualifications, experience and on payment of such fees as may be prescribed to record the evidence of the child.

Chapter IX
Miscellaneous

39. Guidelines for child to take assistance of experts, etc.

Subject to such rules as may be made in this behalf, the State Government shall prepare guidelines for use of non-governmental organisations, professionals and experts or persons having knowledge of psychology, social work, physical health, mental health and child development to be associated with the pre-trial and trial stage to assist the child.

40. Right of child to take assistance of legal practitioner:

Subject to the proviso to Sec. 301 of the Code of Criminal Procedure, 1973 (2 of 1974) the family or the guardian of the child shall be entitled to the assistance of a legal counsel of their choice for any offence under this Act: Provided that if the family or the guardian of the child are unable to afford a legal counsel, the Legal Services Authority shall provide a lawyer to them.

41. Provisions of Secs. 3 to 13 not to apply in certain cases:

The provisions of Secs. 3 to 13 (both inclusive) shall not apply in case of medical examination or medical treatment of a child when such medical examination or medical treatment is undertaken with the consent of his parents or guardian.

42. Alternative punishment:

Where an act or omission constitute an offence punishable under this Act and also under any other law for the time being in force, then, notwithstanding anything contained in any law for the time being in force, the offender found guilty of such offence shall be liable to punishment only under such law or this Act as provides for punishment which is greater in degree.

43. Public awareness about Act:

The Central Government and every State Government, shall take all measures to ensure that

a. the provisions of this Act are given wide publicity through media including the television, radio and the print media at regular intervals to make the general public, children as well as their parents and guardians aware of the provisions of this Act;
b. the officers of the Central Government and the State Governments and other concerned persons (including the police officers) are imparted periodic training on the matters relating to the implementation of the provisions of the Act.

44. Monitoring of implementation of Act:

a. The National Commission for Protection of Child Rights constituted under Sec. 3, or as the case may be, the State Commission for Protection of Child Rights constituted under Sec. 17, of the Commissions for Protection of Child Rights Act 2005 (4 of 2006), shall, in addition to the functions assigned to them under that Act also monitor the implementation of the provisions of this Act in such manner as may be prescribed.
b. The National Commission or, as the case may be, the State Commission, referred to in Sub-section (1), shall, while inquiring into any matter relating to any offence under this Act have the same powers as are vested in it under the Commissions for Protection of Child Rights Act 2005 (4 of 2006).
c. The National Commission or, as the case may be, the State Commission, referred to in Sub-section (1), shall, also include, its activities under this section, in the annual report referred to in Sec. 16 of the Commissions for Protection of Child Rights Act 2005 (4 of 2006).

45. Power to make rules:

a. The Central Government may, by notification in the Official Gazette, make rules for carrying out the purposes of this Act.
b. In particular, and without prejudice to the generality of the foregoing powers, such rules may provide for all or any of the following matters, namely:

i. the qualifications and experience of, and the fees payable to, a translator or an interpreter, a special educator or any person familiar with the manner of communication of the child or an expert in that field, under Sub-section (4) of Sec. 19; Sub-sections (2) and (3) of Sec. 26 and Sec. 38.
ii. care and protection and emergency medical treatment of the child under Sub-section (5) of Sec. 19.
iii. the payment of compensation under Sub-section (8) of Sec. 33.
iv. the manner of periodic monitoring of the provisions of the Act under Sub-section (1) of Sec. 44.

c. Every rule made under this section shall be laid, as soon as may be after it is made, before each House of Parliament, while it is in session, for a total period of thirty days which may be comprised in one session or in two or more successive sessions, and if, before the expiry of the session immediately following the session or the successive sessions aforesaid, both Houses agree in making any modification in the rule or both Houses agree that the rule should not be made, the rule shall thereafter have effect only in such modified form or be of no effect, as the case may be; so, however, that any such modification or annulment shall be without prejudice to the validity of anything previously done under that rule.

46. Power to remove difficulties:

a. If any difficulty arises in giving effect to the provisions of this Act the Central Government may, by order published in the Official Gazette, make such provisions not inconsistent with the provisions of this Act as may appear to it to be necessary or expedient for removal of the difficulty: Provided that no order shall be made under this section after the expiry of the period of two years from the commencement of this Act.
b. Every order made under this section shall be laid, as soon as may be after it is made, before each House of Parliament.

The Schedule (See Section 2(c))

Armed forces and security forces constituted under:

a. The Air Force Act 1950 (45 of 1950)
b. The Army Act 1950 (46 of 1950)
c. The Assam Rifles Act 2006 (47 of 2006)
d. The Bombay Home Guard Act 1947 (3 of 1947)
e. The Border Security Force Act 1968 (47 of 1968)
f. The Central Industrial Security Force Act 1968 (50 of 1968)
g. The Central Reserve Police Force Act 1949 (66 of 1949)
h. The Coast Guard Act 1978 (30 of 1978)
i. The Delhi Special Police Establishment Act 1946 (25 of 1946)
j. The Indo-Tibetan Border Police Force Act 1992 (35 of 1992)
k. The Navy Act 1957 (62 of 1957)
l. The National Investigation Agency Act 2008 (34 of 2008)
m. The National Security Guard Act1986 (47 of 1986)
n. The Railway Protection Force Act 1957 (23 of 1957)
o. The Sashastra Seema Bal Act 2007 (53 of 2007)
p. The Special Protection Group Act 1988 (34 of 1988)
q. The Territorial Army Act 1948 (56 of 1948);
r. The State police forces (including armed constabulary) constituted under the State laws to aid the civil powers of the State and empowered to employ force during internal disturbances or otherwise including armed forces as defined in clause (a) of Sec. 2 of the Armed Forces (Special Powers) Act 1958 (28 of 1958).

Appendix II

IMPORTANT PROVISIONS IN THE ORDINANCE

New Offences

This new Ordinance created some new offences or have expressedly created certain offences which were dealt under related laws. These new offences like, acid attack, sexual harassment, voyeurism, stalking has been incorporated into the Indian Penal Code (IPC).

Sections	*Offences*	*Punishments*	*Notes*
326A	Acid attack	Imprisonment not less than ten years but which may extend to imprisonment for life and with fine which may extend to ten lakh rupees	Gender neutral
326B	Attempt to acid attack	Imprisonment not less than five years but which may extend to seven years, and shall also be liable to fine	Gender neutral
354A	Sexual harassment	Rigorous imprisonment upto five years, or with fine, or with both in case of offence described in clauses (i) and (ii) Imprisonment upto one year, or with fine, or with both in other cases	Gender neutral (i) physical contact and advances involving unwelcome and explicit sexual overtures; or (ii) a demand or request for sexual favours; or (iii) making sexually coloured remarks; or (iv) forcibly showing pornography; or (v) any other unwelcome physical, verbal or non-verbal conduct of sexual nature.
354B	Public disrobing of woman	Imprisonment not less than three years but which may extend to seven years and with fine.	Assaults or uses criminal force to any woman or abets such act with the intention of disrobing or compelling her to be naked in any public place.
354C	Voyeurism	In case of first conviction, imprisonment not less than one year, but which may extend to three years, and shall also be liable to fine, and be punished on a second or subsequent conviction, with imprisonment of either description for a term which shall not be less than three years, but which may extend to seven years, and shall also be liable to fine.	Watching or capturing a woman in "private act", which includes an act of watching carried out in a place which, in the circumstances, would reasonably be expected to provide privacy, and where the victim's genitals, buttocks or breasts are exposed or covered only in underwear; or the victim

Contd.

Contd.

Sections	*Offences*	*Punishments*	*Notes*
			is using a lavatory; or the person is doing a sexual act that is not of a kind ordinarily done in public.
354D	Stalking	Imprisonment not less than one year but which may extend to three years, and shall also be liable to fine	Gender neutral. Whoever follows a person and contacts, or attempts to contact such person to foster personal interaction repeatedly, despite a clear indication of disinterest by such person, or whoever monitors the use by a person of the internet, email or any other form of electronic communication, or watches or spies on a person in a manner that results in a fear of violence or serious alarm or distress in the mind of such person, or interferes with the mental peace of such person, commits the offence of stalking.

Changes in law

Section 370 of Indian Penal Code (IPC) has been substituted with new Secs. 370 and 370A which deals with trafficking of person for exploitation. If a person (a) recruits, (b) transports, (c) harbours, (d) transfers, or (e) receives, a person or persons, by using threats, or force, or coercion, or abduction, or fraud, or deception, or by abuse of power, or inducement for exploitation including prostitution, slavery, forced organ removal, etc. will be punished with imprisonment ranging from atleast 7 years to imprisonment for the remainder of that person's natural life depending on the number or category of persons trafficked.[14] Employment of a trafficked person will attract penal provision as well.[14]

The most important change that has been made is the change in definition of rape under IPC. The word rape has been replaced with sexual assault in Sec. 375, and have added penetrations other than penile penetration an offence. The definition is broadly worded and gender neutral in some aspect, with acts like penetration of penis, or any object or any part of body to any extent, into the vagina, mouth, urethra or anus of another person or making another person do so, apply of mouth or touching private parts constitutes the offence of sexual assault. The section has also clarified that penetration means "penetration to any extent", and lack of physical resistance is immaterial for constituting an offence. Except in certain aggravated situation the punishment will be imprisonment not less than seven years but which may extend to imprisonment for life, and shall also be liable to fine. In aggravated situations, punishment will be rigorous imprisonment for a term which shall not be less than ten years but which may extend to imprisonment for life, and shall also be liable to fine. A new Sec. 376A has been added which states that if a person committing the offence of sexual assault, "inflicts an injury which causes the death of the person or causes the person to be in a persistent vegetative state, shall be punished with rigorous imprisonment for a term which shall not be less than twenty years, but which may extend to imprisonment for life, which shall mean the remainder of that person's natural life, or with death."[15] In case of "gang rape", persons involved regardless of their gender shall be punished with rigorous imprisonment for a term which shall not be less than twenty years, but which may extend to life and shall pay compensation to the victim which shall be reasonable to meet the medical expenses and rehabilitation of the victim.

Certain changes has been introduced in the CrPC and Evidence Act like the recording of statement of the victim, more friendly and easy, character of the victim is irrelevant, presumption of no consent where sexual intercourse is proved and the victim states in the court that there has been no consent, etc.

Criticisms of Ordinance

The Criminal Law (Amendment) Ordinance, 2013 has been strongly criticised by several human rights and womens' rights organisations for not including certain suggestions recommended by the Verma Committee Report like, *marital rape*, reduction of *age of consent*, amending Armed Forces (Special Powers) Act so that no sanction is needed for prosecuting an armed force personnel accused of a crime against woman.[16][17][18] The *Government of India*, replied that it has not rejected the suggestions fully, but changes can be made after proper discussion.[19][20]

References

1. ^ "Lok Sabha passes amendments". *NDTV*. 19 March 2013. Retrieved 4 February 2013.
2. ^ "Lok Sabha passes anti-rape bill". *Hindustan Times*. 19 March 2013. Retrieved 4 February 2013.
3. ^ "Prez Pranab Mukherjee promulgates ordinance on crime against women". *Indian Express*. 3 February 2013. Retrieved 4 February 2013.
4. ^ "President signs ordinance to effect changes in laws against sexual crimes". *India Today*. 3 February 2013. Retrieved 4 February 2013.
5. ^ "IAP condoles death of Delhi gang-rape victim". New Delhi: Zeenews.com. *PTI*. 29 December 2012. *Archived* from the original on 30 December 2012. Retrieved 30 December 2012.
6. ^ Stenhammer, Anne F. (20 December 2012). "UN Women condemns gang rape of Delhi student" (Press release). UN Women. Retrieved 21 December 2012.
7. ^ Joshi, Sandeep (24 December 2012). "Shinde calls meeting of Chief Secretaries, police chiefs to review crime against women". *The Hindu*. Retrieved 27 December 2012.
8. ^ "Justice J S Verma committee submits report on rape laws". *Times of India*. 23 January 2013. Retrieved 4 February 2013.
9. ^ "Failure of governance root cause of crimes against women: Verma committee". *The Hindu*. 23 January 2013. Retrieved 23 January 2013.
10. ^ "Read: Highlights of Justice Verma Committee report". *CNNIBN Live*. 23 January 2013. Retrieved 23 January 2013.
11. ^ "Cabinet clears anti-rape law ordinance, says death sentence for extreme cases". *NDTV*. 1 February 2013. Retrieved 4 February 2013.
12. ^ "We have accepted 90% of Justice Verma panel's recommendations: Law Minister". *NDTV*. 3 February 2013. Retrieved 4 February 2013.
13. ^ http://www.hindustantimes.com/India-news/NewDelhi/Lok-Sabha-passes-anti-rape-bill/Art.1-1028961.aspx
14. ^ *a b* Section 7, Criminal Law (Amendment) Ordinance, 2013
15. ^ Section 8, Criminal Law (Amendment) Ordinance, 2013
16. ^ "Read: Ordinance *vs* Verma commission recommendations". *NDTV*. 1 February 2013. Retrieved 5 February 2013.
17. ^ "Women groups protest anti-rape ordinance". *DNA*. 4 February 2013. Retrieved 5 February 2013.
18. ^ "Despite protest, ordinance on sexual offences promulgated". *The Hindu*. 3 February 2013. Retrieved 5 February 2013.
19. ^ "Open to revisions in anti-rape bill: Govt". *Times of India*. 3 February 2013. Retrieved 5 February 2013.
20. ^ "Govt defends ordinance on sexual crimes". *LiveMint*. 4 February 2013. Retrieved 5 February 2013.

Appendix III

THE CRIMINAL LAW (AMENDMENT) BILL, 2013

In a bill passed by the Lok Sabha on 19 March 2013 which provides for amendment of Indian Penal Code, Indian Evidence Act and Code of Criminal Procedure, 1973 on laws related to sexual offences.[1][2] It was originally an Ordinance promulgated by the President of India, Pranab Mukherjee, on 3 February 2013, in light of the protests in the 2012 Delhi gang rape case.[3][4]

- Introduction
- Important provisions in the Ordinance
  - i. New offences
  - ii. Changes in law
- Criticisms of Ordinance
- References

INTRODUCTION

On 16 December 2012, a female physiotherapy intern[5] was beaten and gang raped in Delhi. She died from her injuries thirteen days later, despite receiving treatment in India and Singapore. The incident generated international coverage and was condemned by the United Nations Entity for Gender Equality and the Empowerment of Women, who called on the Government of India and the Government of Delhi "to do everything in their power to take up radical reforms, ensure justice and reach out with robust public services to make women's lives more safe and secure".[6] Public protests took place in Delhi, where thousands of protesters clashed with security forces. Similar protests took place in major cities throughout the country.

On 22 December 2012, a judicial committee headed by *J. S. Verma*, former *Chief Justice of India*, was appointed by the Central government to submit a report, within 30 days, to suggest amendments to criminal law to sternly deal with sexual assault cases. The Committee submitted its report after 29 days on 23 January 2013, after considering 80,000 suggestions received by them during the period from public in general and particularly eminent jurists, legal professionals, NGOs, women's groups and civil society.[7][8] The report indicated that failures on the part of the Government and Police were the root cause behind crimes against women. Major suggestions of the report included the need to review AFSPA in conflict areas, maximum punishment for rape as life imprisonment and not death penalty, clear ambiguity over control of Delhi Police, etc.[9][10]

The *Cabinet Ministers* on 1 February 2013 approved for bringing an ordinance, for giving effect to the changes in law as suggested by the Verma Committee Report.[11] According to Minister of Law and Justice, *Ashwani Kumar*, 90 percent of the suggestions given by the Verma Committee Report has been incorporated into the Ordinance.[12] The ordinance was subsequently approved by the Lok Sabha to become a Bill on 19 March 2013.[13]

Appendix IV

THE JUVENILE JUSTICE (CARE AND PROTECTION OF CHILDREN) ACT 2000

(Act No. 56 of 2000)
[30th December 2000]

An Act to consolidate and amend the law relating to juveniles in conflict with law and children in need of care and protection, by providing for proper care, protection and treatment by catering to their development needs, and by adopting a child-friendly approach in the adjudication and disposition of matters in the best interest of children and for their ultimate rehabilitation through various institutions established under this enactment.

WHEREAS the Constitution has, in several provisions, including clause (3) of Art. 15, clauses (e) and (f) of Art. 39, Arts. 45 and 47, impose on the State a primary responsibility of ensuring that all the needs of children are met and that their basic human rights are fully protected.

AND WHEREAS, the General Assembly of the United Nations has adopted the Convention on the Rights of the Child on the 20th November, 1989.

AND WHEREAS, the Convention on the Rights of the Child has prescribed a set of standards to be adhered to by all State parties in securing the best interests of the child.

AND WHEREAS, the Convention on the Rights of the Child emphasises social reintegration of child victims, to the extent possible, without resorting to judicial proceedings.

AND WHEREAS, the Government of India has ratified the Convention on the 11th December, 1992.

AND WHEREAS, it is expedient to re-enact the existing law relating to juveniles bearing in mind the standards prescribed in the Convention on the Rights of the Child, the United Nations Standard Minimum Rules for the Administration of Juvenile Justice, 1985 (the Beijing rules), the United Nations Rules for the Protection of Juveniles Deprived of their Liberty (1990), and all other relevant international instruments.

Be it enacted by Parliament in the Fifty-first Year of the Republic of India as follows:

Chapter I

Preliminary

1. **Short title, extent and commencement:**
   1. This Act may be called the Juvenile Justice (Care and Protection of Children) Act 2000.
   2. It extends to the whole of India except the State of Jammu and Kashmir.
   3. It shall come into force on such date as the Central Government may, by notification in the Official Gazette, appoint.
2. **Definitions: In this Act unless the context otherwise requires:**
   a. "advisory board" means a Central or a state advisory board or a district and city level advisory board, as the case may be, constituted under Sec. 62

   b. "begging" means:

      i. soliciting or receiving alms in a public place or entering into any private premises for the purpose of soliciting or receiving alms, whether under any pretence.

      ii. exposing or exhibiting with the object of obtaining or extorting alms, any sore, wound, injury, deformity or disease, whether of himself or of any other person or of an animal.

   c. "Board" means a Juvenile Justice Board constituted under Sec. 4.

   d. "child in need of care and protection" means a child.

      i. who is found without any home or settled place or abode and without any ostensible means of subsistence.

      ii. who resides with a person (whether a guardian of the child or not) and such person
         - has threatened to kill or injure the child and there is a reasonable likelihood of the threat being carried out, or
         - has killed, abused or neglected some other child or children and there is a reasonable likelihood of the child in question being killed, abused or neglected by that person.

      iii. who is mentally or physically challenged or ill children or children suffering from terminal diseases or incurable diseases having no one to support or look after.

      iv. who has a parent or guardian and such parent or guardian is unfit or incapacitated to exercise control over the child.

      v. who does not have parent and no one is willing to take care of or whose parents have abandoned him or who is missing and run away child and whose parents cannot be found after reasonable inquiry.

      vi. who is being or is likely to be grossly abused, tortured or exploited for the purpose of sexual abuse or illegal acts.

      vii. who is found vulnerable and is likely to be inducted into drug abuse or trafficking.

      viii. who is being or is likely to be abused for unconscionable gains.

ix. who is victim of any armed conflict, civil commotion or natural calamity.

e. "children's home" means an institution established by a State Government or by voluntary organisation and certified by that Government under Sec. 34.

f. "Committee" means a Child Welfare Committee constituted under Sec. 29.

g. "competent authority" means in relation to children in need of care and protection a Committee and in relation to juveniles in conflict with law a Board.

h. "fit institution" means a governmental or a registered non-governmental organisation or a voluntary organisation prepared to own the responsibility of a child and such organisation is found fit by the competent authority.

i. "fit person" means a person, being a social worker or any other person, who is prepared to own the responsibiliy of a child and is found fit by the competent authority to receive and take care of the child.

j. "guardian", in relation to a child, means his natural guardian or any other person having the actual charge or control over the child and recognised by the competent authority as a guardian in course of proceedings before that authority.

k. "juvenile" or "child" means a person who has not completed eighteenth year of age.

l. "juvenile in conflict with law" means a juvenile who is alleged to have committed an offence.

m. "local authority" means Panchayats at the village and Zila Parishad at the district level and shall also include a Municipal Committee or Corporation or a Cantonment Board or such other body legally entitled to function as local authority by the Government.

n. "narcotic drug" and "psychotropic substance" shall have the meanings respectively assigned to them in the Narcotic Drugs and Psychotropic Substances Act 1985 (61 of 1985).

o. "observation home" means a home established by a State Government or by a voluntary organisation and certified by that State Government under Sec. 8 as an observation home for the juvenile in conflict with law.

p. "offence" means an offence punishable under any law for the time being in force.

q. "place of safety" means any place or institution (not being a police lock-up or jail), the person incharge of which is willing temporarily to receive and take care of the juvenile and which, in the opinion of the competent authority, may be a place of safety for the juvenile.

r. "prescribed" means prescribed by rules made under this act.

s. "Probation officer" means an officer appointed by the State Government as a probation officer under the Probation of Offenders Act 1958 (20 of 1958).

t. "public place" shall have the meaning assigned to it in the Immoral Traffic (Prevention) Act 1956 (104 of 1956).

u. "shelter home" means a home or a drop-in-centre set up under Sec. 37.

v. "special home" means an institution established by a State Government or by a voluntary organisation and certified by that Government under Sec. 9; "special juvenile police unit" means a unit of the police force of a State designated for handling of juveniles or children under Sec. 63.

w. "State Government", in relation to a Union territory, means the Administrator of that Union territory appointed by the President under Art. 239 of the Constitution.

x. all words and expressions used but not defined in this Act and defined in the Code of Criminal Procedure, 1973 (2 of 1974), shall have the meanings respectively assigned to them in that code.

3. **Continuation of inquiry in respect of juvenile who has ceased to be a juvenile:** Where an inquiry has been initiated against a juvenile in conflict with law or a child in need of care and protection and during the course of such inquiry the juvenile or the child ceases to be such, then, notwithstanding anything contained in this Act or in any other law for the

time being in force, the inquiry may be continued and orders may be made in respect of such person as if such person had continued to be a juvenile or a child.

Chapter II
Juvenile in Conflict with Law

4. **Juvenile justice board:**
   a. Notwithstanding anything contained in the Code of Criminal Procedure, 1973 (2 of 1974), the State Government may, by notification in the Official Gazette, constitute for a district or a group of districts specified in the notification, one or more Juvenile Justice Boards for exercising the powers and discharging the duties conferred or imposed on such Boards in relation to juveniles in conflict with law under this act.
   b. A Board shall consist of a Metropolitan Magistrate or a Judicial Magistrate of the first class, as the case may be, and two social workers of whom at least one shall be a woman, forming a Bench and every such Bench shall have the powers conferred by the Code of Criminal Procedure, 1973 (2 of 1974), on a Metropolitan Magistrate or, as the case may be, a Judicial Magistrate of the first class and the Magistrate on the Board shall be designated as the principal Magistrate.
   c. No Magistrate shall be appointed as a member of the Board unless he has special knowledge or training in child psychology or child welfare and no social worker shall be appointed as a member of the Board unless he has been actively involved in health, education, or welfare activities pertaining to children for at least seven years.
   d. The term of office of the members of the Board and the manner in which such member may resign shall be such as may be prescribed.
   e. The appointment of any member of the Board may be terminated after holding inquiry, by the State Government, if:
      i. he has been found guilty of misuse of power vested under this act.
      ii. he has been convicted of an offence involving moral turpitude, and such conviction has not been reversed or he has not been granted full pardon in respect of such offence.
      iii. he fails to attend the proceedings of the Board for consecutive three months without any valid reason or he fails to attend less than three-fourth of the sittings in a year.
5. **Procedure, etc. in relation to board:**
   a. The Board shall meet at such times and shall, observe such rules of procedure in regard to the transaction of business at its meetings, as may be prescribed.
   b. A child in conflict with law may be produced before an individual member of the Board, when the Board is not sitting.
   c. A Board may act notwithstanding the absence of any member of the Board, and no order made by the Board shall be invalid by reason only of the absence of any member during any stage of proceedings: Provided that there shall be at least two members including the principal Magistrate present at the time of final disposal of the case.
   d. In the event of any difference of opinion among the members of the Board in the interim or final disposition, the opinion of the majority shall prevail, but where there is no such majority, the opinion of the principal Magistrate, shall prevail.
6. **Powers of juvenile justice board:**
   a. Where a Board has been constituted for any district or a group of districts, such Board shall, notwithstanding anything contained in any other law for the time being in force but *save as otherwise* expressly provided in this Act have power to deal exclusively with all proceedings under this Act relating to juvenile in conflict with law.
   b. The powers conferred on the Board by or under this Act may also be exercised by the High Court and the Court of Session, when the proceedings comes before them in appeal, revision or otherwise.

7. Procedure to be followed by a Magistrate not empowered under the Act:

a. When any Magistrate not empowered to exercise the powers of a Board under this Act is of the opinion that a person brought before him under any of the provisions of this Act (other than for the purpose of giving evidence), is a juvenile or the child, he shall without any delay record such opinion and forward the juvenile or the child, and the record of the proceeding to the competent authority having jurisdiction over the proceeding.

b. The competent authority to which the proceeding is forwarded under Sub-section (1) shall hold the inquiry as if the juvenile or the child had originally been brought before it.

8. Observation homes:

a. Any State Government may establish and maintain either by itself or under an agreement with voluntary organisations, observation homes in every district or a group of districts, as may be required for the temporary reception of any juvenile in conflict with law during the pendency of any inquiry regarding them under this Act.

b. Where the State Government is of opinion that any institution other than a home established or maintained under Sub-section (1), is fit for the temporary reception of juvenile in conflict with law during the pendency of any inquiry regarding them under this Act it may certify such substitution as an observation home for purposes of this Act.

c. The State Government may, by rules made under this Act provide for the management of observation homes, including the standards and various types of services to be provided by them for rehabilitation and social integration of a juvenile, and the circumstances under which, and the manner in which, the certification of an observation home may be granted or withdrawn.

d. Every juvenile who is not placed under the charge of parent or guardian and is sent to an observation home shall be initially kept in a reception unit of the observation home for preliminary inquiries, care and classification for juveniles according to his age group, such as seven to twelve years, twelve to sixteen years and sixteen to eighteen years, giving due considerations to physical and mental status and degree of the offence committed, for further induction into observation home.

9. Special homes:

a. Any State Government may establish and maintain either by itself or under an agreement with voluntary organisations, special homes in every district or a group of districts, as may be required for reception and rehabilitation of juvenile in conflict with law under this Act.

b. Where the State Government is of opinion that any institution other than a home established or maintained under Sub-section (1), is fit for the reception of juvenile in conflict with law to be sent there under this Act it may certify such institution as a special home for the purposes of this Act.

c. The State Government may, by rules made under this Act provide for the management of special homes, including the standards and various types of services to be provided by them which are necessary for re-socialisation of a juvenile, and the circumstances under which and the manner in which, the certification of a special home may be granted or withdrawn.

d. The rules made under Sub-section (3) may also provide for the classification and separation of juvenile in conflict with law on the basis of age and the nature of offences committed by them and his mental and physical status.

10. Apprehension of juvenile in conflict with law:

a. As soon as a juvenile in conflict with law is apprehended by police, he shall be placed under the charge of the special juvenile police unit or the designated police officer who shall immediately report the matter to a member of the Board.

b. The State Government may make rules consistent with this Act:
   i. to provide for persons through whom (including registered voluntary organisations) any juvenile in conflict with law may be produced before the Board.
   ii. to provide the manner in which such juvenile may be sent to an observation home.

11. Control of custodian over juvenile: Any person in whose charge a juvenile is placed in pursuance of this Act shall, while the order is in force have the control over the juvenile as he would have if he were his parents, and shall be responsible for his maintenance, and the juvenile shall continue in his charge for the period stated by competent authority, notwithstanding that he is claimed by his parents or any other person.

12. Bail of juvenile:

a. When any person accused of a bailable or non-bailable offence, and apparently a juvenile, is arrested or detained or appears or is brought before a Board, such person shall, notwithstanding anything contained in the Code of Criminal Procedure, 1973 (2 of 1974) or in any other law for the time being in force, be released on bail with or without surety but he shall not be so released if there appear reasonable grounds for believing that the release is likely to bring him into association with any known criminal or expose him to moral, physical or psychological danger or that his release would defeat the ends of justice.

b. When such person having been arrested is not released on bail under Sub-section (1) by the officer incharge of the police station, such officer shall cause him to be kept only in an observation home in the prescribed manner until he can be brought before a Board.

c. When such person is not released on bail under Sub-section (1) by the Board it shall, instead of committing him to prison, make an order sending him to an observation home or a place of safety for such period during the pendency of the inquiry regarding him as may be specified in the order.

13. Information to parent, guardian or probation officer: Where a juvenile is arrested, the officer incharge of the police station or the special juvenile police unit to which the juvenile is brought shall, as soon as may be after the arrest, inform:

a. the parent or guardian of the juvenile, if he can be found, of such arrest and direct him to be present at the Board before which the juvenile will appear; and

b. the probation officer of such arrest to enable him to obtain information regarding the antecedents and family background of the juvenile and other material circumstances likely to be of assistance to the Board for making the inquiry.

14. Inquiry by board regarding juvenile: Where a juvenile having been charged with the offence is produced before a Board, the Board shall hold the inquiry in accordance with the provisions of this Act and may make such order in relation to the juvenile as it deems fit:

Provided that an inquiry under this section shall be completed within a period of four months from the date of its commencement, unless the period is extended by the Board having regard to the circumstances of the case and in special cases after recording the reasons in writing for such extension.

15. Order that may be passed regarding juvenile:

a. Where a Board is satisfied with inquiry that a juvenile has committed an offence, then notwithstanding anything to the contrary contained in any other law for the time being in force, the Board may, if it thinks so fit:
   i. allow the juvenile to go home after advice or admonition following appropriate inquiry against and counselling to the parent or the guardian and the juvenile.

ii. direct the juvenile to participate in group counselling and similar activities.
iii. order the juvenile to perform community service.
iv. order the parent of the juvenile or the juvenile himself to pay a fine, if he is over fourteen years of age and earns money.
v. direct the juvenile to be released on probation of good conduct and placed under the care of any parent, guardian or other fit person, on such parent, guardian or other fit person executing a bond, with or without surety, as the Board may require, for the good behavior and well-being of the juvenile for any period not exceeding three years.
vi. direct the juvenile to be released on probation of good conduct and placed under the care of any fit institution for the good behavior and well-being of the juvenile for any period not exceeding three years.
vii. make an order directing the juvenile to be sent to a special home:
    - in the case of juvenile, over seventeen years but less than eighteen years of age for a period of not less than two years;
    - in case of any other juvenile for the period until he ceases to be a juvenile: Provided that the Board may, if it is satisfied that having regard to the nature of the offence and the circumstances of the case it is expedient so to do, for reasons to be recorded, reduce the period of stay to such period as it thinks fit.

b. The Board shall obtain the social investigation report on juvenile either through a probation officer or a recognised voluntary organisation or otherwise, and shall take into consideration the findings of such report before passing an order.
c. Where an order under clause (d), clause (e) or clause (f) of Sub-section (1) is made, the Board may, if it is of opinion that in the interests of the juvenile and of the public, it is expedient so to do, in addition make an order that the juvenile in conflict with law shall remain under the supervision of a probation officer named in the order during such period, not exceeding three years as may be specified therein, and may in such supervision order impose such conditions as it deems necessary for the due supervision of the juvenile in conflict with law: Provided that if at any time afterwards it appears to the Board on receiving a report from the probation officer or otherwise, that the juvenile in conflict with law has not been of good behavior during the period of supervision or that the fit institution under whose care the juvenile was placed is no longer able or willing to ensure the good behavior and well-being of the juvenile, it may, after making such inquiry as it deems fit, order the juvenile in conflict with law to be sent to a special home.
d. The Board shall while making a supervision order under Sub-section (3), explain to the juvenile and the parent, guardian or other fit person or fit institution, as the case may be, under whose care the juvenile has been placed, the terms and conditions of the order shall forthwith furnish one copy of the supervision order to the juvenile, the parent, guardian or other fit person or fit institution, as the case may be, the sureties, if any, and the probation officer.

16. Order that may not be passed against juvenile:

a. Notwithstanding anything to the contrary contained in any other law for the time being in force, no juvenile in conflict with law shall be sentenced to death or life imprisonment, or committed to prison in default of payment of fine or in default of furnishing security: Provided that where a juvenile who has attained the age of sixteen years has committed an offence and the Board is satisfied that the offence committed is of so serious nature or that his conduct and behavior have been such that it would not be in his interest or in the interest of other juvenile in a special home to send him to such special home and that none of the other measures provided under this Act is suitable or sufficient, the Board may order the juvenile in conflict with law to be kept in such place of safety and in such manner as it thinks fit and shall report the case for the order of the State Government.

b. On receipt of a report from a Board under Sub-section (1), the State Government may make such arrangement in respect of the juvenile as it deems proper and may order such juvenile to be kept under protective custody at such place and on such conditions as it thinks fit: Provided that the period of detention so ordered shall not exceed the maximum period of imprisonment to which the juvenile could have been sentenced for the offence committed.

17. **Proceeding under Chapter VIII of the Code of Criminal Procedure not component against juvenile:** Notwithstanding anything to the contrary contained in the Code of Criminal Procedure, 1973 (2 of 1974) no proceeding shall be instituted and no order shall be passed against the juvenile under Chapter VIII of the said Code.

18. **No joint proceeding of juvenile and person not a juvenile:**

a. Notwithstanding anything contained in Sec. 223 of the Code of Criminal Procedure, 1973 (2 of 1974) or in any other law for the time being in force, no juvenile shall be charged with or tried for any offence together with a person who is not a juvenile.

b. If a juvenile is accused of an offence for which under Sec. 223 of the Code of Criminal Procedure, 1973 (2 of 1974) or any other law for the time being in force, such juvenile and any person who is not a juvenile would, but for the prohibition contained in Sub-section (1), have been charged and tried together, the Board taking cognizance of that offence shall direct separate trials of the juvenile and the other person.

19. **Removal of disqualification attaching to conviction:**

a. Notwithstanding anything contained in any other law, a juvenile who has committed an offence and has been dealt with under the provisions of this Act shall not suffer disqualification, if any, attaching to a conviction of an offence under such law.

b. The Board shall make an order directing that the relevant records of such conviction shall be removed after the expiry of the period of appeal or a reasonable period as prescribed under the rules, as the case may be.

20. **Special provision in respect of pending cases:** Notwithstanding anything contained in this Act all proceedings in respect of a juvenile pending in any court in any area on the date on which this Act comes into force in that area, shall be continued in that court as if this Act had not been passed and if the court finds that the juvenile has committed an offence, it shall record such finding and instead of passing any sentence in respect of the juvenile, forward the juvenile to the Board which shall pass orders in respect of that juvenile in accordance with the provisions of this Act as if it had been satisfied with inquiry under this Act that a juvenile has committed the offence.

21. **Prohibition of publication of name, etc. of juvenile involved in any proceeding under the Act:**

a. No report in any newspaper, magazine, news-sheet or visual media of any inquiry regarding a juvenile in conflict with law under this Act shall disclose the name, address or school or any other particulars calculated to lead to the identification of the juvenile nor shall any picture of any such juvenile be published: Provided that for reasons to be recorded in writing the authority holding the inquiry may permit such disclosure, if in its opinion such disclosure is in interest of the juvenile.

b. Any person contravening the provisions of Sub-section (1) shall be punishable with fine, which may extend to one thousand rupees.

22. Provision in respect of escaped juvenile: Notwithstanding anything to the contrary contained in any other law for the time being in force, any police officer may take charge without warrant of a juvenile in conflict with law who has escaped from a special home or an observation home or from the care of a person under whom he was placed under this Act and shall be sent back to the special home or the observation home or that person, as the case may be; and no proceeding shall be instituted in respect of the juvenile by reason of such escape, but the special home, or the observation home or the person may, after giving the information to the Board which passed the order in respect of the juvenile, take such steps in respect of the juvenile as may be deemed necessary under the provisions of this Act.

23. Punishment for cruelty to juvenile or child: Whoever, having the actual charge of, or control over, a juvenile or the child, assaults, abandons, exposes or willfully neglects the juvenile or causes or procures him to be assaulted, abandoned, exposed or neglected in a manner likely to cause such juvenile or the child unnecessary mental or physical suffering shall be punishable with imprisonment for a term which may extend to six months, or fine, or with both.

24. Employment of juvenile or child for begging:

a. Whoever employs or uses any juvenile or the child for the purpose or causes any juvenile to beg shall be punishable with imprisonment for a term which may extend to three years and shall also be liable to fine.
b. Whoever, having the actual charge of, or control over, a juvenile or the child abets the commission of the offence punishable under Sub-section (1), shall be punishable with imprisonment for a term which may extend to one year and shall also be liable to fine.

25. Penalty for giving intoxicating liquor or narcotic drug or psychotropic substance to juvenile or child: Whoever gives, or causes to be given, to any juvenile or the child any intoxicating liquor in a public place or any narcotic drug or psychotropic substance except upon the order of duly qualified medical practitioner or in case of sickness shall be punishable with imprisonment for a term which may extend to three years and shall be liable to fine.

26. Exploitation of juvenile or child employee: Whoever ostensibly procures a juvenile or the child for the purpose of any hazardous employment keeps him in bondage and withholds his earnings or uses such earnings for his own purposes shall be punishable with imprisonment for a term which may extend to three years and shall be liable to fine.

27. Special offences: The offences punishable under Secs. 23, 24, 25 and 26 shall be cognizable.

28. Alternative punishment: Where an act or omission constitute an offence punishable under this Act and also under any other Central or State Act then, notwithstanding anything contained in any law for the time being in force, the offender found guilty of such offences shall be liable to punishment only under such Act as provides for punishment which is greater in degree.

Chapter III
Child in Need of Care and Protection

29. Child Welfare Committee:

a. The State Government may, by notification in Official Gazette, constitute for every district or group of districts, specified in the notification, one or more Child Welfare Committees for exercising the powers and discharge the duties conferred on such Committees in relation to child in need of care and protection under this Act.
b. The Committee shall consist of a Chairperson and four other members as the State Government may think fit to appoint, of whom at least one shall be a woman and another, an expert on matters concerning children.
c. The qualifications of the Chairperson and the members, and the tenure for which they may be appointed shall be such as may be prescribed.

d. The appointment of any member of the Committee may be terminated, after holding inquiry, by the State Government, if:
   i. he has been found guilty of misuse of powers vested under this Act.
   ii. he has been convicted of an offence involving moral turpitude, and such conviction has not been reversed or he has not been granted full pardon in respect of such offence.
   iii. he fails to attend the proceedings of the Committee for consecutive three months without any valid reason or he fails to attend less than three-fourth of the sittings in a year.

e. The Committee shall function as a Bench of Magistrates and shall have the powers conferred by the Code of Criminal Procedure, 1973 (2 of 1974) on a Metropolitan Magistrate or, as the case may be, a Judicial Magistrate of the first class.

30. Procedure, etc. in relation to Committee:

a. The Committee shall meet at such times and shall observe such rules of procedure in regard to the transaction of business in its meetings, as may be prescribed.

b. A child in need of care and protection may be produced before an individual member for being placed in safe custody or otherwise when the Committee is not in session.

c. In the event of any difference of opinion among the members of the Committee at the time of any interim decision, the opinion of the majority shall prevail but where there is no such majority the opinion of the Chairperson shall prevail.

d. Subject to the provisions of Sub-section (1), the Committee may act, notwithstanding the absence of any member of the Committee, and no order made by the Committee shall be invalid by reason only of the absence of any member during any stage of the proceeding.

31. Powers of committee:

a. The Committee shall have the final authority to dispose off cases for the care, protection, treatment, development and rehabilitation of the children as well as to provide for their basic needs and protection of human rights.

b. Where a Committee has been constituted for any area, such Committee shall, notwithstanding anything contained in any other law for the time being in force but *save as otherwise* expressly provided in this Act have the power to deal exclusively with all proceedings under this Act relating to children in need of care and protection.

32. Production before committee:

a. Any child in need of care and protection may be produced before the Committee by one of the following persons:
   i. any police officer or special juvenile police unit or a designated police officer;
   ii. any public servant;
   iii. childline, a registered voluntary organisation or by such other voluntary organisation or an agency as may be recognised by the State Government;
   iv. any social worker or a public spirited citizen authorised by the State Government; or
   v. by the child himself.

b. The State Government may make rules consistent with this Act to provide for the manner of making the report to the police and to the Committee and the manner of sending and entrusting the child to children's home pending the inquiry.

33. Inquiry:

a. On receipt of a report under Sec. 32, the Committee or any police officer or special juvenile police unit or the designated police officer shall hold an inquiry in the prescribed manner and the Committee, on its own or on the report from any person or agency as mentioned in Sub-section (1) of Sec. 32, may pass an order to send the child to the children's home for speedy inquiry by a social worker or child welfare officer.

b. The inquiry under this section shall be completed within four months of the receipt of the order or within such shorter period as may be fixed by the Committee: Provided that the time for the submission of the inquiry report may be extended by such period as the Committee may, having regard to the circumstances and for the reasons recorded in writing, determine.

c. After the completion of the inquiry if the Committee is of the opinion that the said child has no family or ostensible support, it may allow the child to remain in the children's home or shelter home till suitable rehabilitation is found for him or till he attains the age of eighteen years.

34. Children's homes:

a. The State Government may establish and maintain either by itself or in association with voluntary organisations, children's homes, in every district or group of districts, as the case may be, for the reception of child in need of care and protection during the pendency of any inquiry and subsequently for their care, treatment, education, training, development and rehabilitation.

b. The State Government may, by rules made under this Act provide for the management of children's homes including the standard and the nature of services to be provided by them, and the circumstances under which, and the manner in which, the certification of a children's home or recognition to a voluntary organisation may be granted or withdrawn.

35. Inspection:

a. The State Government may appoint inspection committees for the children's homes (hereinafter referred to as the inspection committees) for the State, a district and city, as the case may be, for such period and for such purposes as may be prescribed.

b. The inspection committee of a State, district or of a city shall consist of such number of representatives from the State Government, local authority, committee, voluntary organisations and such other medical experts and social workers as may be prescribed.

36. Social auditing: The Central Government or State Government may monitor and evaluate the functioning of the children's homes at such period and through such persons and institutions as may be specified by that Government.

37. Shelter homes:

a. The State Government may recognise, reputed and capable voluntary organisations and provide them assistance to set up and administer as many shelter homes for juveniles or children as may be required.

b. The shelter homes referred in Sub-section (1) shall function as drop-in-centres for the children in the need of urgent support who have been brought to such homes through such persons as are referred to in Sub-section (1) of Sec. 32.

c. As far as possible, the shelter homes shall have such facilities as may be prescribed by the rules.

38. Transfer:

a. If during the inquiry it is found that the child hails from the place outside the jurisdiction of the Committee, the Committee shall order the transfer of the child to the competent authority having jurisdiction over the place of residence of the child.

b. Such juvenile or the child shall be escorted by the staff to the home in which he is lodged originally.

c. The State Government may make rules to provide for the travelling allowance to be paid to the child.

39. Restoration:

a. Restoration of and protection to a child shall be the prime objective of any children's home or the shelter home.

b. The children's home or a shelter home, as the case may be, shall take such steps as are considered necessary for the restoration of and protection to a child deprived of his family environment temporarily or permanently where such child is under the care and protection of a children's home or a shelter home, as the case may be.

c. The Committee shall have the powers to restore any child in need of care and protection to his parent, guardian, fit person or fit institution, as the case may be, and give them suitable directions.

Explanation: *For the purposes of this section "restoration of child" means restoration to:*

a. parents
b. adopted parents
c. foster parents

Chapter IV
Rehabilitation and Social Reintegration

40. Process of rehabilitation and social reintegration: The rehabilitation and social reintegration of a child shall begin during the stay of the child in a children's home or special home and the rehabilitation and social reintegration of children shall be carried out alternatively by: (i) adoption, (ii) foster care, (iii) sponsorship, and (iv) sending the child to an after-care organisation.

41. Adoption:

a. The primary responsibility for providing care and protection to children shall be that of his family.
b. Adoption shall be resorted to for the rehabilitation of such children as are orphaned, abandoned, neglected and abused through institutional and non-institutional methods.
c. In keeping with the provisions of the various guidelines for adoption issued from time to time by the State Government, the Board shall be empowered to give children in adoption and carry out such investigations as are required or giving children in adoption in accordance with the guidelines issued by the State Government from time to time in this regard.
d. The children's homes or the State Government run institutions for orphans shall be recognised as an adoption agencies both for scrutiny and placement of such children for adoption in accordance with the guidelines issued under Sub-section (3).
e. No child shall be offered for adoption:
   i. until two members of the Committee declare the child legally free for placement in the case of abandoned children,
   ii. till the two months period for reconsideration by the parent is over in the case of surrendered children, and
   iii. without his consent in the case of a child who can understand and express his consent.
f. The Board may allow a child to be given in adoption:
   i. to a single parent, and
   ii. to parents to adopt a child of same sex irrespective of the number of living biological sons or daughters.

42. Foster care:

a. The foster care may be used for temporary placement of those infants who are ultimately to be given for adoption.
b. In foster care, the child may be placed in another family for a short or extended period of time, depending upon the circumstances where the child's own parent usually visit regularly and eventually after the rehabilitation, where the children may return to their own homes.
c. The State Government may make rules for the purposes of carrying out the scheme of foster care programme of children.

43. Sponsorship:

a. The sponsorship programme may provide supplementary support to families, to children's homes and to special homes to meet medical, nutritional, educational and other needs of the children with a view to improving their quality of life.
b. The State Government may make rules for the purposes of carrying out various schemes of sponsorship of children, such as individual to individual sponsorship, group sponsorship or community sponsorship.

44. After-care organisation: The State Government may, by rules made under this Act provide:

a. for the establishment or recognition of after-care organisations and the functions that may be performed by them under this Act.
b. for a scheme of after-care programme to be followed by such after-care organisations for the purpose of taking care of

juveniles or the children after they leave special homes, children homes and for the purpose of enabling them to lead an honest, industrious and useful life.

c. for the preparation or submission of a report by the probation officer or any other officer appointed by that Government in respect of each juvenile or the child prior to his discharge from a special home, children's home, regarding the necessity and nature of after-care of such juvenile or of a child, the period of such after-care, supervision thereof and for the submission of report by the probation officer or any other officer appointed for the purpose, on the progress of each juvenile or the child.

d. for the standards and the nature of services to be maintained by such after care organisations.

e. for such other matters as may be necessary for the purpose of carrying out the scheme of after-care programme for the juvenile or the child: Provided that any rule made under this section shall not provide for such juvenile or child to stay in the after-care organisation for more than three years: Provided further that a juvenile or child over seventeen years of age but less than eighteen years of age would stay in the after-care organisation till he attains the age of twenty years.

45. **Linkages and co-ordination:** The State Government may make rules to ensure effective linkages between various governmental, non-governmental, corporate and other community agencies for facilitating the rehabilitation and social reintegration of the child.

Chapter V

Miscellaneous

46. **Attendance of parent or guardian of juvenile or child:** Any competent authority before which a juvenile or the child is brought under any of the provisions of this Act may, whenever it so thinks fit, require any parent or guardian having the actual charge of or control over the juvenile or the child to be present at any proceeding in respect of the juvenile or the child.

47. **Dispensing with attendance of juvenile or child:** If, at any stage during the course of an inquiry, a competent authority is satisfied that the attendance of the juvenile or the child is not essential for the purpose of inquiry, the competent authority may dispense with his attendance and proceed with the inquiry in the absence of the juvenile or the child.

48. **Committal to approved place of juvenile or child suffering from dangerous diseases and his future disposal:**

a. When a juvenile or the child who has been brought before a competent authority under this Act is found to be suffering from a disease requiring prolonged medical treatment or physical or mental complaint that will respond to treatment, the competent authority may send the juvenile or the child to any place recognised to be an approved place in accordance with the rules made under this Act for such period as it may think necessary for the required treatment.

b. Where a juvenile or the child is found to be suffering from leprosy, sexually transmitted disease, hepatitis B, open cases of tuberculosis and such other diseases or is of unsound mind, he shall be dealt with separately through various specialised referral services or under the relevant laws as such.

49. **Presumption and determination of age:**

a. Where it appears to a competent authority that person brought before it under any of the provisions of this Act (otherwise than for the purpose of giving evidence) is a juvenile or the child, the competent authority shall make due inquiry so as to the age of that person and for that purpose shall take such evidence as may be necessary (but not an affidavit) and shall record a finding whether the person is a juvenile or the child or not, stating his age as nearly as may be.

b. No order of a competent authority shall be deemed to have become invalid merely by any subsequent proof that the person in respect of whom the order has been made is not a juvenile or the child, and the age recorded by the competent authority to be the age of person so brought before it, shall for the purpose of this Act be deemed to be the true age of that person.

50. **Sending a juvenile or child outside jurisdiction:** In the case of a juvenile or the child, whose ordinary place of residence lies outside the jurisdiction of the competent authority before which he is brought, the competent authority may, if satisfied after due inquiry that it is expedient so to do, send the juvenile or the child back to a relative or other person who is fit and willing to receive him at his ordinary place of residence and exercise proper care and control over him, notwithstanding that such place of residence is outside the jurisdiction of the competent authority; and the competent authority exercising jurisdiction over the place to which the juvenile or the child is sent shall in respect of any matter arising subsequently have the same powers in relation to the juvenile or the child as if the original order had been passed by itself.

51. **Reports to be treated as confidential:** The report of the probation officer or social worker considered by the competent authority shall be treated as confidential: Provided that the competent authority may, if it so thinks fit, communicate the substance thereof to the juvenile or the child or his parent or guardian and may give such juvenile or the child,parent or guardian an opportunity of producing such evidence as may be relevant to the matter stated in the report.

52. **Appeals:**

    a. Subject to the provisions of this section, any person aggrieved by an order made by a competent authority under this Act may, within thirty days from the date of such order, prefer an appeal to the Court of Session: Provided that the Court of Session may entertain the appeal after the expiry of the said period of thirty days if it is satisfied that the appellant was prevented by sufficient cause from filing the appeal in time.

    b. No appeal shall lie from:

        i. any order of acquittal made by the Board in respect of a juvenile alleged to have committed an offence; or

        ii. any order made by a Committee in respect of a finding that a person is not a neglected juvenile.

    c. No second appeal shall lie from any order of the Court of Session passed in appeal under this section.

53. **Revision:** The High Court may, at any time, either of its own motion or on an application received in this behalf, call for the record of any proceeding in which any competent authority or Court of Session has passed an order for the purpose of satisfying itself as to the legality or propriety of any such order and may pass such order in relation thereto as it thinks fit: Provided that the High Court shall not pass an order under this section prejudicial to any person without giving him a reasonable opportunity of being heard.

54. **Procedure in inquiries, appeals and revision proceedings:**

    a. *Save as otherwise* expressly provided by this Act a competent authority while holding any inquiry under any of the provisions of this Act shall follow such procedure as may be prescribed and subject thereto, shall follow, as far as may be, the procedure laid down in the Code of Criminal Procedure, 1973 (2 of 1974) for trials in summons cases.

    b. *Save as otherwise* expressly provided by or under this Act the procedure to be followed in hearing appeals or revision proceedings under this Act shall be, as far as practicable, in accordance with the provisions of the Code of Criminal Procedure, 1973 (2 of 1974).

55. **Power to amend orders:**

    a. Without prejudice to the provisions for appeal and revision under this Act any competent authority may, on an application received in this behalf, amend any order as to the institution to which a juvenile or the child is to be sent or as to the person under whose care or supervision a juvenile or the child is to be placed under this Act: Provided that there shall be at least two members and the parties or its defence present during the course of hearing for passing an amendment in relation to any of its order.

b. Clerical mistakes in orders passed by a competent authority or errors arising therein from any accidental slip or omission may, at any time, be corrected by the competent authority either on its own motion or on an application received in this behalf.

56. **Power of competent authority to discharge and transfer juvenile or child:** The competent authority or the local authority may, notwithstanding anything contained in this Act at any time, order a child in need of care and protection or a juvenile in conflict with law to be discharged or transferred from one children's home or special home to another, as the case may be, keeping in view the best interest of the child or the juvenile, and his natural place of stay, either absolutely or on such conditions as it may think fit to impose: Provided that the total period of stay of the juvenile or the child in a children's home or a special home or a fit institution or under a fit person shall not be increased by such transfer.

57. **Transfer between children's homes, under the Act and juvenile homes, of like nature in different parts of India:** The State Government or the local authority may direct any child or the juvenile to be transferred from any children's home or special home outside the State to any other children's home, special home or institution of a like nature with the prior intimation to the local Committee or the Board, as the case may be, and such order shall be deemed to be operative for the competent authority of the area to which the child or the juvenile is sent.

58. **Transfer of juvenile or child of unsound mind or suffering from leprosy or addicted to drugs:** Where it appears to the competent authority that any juvenile or the child kept in a special home or a children's home or shelter home or in an institution in pursuance of this Act is suffering from leprosy or is of unsound mind or is addicted to any narcotic drug or psychotropic substance, the competent authority may order his removal to a leper asylum or mental hospital or treatment centre for drug addicts or to a place of safety for being kept there for such period not exceeding the period for which he is required to be kept under the order of the competent authority or for such further period as may be certified by the medical officer necessary for the proper treatment of the juvenile or the child.

59. **Release and absence of juvenile or child on placement:**

a. When a juvenile or the child is kept in a children's home or special home and on a report of a probation officer or social worker or of Government or a voluntary organisation, as the case may be, the competent authority may consider, the release of such juvenile or the child permitting him to live with his parent or guardian or under the supervision of any authorised person named in the order, willing to receive and take charge of the juvenile or the child to educate and train him for some useful trade or calling or to look after him for rehabilitation.

b. The competent authority may also permit leave of absence to any juvenile or the child, to allow him, on special occasions like examination, marriage of relatives, death of kith and kin or the accident or serious illness of parent or any emergency of like nature, to go on leave under supervision, for maximum seven days, excluding the time taken in journey.

c. Where a permission has been revoked or forfeited and the juvenile or the child refuses or fails to return to the home concerned or juvenile to which he was directed so to return, the Board may, if necessary, cause him to be taken charge of and to be taken back to the concerned home.

d. The time during which a juvenile or the child is absent from a concerned home in pursuance of such permission granted under this section shall be deemed to be part of the time for which he is liable to be kept in the special home: Provided that when a juvenile has failed to return to the special home on the permission being revoked or forfeited, the time which lapses after his failure so to return shall be excluded in computing the time during which he is liable to be kept in the institution.

60. Contribution by parents:

a. The competent authority which makes an order for sending a juvenile or the child to a children's home or to a special home or placing the juvenile under the care of a fit person or fit institution may make an order requiring the parent or other person liable to maintain the juvenile or the child to contribute to his maintenance, if able to do so, in the prescribed manner according to income.

b. The competent authority may direct, if necessary, the payment to be made to poor parent or guardian by the Superintendent or the Project Manager of the home to pay such expenses for the journey of the inmate or parent or guardian or both, from the home to his ordinary place of residence at the time of sending the juvenile as may be prescribed.

61. Fund:

a. The State Government or local authority may create a Fund under such name as it thinks fit for the welfare and rehabilitation of the juvenile or the child dealt with under this Act.

b. There shall be credited to the Fund such voluntary donations, contributions or subscriptions as may be made by any individual or organisation.

c. The Fund created under Sub-section (1) shall be administered by the State advisory board in such manner and for such purposes as may be prescribed.

62. Central, State, district and city advisory boards:

a. The Central Government or a State Government may constitute a Central or State Advisory boad, as the case may be, to advise that Government on matter relating to the establishment and maintenance of the homes, mobilisation of resources, provision of facilities for education, training and rehabilitation of child in need of care and protection and juvenile in conflict with law and co-ordination among the various official and non-official agencies concerned.

b. The Central or State advisory board shall consist of such persons as the Central Government or the State Government, as the case may be, may think fit and shall include eminent social workers, representatives of voluntary organisations in the field of the child welfare corporate sector, academicians, medical professionals and the concerned Department of the State Government.

c. The district or city level inspection committee constituted under Sec. 35 of this Act shall also function as the district or city advisory board.

63. Special juvenile police unit:

a. In order to enable the police officers who frequently or exclusively deal with juveniles or are primarily engaged in the prevention of juvenile crime or handling of the juveniles or children under this Act to perform their functions more effectively, they shall be specially instructed and trained.

b. In every police station at least one officer with aptitude and appropriate training and orientation may be designated as the 'juvenile or the child welfare officer' who will handle the juvenile or the child in co-ordination with the police.

c. Special juvenile police unit, of which all police officers designated as above, to handle juveniles or children will be members, may be created in every district and city to coordinate and to upgrade the police treatment of the juveniles and the children.

64. Juvenile in conflict with law undergoing sentence at commencement of this Act: In any area in which this Act is brought into force, the State Government or the local authority may direct that a juvenile in conflict with law who is undergoing any sentence of imprisonment at the commencement of this Act shall, in lieu of undergoing such sentence, be sent to a special home or kept in fit institution in such manner as the State Government or the local authority thinks fit for the remainder of the period of the sentence; and the provisions of this Act shall apply to the juvenile as if he had been ordered by the Board to be sent to such special home or institution or, as the case may be, ordered to be kept under protective care under Sub-section (2) of Sec. 16 of this Act.

65. Procedure in respect of bonds: Provisions of Chapter XXXIII of the Code of Criminal Procedure, 1973 (2 of 1974) shall, as far as nay be, apply to bonds taken under this Act.

66. Delegation of powers: The State Government may, by the general order, direct that any power exercisable by it under this Act shall, in such circumstances and under such conditions, if any, as may be prescribed in the order, be exercisable also by an officer subordinate to that Government or the local authority.

67. Protection of action taken in good faith: No suit or legal proceedings shall lie against the State Government or voluntary organisation running the home or any officer and the staff appointed in pursuance of this Act in respect of anything which is in good faith done or intended to be done in pursuance of this Act or of any rules or order made thereunder.

68. Power to make rules:

a. The State Government may, by notification in the Official Gazette,make rules to carry out the purposes of this Act.

b. In particular, and without prejudice to the generality of the foregoing powers, such rules may provide for all or any of the following matters, namely:

i. the term of office of the members of the Board, and the manner in which such member may resign under Sub-section (4) of Sec. 4.

ii. the time of the meetings of the Board and the rules of procedure in regard to the transaction of business at its meeting under Sub-section (1) of Sec. 5.

iii. the management of observation homes including the standards and various types of services to be provided by them and the circumstances in which and the manner in which, the certification of the observation home may be granted or withdrawn and such other matters as are referred to in Sec. 8.

iv. the management of special home including the standards and various types of services to be provided by them and the circumstances in which and the manner in which, the certification of the special home may be granted or withdrawn and such other matters as are referred to in Sec. 9.

v. persons by whom any juvenile in conflict with law may be produced before the Board and the manner of sending such juvenile to an observation home under Sub-section (2) of Sec. 10.

vi. matters relating to removal of disqualifications attaching to conviction of a juvenile under Sec. 19.

vii. the qualifications of the Chairperson and members, and the tenure for which they may be appointed under Sub-section (3) of Sec. 29.

viii. the time of the meetings of the Committee and the rules of procedure in regard to the transaction of business at its meeting under Sub-section (1) of Sec. 30.

ix. the manner of making the report to the police and to the Committee and the manner of sending and entrusting the child to children's home pending the inquiry under Sub-section (2) of Sec. 32.

x. the management of children's homes including the standards and nature of services to be provided by them, and the manner in which certification of a children's home or recognition to a voluntary organisation may be granted or withdrawn under Sub-section (2) of Sec. 34.

xi. appointment of inspection committees for children's homes, their tenure and purposes for which inspection committees may be appointed and such other matters as are referred to in Sec. 35.

xii. facilities to be provided by the shelter homes under Sub-section (3) of Sec. 37.

xiii. for carrying out the scheme of foster care programme of children under Sub-section (3) of Sec. 42.

xiv. for carrying out various schemes of sponsorship of children under Sub-section (2) of Sec. 43.

xv. matters relating to after-care organisation under Sec. 44.

xvi. for ensuring effective linkages between various agencies for facilitating rehabilitation and social integration of the child under Sec. 45.

xvii. the purposes and the manner in which the fund shall be administered under Sub-section (3) of Sec. 61.

xviii. any other matter which is required to be or may be, prescribed.

c. Every rule made by a State Government under this Act shall be laid, as soon as may be after it is made, before the Legislature of that State.

69. Repeal and savings:

a. The Juvenile Justice Act 1986 (53 of 1986) is hereby repealed.

b. Notwithstanding such repeal, anything done or any action taken under the said Act shall be deemed to have been done or taken under the corresponding provisions of this Act.

70. Power to remove difficulties:

a. If any difficulty arises in giving effect to the provisions of this Act the Central Government may, by order, not inconsistent with the provisions of this Act remove the difficulty: Provided that no such order shall be made after the expiry of the period of two years from the commencement of this Act.

b. However, order made under the section shall be laid, as soon as may be after it is made, before each House of Parliament.

Bibliography

1. (1983) 2 SCC 308
2. (1986) 3 SCC 632, Vide order date 15.4.1986
3. (1989) SUPP 1 SCC 644
4. (1994) 3 Supp SCC 374
5. (2002) 3 SCC 31
6. (2002) 3 SCC 31
7. 1963 (2) Cri L J 329: AIR 1963 SC 1295.
8. 1975 Cri L J 1111: AIR 1975 SC 1378.
9. 2010 Cri L J 94 (Del)
10. 2010 Cri L J 94 (Del)
11. 2010 Cri LJ 94 (Del)
12. 2010 Cri LJ 94 (Del)
13. 2010 Cri LJ 94 (Del)
14. 2010 Cri LJ 94 (Del)
15. 2010 Cri LJ 94 (Del)
16. 2010 Cri LJ 94 (Del)
17. 2010 Cri LJ 94 (Del)
18. 2010 Cri LJ 94 (Del)
19. 2010 Cri LJ 94 (Del)
20. 2010 Cri LJ 94 (Del)
21. A peculiar feature of this case was that completely contradictory affidavits had been filed by two wings of Union of India. The Minister of Home Affairs argued that the impugned provision was necessary for effective treatment and prevention of HIV/AIDS while both the Ministry of Health and Family Welfare and the National AIDS Control Organization (NACO) submitted affidavits contrary to that which supported the petitioner's contention.
22. Abel GG, Osborn C. The paraphilias: The extent and nature of sexually deviant and criminal behavior. Psychiatr Clin North Am 15:675, 1992.
23. Siddique Ahman. Criminology, problem and perspectives, Lucknow, E B Company, Fourth Ed p 448.
24. Aigner G, Centerwall E (1983). Barnens Karleksliv. Prisms/RFSU.
25. AIR 1983 SC 339
26. AIR 1995 SC 264
27. AIR 1997 SC 568
28. AIR 2003 SC 3450
29. AIR 2008 SC (Supp) 1
30. AIR 2008 SC 663
31. Ajoy Ghosh Story, Justice Anand AS (Rtd). The Tribune, Dec 20, 2003
32. American Psychological Association, "Violence and youth: Psychology's response", summary report of the APA Commission on Violence and Youth (Washington DC, 1993).
33. Araji SK (1997). Sexually aggressive children—coming to understand them. Sage publications. London.
34. Article 32 is the right to move the Supreme by appropriate proceedings for the enforcement of the rights.
35. As observed by their parents, Manuscript.
36. Thakur Ashok Kumar *vs* Union of India, supra 30.
37. Azheimer's Association, 2012 Alzheimer's

Disease Facts and Figures, Alzheimer's and Dementia, Volume 8, Issue 2.A

38. Bailey S 1996. Adolescents who murder. Journal of Adolescence 19: 19–39.
39. Adons Bert N and Sydie RA. Sociological Theory, p 98 2002, Vistaar publications, New Delhi.
40. Boyer WF, Bakalar NH, Lake CR. Anticholinergic prophylaxis of acute haloperidol-induced acute dystonic reactions. J Clin Psychopharmacol 7: 264, 1987. Fauman BJ: Other psychiatric emergencies. In Comprehensive textbook of psychiatry, Ed 6, Kaplan HI, Sadock BJ, editors, p 1752. Williams and Wilkins, Baltimore, 1995.
41. Bremer JF 1993. The treatment of children and adolescents with aberrant sexual behaviors.
42. Brunner HG, Nelen, Breakefield, Ropers, and van Oost M. Science (1993); 262, 578–58
43. Buckland G and Stevens A (2001). Review of Effective Practice With Young Offenders in mainland Europe, EISS University of Kent at Canterbury, UK
44. Cavanagh Johnson T (1996). Understanding children's sexual behaviors—what's natural and healthy. Booklet issued by Cavanagh Johnson, California, USA.
45. Cavanagh Johnson T, Feldmeth JR (1993). "Sexual behaviors—a continuum". In Gil IE and Johnson T Cavanagh. Sexualized Children (pp 39–52).
46. Center for the protection of women and children "Violence against women and children in Kosova". Regional Conference on Violence against Women and Children in Kosova, Pristina, 30 June to 2 July 2002.
47. Chenna Jagadeeswar *vs* State of Andhra Pradesh, 1988 Cri LJ 549 (AP).
48. Connor Daniel F, 2009. Disruptive Behavior Disorders. In Kaplan and Sadock's Comprehensive Textbook of Psychiatry, 9th Edition. Editors—Sadock, Benjamin J; Sadock, Virginia A; Ruiz, Pedro Lippincott Williams and Wilkins Publishers. New York: pp 3581–3596.
49. Henderson DK and Gillespie RD. A Textbook of Psychiatry, 1956, Eighth Edn, Oxford Medical Publications, University press, London, 714–715.
50. Douglas J, Olshaker M. Obsession. New York: Scribner, 1998. pp 265–269.
51. Douglas J, Olshaker M. The anatomy of motive. New York: Scribner, 1999.
52. Douglas J, Olshaker M. Unabomber: On the trail of America's most-wanted serial killer. New York: Pocket Books, 1996: 105–108.
53. Douglas JE, Burgess AW, Burgess AG, et al. Crime classification manual. New York: Lexington Books, 1992. pp 21–22, 80–85.
54. Eddy M and Reid J (2002). The Antisocial Behavior of The Adolescent Children of Incarcerated parents: A Developmental Perspective, paper presented at US Dept of Health and Human Services Conference.
55. Elliot FA (2000). A neurological perspective of violent behavior. In Fishbein DH (Ed.), The science, treatment, and prevention of antisocial behaviors: Application to the criminal justice system (pp 19–1 to 19–21). Kingston NJ: Civic Research Institute.
56. Eysenck HJ (1996). Personality and crime: Where do we stand? Psychology, Crime, and Law, 2, 143–152.
57. Finkelhor D, Dziuba-Leatherman J. Victimization of children. Am Psychol 1994; 49(3): 173–183.
58. Friedrich WN, Fisher I, Broughton D, Houston M, Shafran CR (1998). "Normative sexual behavior in children: A contemporaty sample". Pediatrics; Vol. 101, no. 4: pp e9.
59. Friedrich WN, Grambsch P, Damon L, Hewitt S, Koverola C, Lang R, Wolfe V, Broughton D (1992). "Child sexual behavior inventory: Normative and clinical comparisons". Psychological Assessment, Vol. 4, no. 3: 303–311.
60. Gagnon JH, Simon W (1973). Sexual conduct — the social sources of human sexuality. Aldine Publ. Company. Chicago.
61. Garn feski N and Okama S (1996). Journal of Adolescence, 19, 503–512.
62. Germany Federal Ministry of the Interior and Federal Ministry of Justice, "First periodical

report on crime and crime control in Germany"...

63. Gil E and Cavanagh Johnson T (1993). Sexualized children—Assessment and treatment of sexualized children and children who molest. Launch press.
64. Gillberg C, Persson E, Grufman M and Themner U (1986). Psychiatric disorders in mildly and severely retarded urban children and adolescents: Epidemiological aspects, Briyidh Journal of Psychiatry 149: 68–74.
65. Gottesman II (1991). Schizophrenia Genesis: The Origin of Madness. New York: Freeman. 012
66. Graves RB, Openshaw DK, Ascione FR and Erikson SL 1996. Demographic and parental characteristics of youthful sexual offenders.
67. Gray AS and Wallace R 1992. Adolescent Sexual Offender Assessment Packet. Orwell, VT: Safer Society press.
68. Hall DK, Mathews F and Pearce J 1998. Factors associated with sexual behavior problems in young sexually abused children. Child Abuse and Neglect 22: 1045–63
69. Harksen *vs* Lane 1998 (1) SA 300 (CC); Prinsloo *vs* Van Der Linde, 1997 (3) SA 1012 (CC); Corbiere *vs* Canda (1999) 2 SCR 203; Romer *vs* Evans, 57 US 620 (1996) Vired *vs* Albetra (1998) 1 SCR 493.
70. Hazelwood RR, Dietz PE, Warren JI. The criminal sexual sadist. In: Hazelwood R, Burgess A, eds. Practical aspects of rape investigation: A multidisciplinary approach, 2nd Ed. Boca Raton: CRC press, 1995: 361–371.
71. Hazelwood RR. Analyzing the rape and profiling the offender. In: Hazelwood R, Burgess A, Eds. Practical aspects of rape investigation: A multidisciplinary approach, 2nd Ed. Boca Raton, Florida, FL: CRC Press, 1995: 155–160.
72. Hillard JR, Editor. Manual of Clinical Emergency Psychiatry, American Psychiatric press, Washington, 1990.
73. Holland A (1997). Forensic psychiatry and learning disability. In Russell, O (Ed.), Seminars in the Psychiatry of Learning Disabilities. London: Gaskell, 259–73.
74. Holmes SE, Slaughter JR and Kashani J (2001). Risk factors in childhood that lead to the development of conduct disorder and antisocial personality disorder. Child Psychiatry and Human Development, 31, 183–193.
75. Howlin P (1997). Autism: Preparing for Adulthood, London: Routledge.
76. http://free thinkers.co.u.k. latest visited on 23/10/2009.(this is the voice of atheism since 1881)
77. http://www.inter-islam.org./Prohibitions/suicide.html. Latest visited on 26/12/09.
78. Hunt A and Dennis (1987). Psychiatric disorder among children with tuberous sclerosis. Developmental Medicine and Child Neurology 29: 190–8.
79. Hunter JA, Lexier LJ, Goodwin DW, Browne PA and Dennis C 1993. Psychosexual.
80. In 1994, South Africa became the first nation to constitutionally safeguard the rights of lesbians and gays. Canada, France, Luxembourg, Holland, Slovenia, Spain, Norway, Denmark, Sweden and New Zealand also have similar laws. In 1996, the US Supreme Court ordered that no State could pass legislation that discriminated against homosexuals.
81. In Hoskot M H *vs* State of Maharashtra, (1978) 3 SCC 544, Hussainara Khatoon and Ors. *vs.* Home Secretary State of Bihar, 1979 Cri LJ 1036: AIR 1979 SC 1360, Sunil Batra *vs* Delhi Admn., 1978 Cri LJ 1741: AIR 1978 SC 1675, Shukla Prem Shankar *vs* Delhi Admn., AIR 1980 SC 1535 : 1980 Cri LJ 930, Mullin Francis Caralie *vs* Administrator, Union Territory of Delhi and others.
82. Indian Journal of Medical Ethics April, June, 1999, 7(2).
83. Johnson J, Smailes E, Cohen P, Kasen S, and Brook JS (2004). "Antisocial Parental Behavior, Problematic Parenting and Aggressive Offspring Behavior During Adulthood; A 25-Year Longitudinal Investigation', in British Journal of Criminology 44: 6, pp 915–930

84. Johnson TC and Feldmeth JR 1993. Sexual behaviors: A continuum. In Gil E and Johnson TC (eds). Sexualised Children: Assessment and Treatment of Sexualised Children and Children who Molest.
85. Joseph J (2001). The Journal of mind and behaviors 22, 179–218.
86. Kendall-Tackett KE, Williams L, Finkelhor D (1993). "The impact of sexual abuse on children: A review and synthesis of recent empirical studies". Psychological Bulletin, 113: 164–180.
87. Langevin R. Biological factors contributing to paraphilic behavior. Psychiatr Ann 22: 307, 1992.
88. Lanning KV. Child molestation: A law enforcement typology. In: Hazelwood R, Burgess A, Eds. Practical aspects of rape investigation: A multidisciplinary approach, 2nd Ed. Boca Raton: CRC press, 1995.
89. Lanning KV. Child molesters: A behavioral analysis for law enforcement officers investigating cases of child sexual exploitation, 3rd Ed. Alexandria, Virginia: National Center for Missing and Exploited Children, December 1992 pp 6–9, 17
90. Lanning KV. Investigative analysis and summary of teaching points. In: Lanning KV, Burgess AW, eds. Child molesters who abduct: Summary of the case in point series. Alexandria, Virginia: National Center for Missing and Exploited Children, 1995.
91. Larsson I, Svedin CG (1999). Sexual behavior in Swedish preschool children.
92. Levine SM and Stava LL. Personality characteristics of sex offenders: A review. Arch Sex Behav 16: 57, 1987.
93. Littell JH, Popa M and Forsythe B (2006). Multisystemic Therapy for Social, Emotional, and Behavioral problems in Youth Aged 10–17 (review), The Cochrane Collaboration, The Cochrane Library 2006, Issue 3.
94. Wolfgang ME, Thornberry TP and Figlio RM. From Boy to Man, from Delinquency to Crime (Chicago, University of Chicago press, 1987).
95. Rama Jois M. Legal and Constitutional History of India at p 407, 1990, Tripathi NM Private Ltd. Bombay.
96. Meegan S Kids and Company. Together for safety, teacher's guide—a comprehensive manual for grades K-5/6, 4th rev. ed.
97. Meyer JK. Paraphilias. In Comprehensive Textbook of Psychiatry, Ed 6, Kaplan H 1, Sadock BJ, editors, p 1334. Williams and Wilkins, Baltimore, 1995.
98. Miles DR and Carey G (1997). Journal of Personality and Social Psychology, 72, 207–217
99. Tsuang Ming T, Stone William S, V Faraone Stephen, 2001. Genes, environment and schizophrenia. British Journal of Psychiatry; 178: s18–24.
100. Monahan J and Shah SA. Dangerousness and commitment of the mentally disordered in the United States. Schizophr Bull 15: 541, 1989.
101. Money J. Forensic sexology: Paraphilic serial rape (biastophilia) and lust murder (erotophonophilia). Am J Psychother 44: 26, 1990
102. Morley K and Hall W (2003). Is there a genetic susceptibility to engage in criminal acts? Australian Institute of Criminology: Trends and Issues in Crime and Criminal Justice, 263, 1–6
103 Morrison B and Ahmed E (2006). Restorative Justice and Civil Society: Emerging practice, Theory and Evidence. Journal of Social Issues 62: 2, 209–215.
104. Munn *vs* Illinois, 94 US 113 (1877); Jane Roe *vs* Henry Wade, 410 US 113 (1973); Bowers Attorney General of Georgia *vs* Hand wicket al, 478 US 186 (1986).
105. Jayan Nithin on January 17, 2011 at 7:08 PM Health Watch.
106. O'Brien G (1999). Traumatic brain damage. In Gillberg C And O'Brien G, eds 9, Developmental Disability and Behavior. London: MacKeith press.
107. Organization of African Unity and UNICEF, "Africa's children, Africa's future", a background sectoral paper prepared for the OAU International Conference on Assistance to African Children, Dakar, 25–27 November 1992.
108. Rathinam P/Patnaik Nagbhushan *vs* Union of India and another, AIR 1994 SC 1844: 1994 Cri LJ 1605.

109. Palmer 2002, cited in Lane et al (2005). Evaluating an Experimental Intensive Juvenile probation program: Supervision and Official Outcomes, Crime and Delinquency 51:1, 26–52).
110. Petition (No. 7560) in Bombay High Court in 1988.
111. Rasmussen K, Storsaeter O and Levander S (1999). Personality disorders, psychopath, and crime in a Norwegian prison population. International Journal of Law and Psychiatry, 22, 91–97.
112. Ressler RK, Burgess AW, Douglas JE. Sexual homicide: Patterns and motives. New York Lexington Books, 1988 pp 17–26; 28–43; 70.
113. Rhee SH and Walolman ID (2002). Psychological Bulletee 128, 490–529.
114. Carson Robert C, Butcher James N, Mineka Susan. Abnormal Psychology and Modern life, 1998, Tenth Edition, p 244 (Longman Publication).
115. Butzlaff Ronald L, Hooley Jill M. Arch Gen Psychiatry. 1998; 55(6): 547–552.
116. Rosenberg RC and Kesselman M. The therapeutic alliance and the psychiatric emergency room. Hosp Community Psychiatry 44: 78, 1993.
117. Rosenfeld A and Wasserman S (1993). "Sexual development in the early school-aged child". Child and adolescent psychiatric clinics of North America, 2; 3: 393–406.
118. Rutter M (1971). "Normal psychosexual Development". Child Psychology and Psychiatry Vol. 11: 259–283.
119. Sanguineti VR and Brooks MO. Factors related to emergency commitment of chronically mentally ill patients who are substance abusers. Hosp Community Psychiatry 43: 237, 1992.
120. Schmitz MF (2003). Influences of race and family environment on child hyperactivity and antisocial behavior. Journal of Marriage and the Family 65: 835–849.
121. Schorr SJ and Richardson D. Psychiatric emergencies. Obstet Gynecol Clin North Am 22: 369, 1995.
122. Scragg P and Shah A (1994). Prevalence of Asperger's syndrome in a secure hospital. British Journal of Psychiatry 16: 679–82.
123. Section 377 reads: Of unnatural offences, whoever voluntarily has carnal intercourse against the order of nature with any man, woman, or animal, shall be punished with imprisonment of either description for a term which may extend to 10 years and also be liable to fine.
124. See; Human Rights Violation Against Sexual Minorities—A Report of PULC Karnataka, Bangalore, 2001; Nag N, Sexual Behavior in India with Risk of HIV/AIDS Transmission, Health Tran. Rev. 1995:5 pp 293–305; AIDS Bhedbhav Virodhi Andolan, Less than Gay: A Citizen's Report on the Status of Homosexuality in India, New Delhi, 1991.
125. Barse Sheela *vs* Union of India (1993) 4 SCC 204.
126. Sirles EA, Araji S, Bosek R (1997). Redirecting Children's Sexually Abusive and Sexually Aggressive Behaviors. Programs and Practices. In (Eds.) Araji SK, Sexually Aggressive Children. Coming to Understand Them: 161–192. Sage Publications.
127. Skuse D, Bentovim A, Hodges J, et al. 1998. Risk factors for the development of sexually abusive behavior in sexually victimised adolescent boys.
128. Sloan PR (2000). Controling our destinus, notre dame: University of Notre Dame Press.
129. Smt. Kaur Gian *vs* State of Punjab, AIR 1966 SC 946.
130. Soderquist M (1995). Jag Kanner mig normal nu! Om samarbete med sexuellt utsatta barn och deras foraldrar. Mareld.
131. Soothill K 1997. Rapists under 14 years in the news. The Howard Journal 36: 367–777.
132. Stalleing Questions and Answers. Washington, DC: The National Center for Victims of Crime, 1995. Available at http://www.ncvc.org/src/main.aspx? dbID=DB.
133. State of Florida, "Key juvenile crime trends and conditions". Available at myflorida.com, the official portal of the State of Florida (see

http://www.djj.state.fl.us/publicsafety/learn/jjcrimetrends.html).

134. Stein DJ, Hollander E, Anthony DT, Schneier FR. Serotonergic medications for sexual obsessions, sexual addictions, and paraphilias. J Clin Psychiatry 53: 267, 1992

135. Tehrani J, and Mednick S (2000). Genetic factors and criminal behavior. Federal Probation 64: 24–28.

136. The American Psychiatric Association (1996). The Diagnostic and Statistical Manual of Mental Disorders 4th Edition (DSM-IV)

137. The Law Commission in its 172nd report has recommended deletion of Sec. 377 IPC. In the report, the Commission, focussed on the need to review the sexual offences and laws, in the light of increased incidents of custodial rape and crime of sexual abuse against youngsters. And inter alia, recommended deleting the section 377 IPC by effecting the recommended amendments in Secs. 375 to 376E of IPC.

138. The submission of NACO and consequently Ministry of Health confirm the case set out by those demanding changes that homosexual community is particularly susceptible to attracting to HIV/AIDS. According to NACO those in the high risk of HIV/AIDS category like homosexual have been found to be mostly reluctant to reveal same sex behavior due to the fear of law enforcement agencies and thus keeping a large section invisible and unreachable and thereby pushing the cases of infection underground making it very difficult for the public worker to even access/assess them.

139. The Wolfendon Committee was required to report on the issue of legal sanctions against homosexual behavior. It observed that the function of criminal law is to preserve public order and decency, to protect the citizen from what is offensive or injurious, and to provide sufficient safeguards against exploitation and corruption of others, particularly those who are especially vulnerable because they are young, weak in body or mind, inexperienced, or in a state of special physical, official, or economic dependence, but not to intervene in the private lives of citizens, or to seek to enforce any particular pattern of behavior, further than is necessary to carry out the purposes we have outlined.

140. Today consensual homosexual acts are illegal in about 70 out of 195 countries of the world. Most of the countries who prohibit same sex are in Asia and Africa.

141. Tueth MJ. Management of behavioral emergencies. Am J Emerg Med 13: 344, 1995.

142. Tueth MJ. Emergencies caused by side effects of psychiatric medications. Am J Emerg Med 12: 212, 1994.

143. United Nations Guidelines for the prevention of Juvenile Delinquency (The Riyadh Guidelines), adopted and proclaimed by General Assembly resolution 45/112 of 14 December 1990, available at.

144. United Nations, "Draft plans of action for the implementation during the period 2001–2005 of the Vienna Declaration on Crime and Justice: Meeting the challenges of the twenty-first century: Report of the Secretary-General", tenth session of the commission on Crime prevention and Criminal Justice, Vienna, 8–17 May 2001 9E/CN.15/2001/5).

145. United Nations, "Draft plans of action for the implementation during the period 2001–2005 of the Vienna Declaration on Crime and Justice: Meeting the challenges of the twenty-first century: Report of the Secretary-General"...

146. United Nations, Center for social Development and Humanitarian Affairs, "The global situation of youth in the 1990s: Trends and prospects" (ST/CSDHA/21) (1993).

147. United Nations, Department of public Information, News Coverage Service, " Need for inter-sectoral approach to fighting crime and illegal drugs stressed in Third Committee debate". Press release: Statement of Dulul Biswas, representative of Bangladesh (4 October 2000) (UNIS/GA/SHC/301).

148. Urban Management Programme, "Street children and gangs in African cities: Guidelines for local authorities"... pp. 26–37.

149. Vizard E, Wynick S, Hawkes C, Woods J and Jenkins J 1996. Juvenile sexual offenders.

150. Vizard E, Monck E and Misch P 1995. Child and adolescent sex abuse perpetrators: A review of the research literature. Journal of Child Psychology and Psychiatry 36: 731–56.
151. Vizard E and Usiskin J 1999. Providing individual psychotherapy for young sexual abusers of other children.
152. World Health Organization (2002): International Statistical Classification of Diseases and Related Health Problems 10th Edition (ICD-10). WP(C) No.7455/2001, Date of decision: 2nd July, 2009 Reported 2010 Cri LJ 94 (Delhi).
153. Writ Petition (Cri) No 73 Of 1982
154. Writ Petition (Cri) No 1777–1778 OF 1983
155. Writ Petition © No 339 OF 1986
156. Writ Petition 357/98 delivered on October 14, 1998.
157. Writ Petition No 1537 of 1984, Bombay.

Index

H

I

J

K

L

M